HEALTH CARE IN CANADA:
A CITIZEN'S GUIDE TO POLICY AND POLITICS

Health Care in Canada examines the challenges faced by the Canadian health care system, a subject of much public debate. In this book Katherine Fierlbeck provides an in-depth discussion of how health care decisions are shaped by politics and why there is so much disagreement over how to fix the system.

Many Canadians point to health care as a source of national pride; others are highly critical of the system's shortcomings and call for major reform. Yet meaningful debate cannot occur without an understanding of how the system actually operates. In this overview, Fierlbeck outlines the basic framework of the health care system with reference to specific areas such as administration and governance, public health, human resources, drugs and drug policy, and mental health. She also discusses alternative models in other countries such as Britain, the United States, and France. As health care becomes increasingly complex, it is crucial that Canadians have a solid grasp of the main issues within both the policy and political environments. With its balanced and accessible assessment of the main political and theoretical debates, *Health Care in Canada* is an essential guide for anyone with a stake in Canada's health system.

KATHERINE FIERLBECK is a professor in the Department of Political Science at Dalhousie University.

KATHERINE FIERLBECK

Health Care in Canada

A Citizen's Guide to Policy and Politics

UNIVERSITY OF TORONTO PRESS
Toronto   Buffalo   London

© University of Toronto Press Incorporated 2011
Toronto Buffalo London
www.utppublishing.com
Printed in Canada

ISBN 978-1-4426-4003-0 (cloth)
ISBN 978-1-4426-0983-9 (paper)

Printed on acid-free paper, 100% post-consumer recycled paper with
vegetable-based inks.

Toronto Italian Studies

Library and Archieves and Canada Cataloguing in Publication

Fierlbeck, Katherine
Health care in Canada : a citizen's guide to policy and politics /
Katherine Fierlbeck.

Includes bibliographical references and index.
ISBN 978-1-4426-4003-0 (bound)   ISBN 978-1-4426-0983-9 (pbk.)

1. Medical care–Canada.   1.Title

RA395.C3F53 2011   362.10971   C2010-907811-X

University of Toronto Press acknowledges the financial assistance to its
publishing program of the Canada Council for the Arts and the Ontario
Arts Council.

 Canada Council   Conseil des Arts   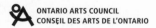 ONTARIO ARTS COUNCIL
for the Arts   du Canada   CONSEIL DES ARTS DE L'ONTARIO

University of Toronto Press acknowledges the financial support of the
Government of Canada through the Canada Book Fund for its publishing
activities.

For Eleanor and Jack
Never stop asking why,
and remember
'because I said so' is never a valid reason
unless it comes from your mother.

Contents

Preface

In December 2008, a writer in the *Globe and Mail Report on Business* stated that 'my wish is that the Canada Health Act be amended so that Canadians have the same freedom to provide and to choose public or private health options that are enjoyed in every other developed country' (Morgan 2008). That provinces can, in fact, introduce private insurance or private services without amending the Canada Health Act was clearly not understood by the writer, the editor, or the fact-checker. They also did not grasp that Canada does *not*, as the article stated, 'outlaw privately funded purchasers of core health services': the government of Canada has no jurisdiction over how health services are funded, and indeed, many of the provinces do not 'outlaw' private health insurance for medically necessary health care at all.

Health care in Canada has an iconic status as a major component of Canadian citizenship, and it rightfully ought to be debated widely in the public realm. We cannot debate health care, however, if we do not understand how health care works. The very complexity of the issues underlying health care and health care reform stymies the attempt to place the discussion over health care reform firmly in the public sphere. Moreover, to the extent that reform is debated with reference to what other countries do, Canadians should also have a good sense of how other countries structure their health care systems. But if the *Report on Business* can't get it right, how are the rest of us to do so?

This book is an explanation of how the Canadian health care system works (and how it doesn't). But it is, more importantly, a discussion of the politics within which the health care system is enmeshed. Health care in Canada is highly political. It plays a major role in federal and provincial elections, constitutional debates, and the articulation of Canadian identity. It figures in debates over trade policy, intergovernmental relations, and even international obligations. Health care touches the quotidian matters of most people's lives: can they see a physician today? Can they afford the drugs they need? What vaccinations should their children receive? What happens when their parents can no longer live independently? Health care is further politicized because of to the impression that it is in crisis and must be radically overhauled. But why are the discussions of solutions so interminable? Why can't health care just be fixed, once and for all?

Rather than simply a description of institutions and processes, this book is a discussion of the political and theoretical debates over health care in Canada. It examines why health care systems face the challenges that we read about in the newspaper, but it also explains why there is so much disagreement over what should be done. Why can't we just end waiting times, if other countries have done so? Why shouldn't we just leave it all up to the market? Or simply hire more doctors? The overarching argument of the book involves two very basic claims: first, health care reform can no longer be discussed simply as a binary choice between 'public' or 'private' options. This was the axis on which health care was debated in the 1980s and 1990s, but it is, for the most part, largely obsolete today. The choices are far more complex. There is more than enough evidence to show that simply privatizing health care is not a viable option. At the same time, a fully public health care system is not sustainable (one-third of Canada's health care spending already is in the private sphere). The harder choices involve selecting various ways of funding and providing health care, and trying to understand how to make all the pieces fit together most effectively.

The second claim is that the contemporary discussion has gone beyond the dyadic public-private debate to whether we face zero-sum choices or positive-sum choices. In other words, will we have to choose between the kinds of qualities we want our health care system to have, or is there a way of changing the way in which things are run so that we can achieve all (or most) of the objectives to which we aspire? Like the health care systems of all modern countries, the ideal Canadian model is premised on the perfect balance between several major components, including cost containment, equity, efficiency, universality, comprehensiveness, and responsiveness. In practice, moving too far in securing one objective (such as choice) will generally undermine one or more of the others (such as cost containment). To a large extent, then, it seems that we face a trade-off between health care goals: we cannot have it all. Or can we?

Those who advocate a positive-sum model argue that the choices aren't so stark. They look at developments in integrating health care services, in data systems, in comparative efficiency research, and in health promotion strategies, and assert that we can have a system with greater choice and efficiency that does not undermine its equity or ability to contain costs.

These discussions have been articulated in the health policy literature for some years now. But they are not easily accessible to the general public. To make reasoned policy choices Canadians must understand how their health care system works and what, therefore, the reform options are. Despite the trend in public administration towards transparency, accountability, and democratic governance, Canadians cannot be expected to engage fully in the debate over health care unless they can comprehend how the system works dynamically in both its policy and political environments. Thus part of the task here is thinking about political interests: who is pushing what option, and for what reasons? Who has an interest in blocking (or delegitimizing) any particular option? The health care system should not simply be seen as a large mechanism with various interlocking cogs and gears, but also as a battlefield of competing interests with varying levels of influence. Even the most sensible health policy will not be enacted if there are powerful agents who don't like it (as health reform in the United States has shown). Identifying some of these interests, and what they have to gain or to lose in any particular health policy debate, should enable us better to evaluate the arguments for or against specific policy options (if, say, Bernie stands to inherit most of Grandma's property, we should probably look hard at his argument to take her off life support).

This book is intended to be a critical overview of the Canadian health care system. It is not simply a description of the system itself, but a discussion of the intellectual debates and political dynamics involved in health care policy. It is not comprehensive: there are a number of important health policy issues that are not included here that could have constituted discrete chapters. These include policy discussions over home care and long-term care; Aboriginal health care and health policy focusing on other vulnerable or unrepresented groups; rural health care; bioethics; orphan diseases; and so on. Many of these issues are briefly mentioned in the context of the larger debates presented in the following chapters.

This book is also about the health care system's intransigence to change, and its capacity for vital reform. One of the most influential works on how to understand the dynamics of change in health care is

Carolyn Hughes Tuohy's *Accidental Logics: The Dynamics of Change in the Health Care Arena in the United States, Britain, and Canada*, which examines health care policy from the perspective of 'historical institutionalism.' This perspective holds that all policy decisions are constrained by the institutional environment within which they are articulated. Health care in Canada, for example, is constrained by a federal system, in which sustained political agreement must be achieved by numerous political actors, often with competing interests, before any significant political change can occur. This explains why so little radical change took place in the past several decades. In contrast, the health care system in the United Kingdom is much more centralized, and has been subject to a number of significant policy reforms throughout the past two decades.

Tuohy points out that this trajectory of 'path dependency' can, however, be recalibrated by 'windows of opportunity' which open at certain times: a pattern of timing that derives 'from factors in the broader political system, not the health care arena itself' (Tuohy 1999: 6). Like most social science, this model is better at explaining why changes happened in the past than at predicting how they will manifest themselves in the future. It is, nevertheless, helpful in obliging us to understand that health policy reform is not purely arbitrary or historically determined, but rather strategic and political. Health policy analysts saw the election of Barack Obama as a critical juncture in shaping health policy in the United States – until the collapse of the banking system in 2009. As this window of opportunity began to close, American political debate became an intense struggle to see what possible changes could be achieved (or prevented). The result was much less than proponents of reform had hoped for, but it was reform nonetheless. Thus, health care policy is constructed and constricted.

A similar debate exists in Canada: the issue of sustainability in a period of economic contraction forces us to think ever more clearly about how long we can go without fundamental reform, while the abysmal health record of the United States makes us realize that the simple debate of public versus private is no longer tenable. The health care system must be fixed; but the shape it should take is unclear. For those confused about why the system is so difficult to fix, this book is a guide for the perplexed. It does not offer simple solutions; it explains why they do not exist. But for those wishing to make changes, it is a road map of how the system is truly an interlinking set of paths, processes, and power struggles.

If health care systems are highly political, so is the study of health care systems. I received a grant to write a book on the politics of health care in 1992. Had I done so then, instead of tending other gardens, it would have been a much different book. It would also have been less interesting (and much thinner). The economic turmoil of the 1990s meant that many of the developments in health policy were discouraging ones. While the seeds of change were sown in this dismal field, it was the economic expansion and theoretical innovation that occurred thereafter that made health policy such an engrossing subdiscipline. Once primarily the province of economics, health policy has become a truly multidisciplinary field of study. Debates once grounded firmly within economics and interest-group politics now encompass ideas presented in public administration, sociology, comparative politics, law, philosophy, and other disciplines.

It is difficult to write about the politics of health care in the present tense. Practices and institutions become quickly outdated, and changes of government also bring changes in policy direction. Merely describing how the system works entails working on shifting sands. What remains constant is the resolutely political nature of the broad debate over health care. This is as true for the *study* of health politics as it is for health care itself. Even as the study of health care becomes more multidisciplinary, funding for the study of health politics has been removed from the sphere of the social sciences (Science and Humanities Research Council of Canada, SHRCC) and relocated to that of the medical sciences (Canadian Institutes of Health Research, CIHR). In 1992, a researcher wishing to investigate the political dynamics underlying health politics would apply for funding from a research agency designed to encourage the analysis of power dynamics underlying contemporary social relations. That the results of such investigations might be exasperating, irritating, or threatening to those holding the balance of power was not only accepted, but generally counted in one's favour. In 2010, a social scientist engaged in the examination of political dynamics within the field of health care would have no option but to compete for funding with medical researchers, who generally operate within a completely different intellectual culture. This is one that largely builds on the status quo rather than opposes it. It is also one that does not tend to ask whose interests are being served by following one direction rather than another. Scientific neutrality, not the bias of scepticism, is the intellectual baseline. But this does not mean that the structure of scientific research is itself necessarily apolitical. Given that CIHR has explicitly articulated the commercialization of health research as one of its fundamental goals and that senior drug company executives are involved in governing this funding body, for example, one is led to wonder about the extent to which any research project that questioned the appropriateness of health care commercialization would be given serious consideration.

The critical evaluation of the Canadian health care system may or may not be affected by the way in which researchers are funded. But the first step in developing any accountable and responsive system is simply having a solid understanding of how the system works. As health care becomes increasingly complex, it is important to ensure that everyone with a stake in the health care system – either as decision maker, health care consumer, health care provider, or taxpayer – is able to understand why things work the way they do, what the obstacles are to change, and what the potential trade-offs are for competing policy directions. I am most fortunate and grateful to have received the advice and criticism from colleagues across a number of disciplines, not only in political science but also in public administration, medicine, law, nursing, pharmacy, and medical anthropology. I would also like to acknowledge the assistance of individuals within various branches of Health Canada (specifically Public Health Agency of Canada, Patented Medicines Prices Review Board, and Health Products and Food Branch), as well as officials within provincial departments of health who took the time thoughtfully to explain how their particular corner of the health care field worked. The patience and professionalism of those at the University of Toronto Press have been exemplary; they are a pleasure to work with. Special thanks are due also to Peter Aucoin, Kate Baltais, Sarah Binder, Gerry Boychuk, Louise Carbert, Annette Daley, Jocelyn Downie, Mary Fierlbeck, Albert Fierlbeck, Gordon Forsyth, Judy Garber, Adam Gibson, Elaine Gibson, Janice Graham, Barb Greschner, Jim Houston, Paula McKay, Norma Kinnear, Jeff Scott, Ingrid Sketris, Steven Tomblin, Gail Tomblin-Murphy and, of course, all of the anonymous reviewers who provided so much thoughtful and constructive advice.

Abbreviations

ACCESS	A Convention on the Canadian Economic and Social Systems
ACHDHR	Federal/Provincial/Territorial Advisory Committee on Health Delivery and Human Resources
ACO	accountable care organization (U.S.)
ACT	assertive community treatment
AHIP	America's health insurance plans
ALLHAT	Antihypertensive and Lipid-Lowering Treatment to Prevent Heart Attack Trial
AMSA	American Medical Student Association
BSE	bovine spongiform encephalopathy
CADTH	Canadian Agency for Drugs and Technologies in Health
CER	comparative effectiveness research
CGPA	Canadian Generic Pharmaceutical Association
CHA	Canada Health Act
CHB	community health board
CHC	community health council
CHI	Commission for Health Improvement (U.K.)
CHSRF	Canadian Health Services Research Foundation
CHST	Canada Health and Social Transfer
CIHI	Canadian Institute for Health Information
CIHR	Canadian Institutes of Health Research
CME	continuing medical education
CMHA	Canadian Mental Health Association
CMU	Couverture Maladie Universelle (Universal Health Coverage Act, France)
CMU-C	Couverture Maladie Universelle Complémentaire (France)
CNIB	Canadian National Institute for the Blind

COMPAS	Canadian Optimal Medication Prescribing and Utilization Service
CPHI	Canadian Population Health Initiative
CPHO	chief public health officer
DFAIT	Department of Foreign Affairs and International Trade
DGF	diagnostic-group financing
DHA	district health authority
DRG	diagnostic-related group
DSEN	Drug Safety and Effectiveness Network
EMA	European Medicines Agency
EPF	Established Program Financing
EU	European Union
FDA	Food and Drug Administration (U.S.)
FDAAA	Food and Drug Administration Amendments Act
FFS	fee for service
FMAP	federal medical assistance percentage (U.S.)
FP	for profit
GATS	General Agreement on Trade in Services
GDP	gross domestic product
GP	general practitioner
GSK	GlaxoSmithKline
HAS	Haute Authorité de Santé (France)
HCC	Health Council of Canada
hcs	health care spending
HiAP	Health in All Policies (EU)
HIE	health insurance experiment
HMO	Health Maintenance Organization
HSRC	Health Services Restructuring Commission
ISRCTN	International Standard Randomized Controlled Trial Number Register
IT	information technology
KOL	key opinion leader
LHIN	local health integration networks (Ontario)
MD	medical doctor
MHCC	Mental Health Commission of Canada
MHITF	Mental Health Implementation Task Force (Ontario)
NAFTA	North American Free Trade Agreement
NDP	New Democratic Party
NFP	not for profit
NHS	National Health Service (U.K.)

NICE	National Institute for Clinical Effectiveness (U.K.)
NIH	National Institutes of Health (U.S.)
NOC/c	conditional notice of compliance
NPDUIS	National Prescription Drug Utilization Information System
NPM	new public management
OECD	Organization for Economic Co-operation and Development
OHA	Ontario Hospital Association
OHIP	Ontario Health Insurance Plan
OMA	Ontario Medical Association
P4P	pay for performance
PACs	political action committees (U.S.)
PBS	Pharmaceutical Benefits Scheme (Australia)
PCG	primary care group (U.K.)
PCT	primary care trust (U.K.)
PFP	private for-profit
PHAC	Public Health Agency of Canada
PhRMA	Pharmaceutical Research and Manufacturers of America (U.S.)
PHU	public health unit
PMPRB	Patented Medicines Prices Review Board
PNFP	private not-for-profit
PPACA	Patient Protection and Affordable Care Act (U.S.)
PPP (or P3)	public-private partnership; also purchasing power parity
PROCTOR	Public Reporting of Clinical Trials Outcomes and Results
R&D	research and development
RAND/HIE	Research and Development Corporation / Health Insurance Experiment
RHA	regional health authority
RN	registered nurse
Rx&D	Canada's research-based pharmaceutical companies
SARS	severe acute respiratory syndrome
SDOH	social determinants of health
SHI	statutory health insurance
TPD	Therapeutic Products Directorate
VA	Veterans Affairs, Department of (U.S.)
VHA	Veterans Health Administration (U.S.)
WHO	World Health Organization
WMD	wet macular degeneration

HEALTH CARE IN CANADA:
A CITIZEN'S GUIDE TO POLICY AND POLITICS

1   Funding Health Care

Revisiting the 'Golden Mean'

The good life, Aristotle argued, depended on finding proper equilibrium. Too much courage led to rash behaviour; too little made one a coward. Too much amiability produced obsequiousness; too little, irascibility. That such excess is undesirable was clear; the difficulty, he noted, was in knowing exactly how far to move in any given situation. This Aristotelian model is useful for thinking about health care funding: extremes are dangerous, but the exact balance between extremes – the 'golden mean' – is much more difficult to determine.

There are a number of desirable qualities in any health care system: these include cost containment, efficiency, equity, universality, comprehensiveness, and responsiveness. The attainment of all these qualities is the ideal objective of health policy. The problem is that the more we move to secure one goal, the more we can undermine one or several others. The real challenge, as Aristotle suggests, is to understand how we ought to balance these qualities. Aristotle's complete doctrine of the mean was quite complicated, yet it comprised only three pillars. Health policy has to balance at least six. Thus the calculations and trade-offs involved can be very complex and, as Aristotle suggested, depend very much on the particular personality of the individual (or polity) involved.

What are these pillars of health care? *Cost containment* is the capacity of a system to control expenditure. This is frequently tied into discussions of 'sustainability' (which is a much fuzzier concept). Public systems are generally better at cost containment, especially if the governments are highly centralized, as decision makers have more control over expenditure. But demand-based forms of cost containment also exist: these include any mechanisms to discourage health consumers from using services (or, at least, to encourage them to use services efficiently). 'Gatekeeping,' in which all initial consultations must be made by general practitioners (GPs) rather than more expensive consultants, is one example. User fees, where people must share the cost of a service, are another. All of these strategies, as we will see, have implications for the *other* objectives. Discussions of cost containment should focus on how well all forms of spending – public and private – are controlled. 'Containing' government spending on health care by allowing individuals to purchase health care in the marketplace, for example, is not containment at all, but merely cost-shifting, and usually results in even higher levels of spending.

Efficiency refers to the amount and quality of goods and services provided relative to the amount of money spent. The provision of health services is efficient if you don't pay more than you have to for goods and services, and if you don't utilize what you don't really need. A health care system can be quite successful at cost containment but still be inefficient: it could, for example, spend less money than other similar countries on health care; but if the money earmarked for health care could potentially be providing more goods and services, then the system is still inefficient. This was seen by many to be the case with the National Health Service (NHS) in the United Kingdom before the internal market reforms of the 1990s. At the same time, a country could conceivably have a very high level of public spending on health care, and still maintain a very efficient level of spending (by providing a significant amount of goods and services per dollar spent). Such a system would probably be found within a nation where health care was highly socially valued, as the money spent – however efficiently – could nonetheless potentially be used in other areas (such as education, housing, or military funding).

'Efficiency' may seem straightforward, but it is a very tricky concept. In the first place, measures of efficiency depend on *counterfactuals*, or speculations about how things could be otherwise. A health system is considered to be inefficient if it could conceivably be supplying more goods and services with the same amount of money: but whether any particular system *would*, in fact, be able to provide more goods and services with less money *if* it were run differently is conjectural. There are also the potent questions of what ought to be fair reimbursement for goods and services (such as physician services or pharmaceuticals), and what constitutes 'need' (are fertility treatments, e.g., based on medical need or subjective desire?). Moreover, there are different ways of understanding efficiency. 'Allocative efficiency' is a concept that assumes that an efficient distribution is one in which only those individuals who *really want* something (and thus are willing to pay for it) will receive it (for a more technical discussion, see Evans 2002). As poorer individuals will be less likely to spend 30 dollars on a consultation with a physician, they are considered to be 'less willing' to pay for it, and their decision not to seek medical advice is, according to this model of market economics, a gain in efficiency. From an epidemiological (or public health) perspective, however, if the patient who does not seek treatment becomes progressively sicker and requires much more expensive treatment in emergency and surgical wards, this is a very inefficient way to run a health care system. This issue is highlighted by the case of a 12-year-old boy in Baltimore whose family could not afford to have his tooth removed by a dentist. When bacteria from the abscessed tooth spread to his brain, he was rushed to the hospital for emergency surgery and spent six weeks in hospital at the cost of U.S.$250,000. Even after this intervention, the boy died (Alakeson 2008: 720–2).

The third pillar of a health care system is *equity*. To a large extent, whether equity is important at all in the provision of health care depends on the values of the jurisdiction responsible for delivering health care. Those who believe that access to health care is a marker of citizenship hold that all individuals should have reasonably similar access to health services regardless of income (or gender, race, age, or region). Those who hold that health services are commodities that should be available to those who can afford them will see equity in health care as much less important. Many European countries articulate a strong sense of social solidarity, which holds that all citizens have a collective responsibility for the less well-off, and access to health care (and other social resources) in these countries is generally indicative of greater equity. Like efficiency, equity can be interpreted in different ways. In health care funding debates, equity generally refers to equitable access to health care by those who are in need of it, regardless of income (vertical equity). But it is possible to base discussions of equity on consumption of resources (horizontal equity): those who consume more health care should pay more; those who use less should be able to pay less. This was the logic, for example, for the poll taxes Prime Minister Thatcher implemented in Great Britain in the early 1990s.

Equity becomes especially contentious in debates over health care when its perceived costs become too high. In Canada, the sense of fairness underlying the idea of 'one-tier' health care becomes weakened when long waiting lists for surgery, GP consultations, and emergency services are seen to be a consequence of a public system. But exactly what is meant by equity in 'health care' is notoriously vague: for example, all Canadians who have a heart attack will receive full treatment for it, regardless of income. This access is not inconsiderable, as the average cost of treatment for a heart attack in the United States is about U.S.$110,405. Statistically, however, one can discern differences in the quality of care for heart-attack patients not only across provinces but also across regions *within* provinces. There is also a discrepancy between the way in which men and women suffering heart attacks are treated. Moreover, there is a vast inequity between Canadians suffering different kinds of illnesses, as all medically necessary hospital treatments are covered by public insurance in Canada, but often prescription drugs in many provinces are not. Thus individuals with illnesses that are addressed in hospitals face no out-of-pocket costs; while Canadians whose illnesses are treated by drugs on an outpatient basis must, in many cases, bear these costs themselves. Likewise, Canadians whose health conditions require buying expensive medical devices (from reading glasses to syringes to oxygen canisters) or services like physiotherapy may feel there is little 'equity' in the Canadian health care system.

Universality and *comprehensiveness* are terms that generally are used to describe the system of health insurance rather than the health care system per se. But because the two systems are so closely interlinked it is worth briefly touching on both terms. Universality is a weaker form of equity. Universality is an objective that has, for the most part, been achieved in all developed countries (with the United States finally making a commitment in 2010 to move towards universal coverage). Universality, however, is a relatively fuzzy concept, as it simply means that all residents of a jurisdiction are covered by some form of health insurance that gives them reasonable access to necessary health services. But God and the devil are in the details: these forms of health insurance can vary widely, and much is left unsaid in what, exactly, is required by the term 'reasonable access.' There is also no stipulation that all access has to be equitable: some individuals can have access to better or faster health care, and their particular forms of health insurance can be widely divergent. This is where the term *comprehensiveness* becomes relevant. Health insurance, whether public or private, that covers only certain kinds of services (primary care, hospital care) and not others (drugs and devices, long-term care, dental and optical, physiotherapy, and so on) is less comprehensive than insurance that covers all of these. Often (but not necessarily) there is a trade-off between comprehensiveness and cost control, or comprehensiveness and equity. How comprehensive is Canadian health care? Not very. The Canada Health Act does stipulate that health care insurance must be 'comprehensive,' but this refers only to medically necessary services that are provided within hospitals, and not on an outpatient basis (provinces are free to cover outpatient services if they choose to do so, but they are not required to). Moreover, the definition of 'medically necessary' is notably arbitrary: it is up to provinces to decide this for themselves, and this is often a political decision. It could not be otherwise: with the current scope and volume of services, products, and technologies available to treat ailments, the expectation that all treatments must be provided to all individuals publically is simply not economically feasible. This is why extremely expensive treatments that benefit a very small number of people are often not covered, despite the apparent evidence that, to these people, such treatment would seem to be 'medically necessary.' Whether a system offers 'comprehensive' health care also depends on the kinds of barriers limiting access to (theoretically existing) services: all Canadians have access to hip replacements, but they face barriers established by waiting times; Americans' access to hip replacements has been limited by economic barriers.

A sixth pillar is playing an increasingly important role in the provision of health care. As the selection of services, drugs, and technology increases, and as patients become seen as consumers, much more attention is being placed on the degree of choice available to health care users. To many individuals, the ability to have a say over what kinds of services they receive, who provides them, and where and when they are provided is important not only because of the sense of autonomy that it fosters, but also because it forces the health care system to be more *responsive* to those it is expected to serve. In this way, 'choice' often involves some form of competition; but not necessarily competition on the free market. In some European systems, for example, the ability to choose between health insurance providers is often a choice between public or private-not-for-profit funders, with private-for-profit insurers comprising a very low proportion of available options. In countries with 'internal markets' (like England), it is the GPs who have greater choices regarding where their patients will receive specialized care: but again, the care options remain largely publicly funded.

The capacity to choose is one factor that seems important in cross-national surveys of satisfaction. It can also be a strongly held social value in certain countries (such as France or the United States), one which is so essential to a critical mass of the population that elected officials are willing to sacrifice other important qualities of health service provision in order to retain it. The ability to offer choice involves costs. In the United Kingdom, for example, choice involving hospitals and admission dates was deemed one of the 'least important aspects' of medical care in a 2006 survey; while in the United States individuals remained much more willing to sacrifice efficient and coordinated care in order to retain their ability to see any doctor at any time (Alakeson 2008: 721). The health care reforms attempted in the United States in the early 1990s failed largely because Americans were told (incorrectly) that a single payer system would severely jeopardize their freedom of choice in all areas of health care. Ironically, the managed care system that developed in the consequent policy vacuum meant that patients' choices became tightly constrained by the privately managed care plan to which they signed on. In France, patients also demand a high degree of choice in payment options and physician services. They enjoy this choice a great deal, but they also pay very highly for it, making France one of the most expensive health care systems in Europe.

In sum, then, we must move away from the simplistic public-private duality as the basis for discussing how health care is to be provided. The debate between 'solidaristic' and 'competitive' models of health care remains as consequential now as ever; but 'private' and 'public' are more usefully seen as mechanisms that can be used to achieve a wide variety of systems. We do need to understand what these public and private mechanisms are in order to consider how they can be used to achieve the particular 'golden mean' best suited for a specific polity at any given time. The attempt to find a perfect balance between all desirable attributes in health policy has been described as a 'holy grail' (e.g., Flood, Stabile, and Tuohy 2008) but, like the quest for the holy grail, the attempt to design a perfect health care system is quixotic (and potentially ruinous). The interesting policy experiments will be those that will be able to protect one element (such as efficiency) without destroying others (such as equity). But the 'best' system will depend ultimately on the collective choices that each society makes for itself.

What Do We Mean by 'Public' and 'Private'?

The discussion over 'public' and 'private' health care in any system must first acknowledge the important distinction between the 'financing' and

Table 1.1. Public and Private Delivery of and Payment for Health Care Services

	Public (Collective) Payment	Private (Individual) Payment
Public sector delivery	Public insurance, public hospitals, and public employees	Public insurance topped up by private user fees
Private sector delivery	Public insurance and privately employed or self-employed providers	Private insurance and privately employed or self-employed providers

the 'delivery' of services. At first glance these categories seem clearly defined; but as one begins to apply them to particular systems the boundaries between them begin to blur considerably. *Financing* refers to the way in which health services are funded (i.e., where the revenue for these services comes from); and *delivery* refers to the 'ownership and motivation of the organizations that are funded from these revenues' (Evans 2002: 4). Private and public financing can in theory work harmoniously with both privately and publicly provided services: self-employed GPs, for example, are *private* practitioners; but they can be paid directly by patients (privately) or be remunerated by government (publicly). Deber (2002: 3) and others have suggested a matrix for understanding how these two components can be combined (see Table 1.1).

At this point things begin to get more difficult.

Ways of Financing Health Care Systems

There are not simply two major models of financing (public and private) but at least four, and these are: *general taxation, social insurance, private insurance,* and *out-of-pocket payment.* Often these components work together in a single health care system. Under a system of health care purely financed by *general taxation,* patients do not pay when receiving treatment, as revenue is collected through various forms of taxation (e.g., some jurisdictions earmark a certain proportion of sales taxes for health care, although most health funding comes from general tax funds). These systems are often referred to as 'public insurance' systems, although social insurance systems (noted below) are often considered to be 'public' systems because they are mandated, not-for-profit, and highly regulated. One advantage of general taxation is its wide tax base, which includes taxation from sources beyond labour income (including rent, interest, and dividends). The large number of people covered under purely public insurance systems means that it is very effective in 'pooling the risks,' as all healthy people subsidize the sick (they cannot, by definition, opt out of general taxation). To the extent that general tax systems are progressive, funding of health care is also progressive. Where there is a public, single-payer system (e.g., government is the only insurer), administrative costs are very low: those requesting reimbursement from the public plan (e.g., GPs) do not have to spend their time filling out numerous forms for different insurance agencies. The main insurer does not have to spend money on advertisements or other inducements to try to win over more customers. There is considerably less regulation, as there is no worry about insurance companies attempting to 'cherry-pick' the healthiest customers to keep their profits up. At the same time, there is no means-testing or other requirement that patients prove their penury in order to receive insurance, as there is with government-sponsored plans targeted only for low-income individuals.

Health care systems based on general taxation are also generally good at overall cost containment: if expenditure is centrally controlled by one department and, formally, one individual (generally the provincial minister of health), then that individual has the discretion to reduce costs when and how she or he sees fit. This was evident in the way in which provinces often quite drastically reduced health care spending in the mid-1990s. It is also perceptible in other countries with general taxation (such as the United Kingdom). One significant concern with systems based on general taxation, however, is 'the substantial information asymmetry that exists between providers and patients and between managers/regulators and patients' (Flood, Stabile, and Tuohy 2008: 11). Because patients (or GPs) do not bear direct responsibility for costs when incurred, there is little direct economic incentive to limit demand; and because those making allocation decisions at the highest level do not know exactly what is needed in every treatment area at each point in time, it is difficult to determine exactly what expenditure levels should be, and how to allocate them. Thus, while Canada, the United Kingdom, and Sweden have been very good in keeping their government expenditure under control compared with other developed countries, they also consistently face charges of 'underfunding' their health care systems as well as problems with waiting lists in certain areas.

Social insurance is a model more common in Europe. Under this system, health insurance is organized around discrete groups (usually based on employment), who can make contributions based on either a flat rate or a rate proportional to income. Most social insurance plans are actually private not-for-profit bodies, but they usually are considered under the category of 'public' financing because they are, by law, not optional: workers are mandated to contribute, and the plans are generally heavily regulated by government. In some countries, such as Germany, people who earn above a certain level of income have been permitted to opt out of their social insurance plan (either contributing to a private plan, or paying out-of-pocket for health care) but since 2009 even high-income earners are required to have some form of health insurance. There is increasing discussion regarding whether Canada should move from a system of general taxation to one based on social insurance (e.g., Flood, Stabile, and Tuohy 2008). It is useful to remember that the European social insurance systems were not established because they were considered to be the best way of financing health care per se, but because they were seen to be politically feasible. The practice of basing health insurance on occupation had its roots in Europe's medieval guild system, which became the basis for late nineteenth- and early-twentieth -century 'friendly societies' and other worker-based systems of social support. Certainly this system of social insurance seems to work reasonably well in the European countries that employ it; but are the merits of a social insurance system so compelling that it ought to replace one based on general taxation?

A major drawback is that social insurance plans are limited by their size: the more plans, the smaller they become, and the less capacity there is to pool the risks. There is also the complexity of administering these plans: in France in 2003, for example, there were 1,444 different private health insurers: 1,275 were *mutuelles* (which also provide statutory health insurance), 51 were provident institutions, and 118 were private for-profit companies. Each category is governed by a separate set of laws. Further, a system based on payroll taxes, by definition, is designed to cover only those people who are employed. Thus France was obliged, in 2000, to implement a new health insurance plan based on general taxation (the *couverture maladie universelle*) for the poorest 10 per cent of French citizens. Social insurance plans, if designed carefully and regulated tightly, can perform relatively well in respect to the criteria noted at the beginning of this chapter but, historical circumstances aside, there seems little reason to pursue a system of social insurance for its own sake. There is slightly more 'information connect' in a social insurance system, compared with one based on general taxation, insofar as individuals can compare their contributions and benefits with those in other plans, and they may recognize how much of their income goes towards health care (most French workers could tell you that about 7 per cent of their salary goes directly into maintaining their health care system, with their employer contributing another 13 per cent). Nonetheless, this has not acted as a damper on demand for health services in France, as the French have a very high utilization rate of services, and they are the highest consumers of prescription drugs in Europe. Most observers have argued that the advantages of a social insurance system are largely political, insofar as members of a discrete occupation may be more willing to bear the burdens of solidarity than members of the general population are (see, e.g., Marmor 2008).

Both *private insurance* and *out-of-pocket* funding are considered to be 'private' financing models, but it must be remembered that both of these entail government involvement in the form of regulation. A health care system based on private insurance must be heavily regulated in order to provide effective coverage, as the demand for profits will lead to the attempt to limit coverage to healthier individuals (at the expense of the sick) and constrain payment for treatment as often as possible. Even out-of-pocket payments cannot exist without regulation (no developed countries, e.g., permit patients to buy organs for transplant on the open market). The advantages and disadvantages of private insurance will be considered in more detail in the next section. Theoretically, the benefits of private insurance are based on its allocative efficiency: goods and services will go to those who most value them. The larger question is the extent to which health care fits into the orthodox model of market efficiency: it does not bother us, for example, that only people who *really* want a toaster will buy one (and will save their income for that purpose, instead of spending it on a kicky pair of new shoes). Should it bother us that anyone who did buy the shoes now cannot afford a GP visit to address what might be strep throat (with possibly severe long-term consequences), or what might just be a cold? Can one act as an informed consumer of health services or insurance with the same ease as one purchases a car? (Consider the following scenario: Hmm, let's see: my odds of contracting breast cancer, with an 87-week total treatment cost of $104,535, given my age, medical history, and lifestyle choices, are probably not worth an extra $125 per year of medical insurance, so I'll choose a plan with lower premiums and less coverage. The likelihood that I'll contract Type 2 diabetes, which costs $5,949 per year for insulin, test strips, syringes, quarterly physician visits, and eye exams, is probably also low, given my weight and diet, despite a high prevalence in North America, so I think I'll forego coverage of it as well. My risk of a stroke ...)

All private insurance is not the same. Countries employ private health insurance for different purposes (see Thomson and Mossialos 2008: 7). In the United States, private insurance is the primary form of coverage (for those who do not qualify for Medicaid, Medicare, Veterans Health Insurance, or the Child Health Insurance Program). In Germany, where the majority of citizens are covered by social insurance, private insurance has a 'substitutive' function, and covers groups that opt out or are excluded from the social insurance funds. Private insurance can also be 'complementary,' and cover services entirely excluded from the public system (as in Belgium) or cover user fees imposed by the public system (as in France). Finally, private insurance can also have a 'supplementary' function, by offering enhanced service options (such as access to faster services, wider treatment options, or aesthetic upgrades in facilities) where basic public coverage already exists (as in Britain).

The disadvantages of private insurance, which will be examined in more detail below, generally focus on its regressive nature (if you have a higher risk of insured conditions, your premiums increase). This means that the sick (and poor, who generally have worse health) will be bearing the economic burden. Another disadvantage comes from the administrative costs involved in sending (and processing) claim forms to numerous insurance agencies. (Canadians should try an experiment: the next time you see your dentist or optometrist, ask them how much time and money they spend processing insurance claims. Then ask your GP.)

To recap, there are four predominant models of health care funding, and these are: general taxation, social insurance, private insurance, and out-of-pocket payments. But the reality is much more complicated, as most countries utilize some combination of these models. New Zealand and the United Kingdom, for example, have parallel or duplicate systems, which means that citizens can choose services from either the public or the private sector. Other countries, such as Germany, have a combination of group-based and private systems. France's social insurance system is combined with both a tax-based public insurance system, for the very poor, and a co-payment system, in which most individuals use private insurance to top up the coverage paid by their social insurance plans (usually about 70 per cent for treatments and 30–65 per cent for drugs.)

It is absolutely imperative to comprehend how health insurance is structured in any country, and to understand not only *how* things are covered, but also *what* is covered. This is especially true for Canada, which is unique among countries in its ability to maintain a clear boundary between services that are publically insured and those that are privately insured (or available for purchase out-of-pocket). Various political and legislative mechanisms (described later in this chapter) have been put into place by provinces in order severely to restrict the growth of a parallel private insurance system similar to that of the United Kingdom. This is why Canadian health care is described as a 'one-tier' system, as opposed to Britain's two-tier model. Proponents see this system as much more equitable because access to 'medically necessary services' is formally independent of income. But the problem is that, for historical reasons, only primary (GP) care and hospital (including diagnostic) services are covered by public insurance. Other goods and services, including prescriptions, optometry, dental care, home care, long-term care, and off-site (non-hospital) mental health care, and physiotherapy are generally not covered, although much depends on each province's health insurance plan. This is why so much of Canada's health care spending is for private care. On average, 73 per cent of all health care spending in member countries of the Organization for Economic Co-operation and Development (OECD) is public sector spending: in some countries, including the United Kingdom, Japan, and the Scandinavian countries, over 80 per cent of health care spending is in the public sector. Canada funds only 70 per cent of its health care sector publicly (OECD 2008: 2). Because so many goods and services that most people would likely view as important, if not essential, are still funded privately, Canada can be criticized as being highly inequitable in its distribution of health care resources (few citizens in France or Germany, for example, have to bear the full cost for filling a drug prescription, an eye examination, or long-term care). Canada's one-tier system of primary and hospital care is thus a sharp two-tier system when other goods and services are considered.

In addition to the practice of combining public and private insurance systems, there are also 'hybrid' models of financing health systems. Evans (2002) discusses five hybrid systems. The first of these are the health care 'premiums' levied by Alberta and British Columbia. These premiums, notes Evans, are more accurately classified as 'poll taxes,' as the Canada Health Act stipulates that provinces must cover *everyone* within their jurisdictions: thus defaulting on one's health care premiums cannot result in refusal of treatment (although it might lead to a penalty). In any case, health care premiums simply end up as part of a province's general revenues. Another hybrid model is the public subsidy of private health insurance. The practice of rebating private insurance premiums to taxpayers has been a strategy pursued in Australia, and is also common in the United States, where over a third of private insurance payments are reimbursed by state subsidies (Shiels and Hogan 1999). This practice encourages wider coverage of socio-economic groups who otherwise might not be able to receive health insurance; but it is also highly regressive, as this kind of tax benefit is worth more the higher one's income is. In recent debates over health reform in the United States, as well as in proposals for Canada by the Fraser Institute (Skinner and Rovere 2008), the public subsidy of private health insurance has been discussed in conjunction with a third mechanism: 'mandation,' or the legal requirement that all individuals contribute to a private plan (although the choice of plan is up to them). Like any system of private insurance, however, it requires careful regulation to ensure that private insurance plans do not refuse to take sick or 'high risk' individuals. The fourth hybrid model suggests linking one's use of health care resources to one's tax bill; and the fifth is the 'medical savings account,' in which families are allocated funds or tax exemptions for use for health care services. Although coverage would not be denied beyond this amount, individuals would be rewarded financially for not using up their allotted funds. While the fourth and the fifth options attempt to limit costs by making users more responsible for costs incurred, they are both also mechanisms that ultimately reward the healthy and penalize the sick.

Ways of Delivering Health Care Services

Health care services can be classified as *public, private not-for-profit,* and *private for-profit* (Deber 2002). Whether health care services are public or private can, unsurprisingly, be determined by looking at the ownership of the undertakings. Increasingly, however, it is becoming more difficult to make a clear distinction about ownership. Moreover, ownership itself tells us relatively little about how an undertaking operates.

Services that are clearly provided by the *public* sector are directly remunerated and are legally liable to the public authority, which (in Canada) can be municipal, regional, provincial, or federal. Most public health offices are run by regional health authorities (RHAs), employ staff who are considered public servants, and are ultimately responsible to the provincial Department of Health (or Department of Public Health, in some provinces.) The public health nurse who checks schoolchildren for head lice and the epidemiologist who examines regional patterns of illness or disease are public employees. In Canada, however, most health care services are provided privately. Most general practitioners and consultant physicians, for example, are privately employed individuals who contract out their services (although some physicians do work on a salaried basis, or for a combination of salary and fees-for-service). They are generally reimbursed by the provincial government for their services, but are not usually employed *by* the state (although some argue that, where there is only a single employer, this is largely a semantic point). Moreover, most general hospitals in Canada are private entities. They are, however, *private not-for-profit* (PNFP) bodies, which means that while they have some independence from government authorities, and they are not organized around the imperative to produce profits, they are usually prohibited from distributing any surpluses as profits should they arise. They recoup costs from funders either through comprehensive contracts or on the basis of services provided: in Canada, hospitals generally receive about 90 per cent of their funding from provincial governments (including federal transfers), often through the intermediary of RHAs. Hospitals are legally liable for their debts, but they usually qualify for government grants and tax exemptions.

A small number of medical clinics in Canada are *private for-profit* (PFP) businesses. Many of these provide 'niche' surgical services, such as cataract or joint replacement surgery. They are run as entrepreneurial endeavours, and have no charitable status. It is important, however, to make the distinction between small for-profit clinics (such as the Shouldice) and large corporate undertakings that generally operate a number of large health care undertakings (such as the Hospital Corporation of America). As most medical institutions in Canada are already privately run (mostly on a NFP basis, but with some small profit-oriented clinics), the debate over the 'privatization' of health care delivery focuses on the role of American-style corporate enterprises that have a responsibility to provide shareholders with profitable returns. The anxiety stems from whether the demands of profit-making will push an enterprise from a quest for efficiency to one of dangerous cost-cutting that may compromise the health of both patients and workers. Again, these are issues that can only be controlled with adequate regulatory instruments; but, as Deber cautions, 'these in turn imply considerable administrative costs and assume that quality is easily measured' (2002: 7).

Like the financing of health care, the provision of health services in practice does not always manifest itself in clear ideal types. One example is public-private partnerships (also called PPPs or P3s). The legacy of balanced-budget legislation, which obliged provinces to rein in capital expenditures, P3s allowed governments to replace crumbling hospital infrastructure without an enormous upfront expenditure. P3 projects are not necessarily cheaper than public sector projects, as governments can generally raise funds at a better rate than private corporations. The legal complexity of P3 projects also means higher legal costs. But as the president of Ontario Infrastructure points out, this can be balanced by the transfer of risk to the private sector: 'We look at the financing of the deal as essentially the thing that incents the private sector to do it fast and do it well, because it is their money on the line and if they miss on something or something happens, the interest clock is ticking on their dime, not ours' (Silversides 2008: 992). In Britain, many hospitals, primary care clinics, and other health care services have been transformed into health care 'trusts.' This means that while these services ultimately remain under the control of the state-run National Health Service, they have been reorganized in a pattern of health care funders and providers which mimics market relationships (see Chapter 9). Another form of interrelationship is the contracting out of services (usually surgical) by public health authorities to private facilitates in order to alleviate waiting lists at hospitals.

How Canada's Health Care System Is Funded

Before one's eyes start glazing over from these descriptions of economic models, it is important to keep in mind that discussions over health care funding are not simply about the allocation of money and the regulation of services, but rather about the interplay of human relations, the resolution of political struggles, and the kinds of values that democratic societies reflect through their public policies. Health care reform, writes one observer, often begins with narratives about cruelty: in Canada's case, this included a 1946 *Globe and Mail* report of a woman in labour who was refused treatment by three successive physicians because of her inability to pay for treatment (Gawande 2009a). Canadians are perhaps more familiar with Tommy Douglas's argument that health care ought to be built on a recognition of human dignity as well as a framework of economic efficiency: 'the time is surely past,' he declared in 1961, 'when people should have to depend on proving need in order to get services that should be the inalienable right of every citizen of a good society. It is all very well for some people to say that there is no stigma or humiliation connected with having to prove need. This is always said by people who know that they are in no danger of having to prove need' (Douglas 2005 [1961]: 122).

Canada's current health care system is often dated back to 1947, when Douglas introduced publicly funded universal hospital insurance in Saskatchewan. Others reference 1972 as the date when a 'fully Canadian' system of health care was finally established. Both dates are correct. Technically, Canada does not have one health care system, but thirteen, as each province and territory has constitutional responsibility for health care within its own jurisdiction (see Chapter 2). While some provinces (such as Ontario) had various publicly funded health programs in place throughout the early twentieth century (Naylor 1992), it was Saskatchewan's 1947 universal hospital insurance plan that served as the model for subsequent provincial hospital insurance plans. By 1957 Ottawa agreed to cost-share this insurance plan with the provinces, and the federal Hospital Insurance and Diagnostic Services Act set out the conditions that provinces would have to meet in order to receive these funds. It was also Saskatchewan that established public insurance for physician services in 1961. Again, Ottawa agreed to cost-share this program for any province that agreed to conform to four basic principles (universality, comprehensiveness, portability, and public administration): thus the 1966 Medical Care Act became the basis for the current Canada Health Act (CHA). By 1972 all provinces and territories were participating in both cost-shared programs with the federal government, and this voluntary coordination of all provinces through federal legislation is what is generally meant by 'the Canadian health care system.'

This complicated relationship between federal, provincial, and territorial governments over health care will be examined more closely in Chapter 2. To understand the current funding system, however, the starting point is the observation that Canada's health care system is a fragmented system *controlled* by the provinces but *coordinated* by the federal government, with the provinces' consent. Most hospital and physician care is publicly insured in Canada (as are most diagnostic tests ordered by physicians), but many medical goods and services are not. Health care services are generally provided by private practitioners who are either reimbursed by public insurance (e.g., most GPs) or by private insurance and out-of-pocket payments (e.g., most dentists). Most hospitals in Canada are private not-for-profit institutions that are funded through a global budget by provincial departments of health, and governed by boards of trustees. While individuals are free to choose their GP (and to switch GPs when they want), all provinces and territories employ a 'gatekeeper' system under which patients have access to specialists only when they are referred by a family physician. Both GPs and specialists are reimbursed by provinces according to fee schedules that are determined in discussion with physicians' professional associations.

Those services that are publicly funded (GP services, hospital care, and diagnostic services performed in hospitals) are paid for out of general revenues. Most funds come from the provinces' respective tax bases, with less than 20 per cent of health care expenditure transferred to the provinces from Ottawa. Two provinces (British Columbia and Quebec) levy 'health care premiums' (Alberta eliminated its health care premium in 2009), although they are more accurately considered 'taxes,' as they go directly into general revenues (rather than into health care programs), and access to publicly insured services is guaranteed to all under the provisions of the CHA regardless of whether premiums are paid. Four provinces (Manitoba, Ontario, Quebec, and Newfoundland) levy 'payroll taxes' but, again, these are not 'true' benefit-linked payroll tax programs like Employment Insurance, Workers' Compensation, or the Canada/Quebec Pension Plans, where only those who enroll can claim benefits. Rather, these health-related payroll taxes go directly into general revenues (rather than into an earmarked fund) and are distributed to all citizens within the province, regardless of whether they have paid the payroll tax.

Goods and services like pharmaceuticals and long-term care are not covered by the CHA. However, many provinces have programs in these areas, and they are funded and provided in different ways. While the CHA does not cover pharmaceuticals, for example, most Canadians do have insurance for pharmaceuticals: in Quebec, for example, workers are 'mandated' (obliged by law) to enroll in private insurance plans for drug coverage (while non-workers are covered by a public plan). Saskatchewan, Manitoba, and British Columbia have income-based pharmacare programs, while other provinces have programs to cover seniors or catastrophic drug needs. Many other Canadians simply have voluntary private drug coverage.

The dynamics of Canadian health care – including the pressures for change and the options for implementing change – are to a large extent determined by legal institutions (pre-eminently the Constitution and the Canada Health Act), economic pressures (such as rising costs and the overall performance of the economy), and various political tensions, including care providers who want 'to open up private payment channels so as to get around public restrictions on prices and servicing patterns' and well-off consumers of care who prefer shifting costs 'from public to private budgets' (Evans 2000: 896) versus voters who demand the maintenance of public insurance, or even the expansion of public insurance to other sectors. These dynamics arise most emphatically in discussions over the exercise and enforcement of the Canada Health Act.

The Canada Health Act

The 1984 Canada Health Act replaced the 1957 Hospital Insurance and Diagnostic Services Act largely because of the shift from a system of 50–50 federal-provincial cost-sharing to a system of block funding established by Ottawa in 1977 (see Chapter 2). Because Ottawa had given the provinces a major tax point transfer in place of direct payment, the federal government no longer had the ability to withhold cash as an effective 'enforcement mechanism' to ensure that provinces met the conditions of universality, comprehensiveness, portability, and public administration set out in the Hospital Insurance and Diagnostic Services Act. By 1979 Ottawa determined that 17.9 per cent of Ontario doctors had opted out of medicare and were engaged in extra-billing their patients (Bégin 2002: 2). As the federal minister of health during this period, Monique Bégin (2002: 2) wrote that, by 1979,'I concluded that extra-billing and user-fees were a case of erosion of the system and that something had to be done. But what and how? The constitutional challenge – controlling provincial institutions and health professionals' behaviour – was not insignificant and was the most important task to address. It took almost three years to find a way and we succeeded thanks to top constitutional experts outside of government. Convincing Cabinet was also a challenge, but on that I will not say more.' That 'something to be done' was Bill C-3, which became the Canada Health Act on 9 April 1984.

The CHA embraces the four principles of the 1957 Hospital Insurance and Diagnostic Services Act, and adds a fifth. These principles –

essentially funding criteria, which have come to represent the 'principles and values that underpin Medicare policy for Canadians' (Marchildon 2005: 24) – are the following:

1. *Public administration:* each provincial plan must be 'administered and operated on a non-profit basis by a public authority, which is accountable to the provincial or territorial government for decision making on benefit levels and services, and whose records and accounts are publicly audited.'
2. *Comprehensiveness:* every plan must 'cover all insured health services provided by hospitals, physicians or dentists (i.e., surgical-dental services that require a hospital setting) and, where the law of the province so permits, similar or additional services rendered by other health care practitioners.'
3. *Universality:* this ensures that 'all insured residents of a province or territory must be entitled to the insured health services provided by the provincial or territorial health care insurance plan on uniform terms and conditions.'
4. *Portability:* Canadians can transfer their coverage between provinces (with no minimum period of residence over three months) and are covered for non-elective services when visiting other provinces.
5. *Accessibility:* provinces must ensure that their citizens 'have reasonable access to insured hospital, medical and surgical-dental services on uniform terms and conditions, unprecluded or unimpeded, either directly or indirectly, by charges (user charges or extra-billing) or other means (e.g., discrimination on the basis of age, health status or financial circumstances).'

Provinces voluntarily adhere to the provisions of the CHA. Because this legislation is federal, it is not binding on the provinces. The provinces *cannot be charged in a court of law* with violating the CHA: that is ultra vires, or beyond the legitimate authority of the federal government. Only two factors maintain provincial compliance with the CHA: the threat of federal clawbacks, and public pressure. The latter is arguably more important than the former. Health Canada notes that 'since the enactment of the *Canada Health Act*, from April 1984 to March 2008, deductions totalling $9,019,499 have been applied against provincial cash contributions in respect of the extra-billing and user charges provisions of the Act. This amount excludes deductions totalling

$244,732,000 that were made between 1984 and 1987 and subsequently refunded to the provinces when extra-billing and user charges were eliminated' (http://www.hc-sc.gc.ca/hcs-sss/pubs/cha-lcs/2008-cha-lcs-ar-ra/index-eng.php#Chapt2). It is useful to keep in mind that the penalties for user fees and extra-billing are outlined in a section of the CHA *separate* from the sections containing the five CHA criteria. Under the former, any instance of extra-billing or user fees will trigger penalties. The federal minister has no discretion in determining whether to impose *these* penalties or not. But such discretion does exist in pursuing perceived violations of the five CHA criteria, and it is noteworthy that no federal minister has ever used this discretion to levy penalties against any province for violating any of these five criteria (for a fuller discussion, see Boychuk 2008a, 2008b).

Currently, Ottawa only provides about 17 per cent of the public spending on health care: the remainder is provided by the provinces (although, as the federal government likes to remind us, this is thanks to the transfer of tax points it gave the provinces in 1977: see Chapter 2). Thus, while the CHA allows Ottawa to deduct a dollar for every dollar of extra-billing or user fees placed on publicly insured services in any province, these penalties can amount to a 'drop in the bucket' for provinces like Alberta.

It is absolutely essential to understand what the CHA can and cannot do: because the CHA is *not binding* on the provinces, provinces are free to establish any blend of private and public insurance they choose (or to eliminate public insurance altogether). They require no permission from Ottawa. Moreover, private health insurance can technically coexist under certain conditions with the CHA. The CHA does not prohibit the private insurance of health care per se, nor does it require that doctors must be 'fully in' or 'fully out' of the public system: these are provincial decisions, supported by provincial laws, made for political reasons by the provinces. Indeed, as Boychuk argues, 'no province allows private funding and insurance for health services to the full extent available under the CHA' (2008b: 1).

Exactly how the CHA is accommodated in each province varies considerably. In most provinces, 'physicians can opt out of the public system and operate wholly in the private sector – but they cannot work in both' (Flood and Choudhry 2002: 15). However, there are exceptions. In Newfoundland, physicians who choose not to be reimbursed directly by the province ('opted-out' doctors) can bill patients whatever they wish, and patients can then ask for reimbursement from the province up to amounts established in the provincial fee schedule (Flood and Archibald 2001: 828). In New Brunswick and Prince Edward Island physicians can both bill patients above provincial rates for some services (although, unlike Newfoundland, without any government reimbursement) and bill the public plan directly for other services (Boychuk 2008b: 19). New Brunswick (but not PEI) permits private insurance for private services that are nonetheless offered through the public system. None of these mechanisms are considered to comprise either 'co-payments' or 'user fees' (which are disallowed under the CHA).

It is important to point out that the health insurance systems of Newfoundland, New Brunswick, and Prince Edward Island are all CHA compliant. Why, then, do other provinces not follow suit? The answer is: politics and population. A much wider latitude for private services and private funding exists in smaller (and poorer) provinces because the population size itself limits the viability of the private health sector. In these provinces, there is simply not a critical mass of individuals who are willing to pay high prices for private services (given the existence of public services that are free at the point of delivery), and therefore, there is little incentive to offer such services. Toronto, Vancouver, and Calgary could likely support such a private market, which is why the laws against private health care are much more restrictive in Ontario, British Columbia, and Alberta.

Provinces generally utilize a combination of mechanisms to discourage private health care. Ontario, for example, simply does not allow its physicians to opt out of the public plan at all (there are about forty-nine physicians operating only in the private sector in Ontario; the practice of opting out was disallowed in 2004, but those already in the private sector were permitted to remain). In provinces where doctors are allowed to opt out, however, physicians may face limits on the amount that they can charge in the private sector (generally only up to the levels set out in the provincial fee schedules), as in the case of Nova Scotia and Manitoba. This means there is little economic incentive for physicians to choose to opt out, despite having the legal ability to do so. In other provinces (including British Columbia, Alberta, Manitoba, PEI, and, to some extent, Quebec), private insurance is not permitted, which gives *patients* less incentive to use private services (as very high potential costs would have to be borne out of pocket).

But why would provinces choose to enact such restrictive legislation if they are not required to do so? One explanation is simply the set of values of the governing party: in British Columbia, for example, the New

Democratic Party (NDP) government actively requested that Ottawa levy penalties in order to give the province a political tool against the practice of extra-billing, leaving the federal minister of health no choice but to do so (Boychuk 2008b: 8–9). It is less clear why provinces such as Ontario and Alberta would continue restrictions on private health care, although the answer is probably some combination of popular support (or lack thereof), the particular distribution of support in a province (the *number of constituencies* in which support for private care palpably exists, as opposed to the total level of support in a province), and the simple 'institutional rule' of laws that were put into place before there was any clear interpretation of precisely what the CHA required of provinces. There is also a theory of political inaction on controversial issues in which politically extreme minorities sandwich an ambivalent electorate, in which cases the priority of governments becomes to avoid such issues as much as possible (Morton 1999).

Grey Areas in Health Care Funding

The relationship between private and public funding mechanisms has become increasingly more complex, and the determination of whether such instances are CHA compliant or not are accordingly more difficult. Two examples can give us more insight into the issues involved in the interplay of public and private treatment in Canada.

NOVA SCOTIA

In March 2008 the Nova Scotia government signed a one million dollar contract with a private surgical firm in order to remove 528 patients from orthopaedic waiting lists. Most operations were to be performed in a private surgical facility by surgeons employed by the company. This led to a public outcry regarding the 'privatization' of health care in Nova Scotia. Was it an example of 'creeping privatization'? Did it violate the CHA? And regardless of answers to either question, was it a good public policy decision?

The funding arrangement is viewed as CHA compliant. Surgeons operating within the hospital are themselves privately employed, as are the GPs who refer patients to them. The hospital itself is a private institution, albeit run on a not-for-profit basis. Individuals *cannot* appear at the surgical clinic and request immediate treatment for which they are willing to pay out-of-pocket. Rather, patients are treated in the same order in which they would have been had the surgeries been performed in the hospital, and they do not incur any direct or out-of-pocket costs.

Was it a good policy decision? Unsurprisingly, that depends on the criteria one uses to evaluate the practice. Provinces argue that these are surgeries that would not otherwise be done. They have reduced some of the waiting times. Critics, however, point out that the profit demanded by private surgical facilities (above and beyond the fees paid to surgeons) is foregone money that could potentially have been used for health care treatment: in the case of Nova Scotia, a quarter of the one million dollar contract went to 'facility fees' (Gillis 2008). This debate is similar to one many individuals face regarding the decision 'to rent, or to buy?' One pays rent money with no equity to show at the end of the day: but it's affordable at the time one needs it, and it permits a greater degree of flexibility if one doesn't know what one's long-term needs will be. Similarly, clinics present a short-term solution to bulges in waiting lists. It does not make sense to invest in a multi-million dollar (not-for-profit) orthopaedic hospital if one anticipates that the pent-up demand is temporary. The problem arises when one begins to depend on such short-term measures over the long term. What if the increased demand for surgery is not temporary? If a health authority loses $250,000 per year paying 'facility fees,' the money, like one's apartment rent, disappears forever from one's budget (as opposed to, say, mortgage payments). Over a ten-year period the lost funds amount to millions. The problem is exacerbated by democratic politics: no provincial government wants a budget dripping with red ink; and massive public investment in expensive medical facilities can make provincial governments appear to be 'spendthrift' in the short term. Political decisions on the 'optics' of funding choices thus figure very closely into decisions on how to pay for health services.

A second criticism of private surgical facilities is that they 'poach' staff from the public system. This includes not only surgeons, but also anaesthetists and nurses. Both groups are in short supply within the Canadian health care system, and there is much concern that removing critical staff from the public system into private facilities will itself lead to surgical cancellations. The private clinic providing surgical services in Nova Scotia was criticized for 'poaching' four operating room nurses from one regional hospital, although the company maintains that it only hires nurses who have 'retired or left' the public sector (Gillis 2008; McLeod 2008). A further issue involves the training of surgical staff. Private facilities are used to perform the minor surgical operations that can be done without complications; this means that hospitals can focus on the more complicated cases. But critics have pointed out that surgeons do not graduate from medical school able to do these complicated cases: they depend on the 'minor' cases to hone their surgical skills over time. Removing more and more of these simple cases from hospitals will raise serious issues about how to train young orthopaedic surgeons.

Another criticism of the use of private facilities by the public health care system is the considerable issue of regulation. Only Alberta and British Columbia have comprehensive regulatory and monitoring systems. Provinces monitor the care given in public medical facilities, but they do not necessarily consider the oversight of private facilities (especially those providing uninsured medical services, such as laser eye surgery or cosmetic procedures) to be their responsibility. In some provinces there are more regulations and restrictions on restaurants than on private surgical facilities. In Ontario, which has over 600 clinics providing 'invasive procedures,' the provincial College of Physicians and Surgeons noted that 'right now, we don't have the authority to approve a facility before it opens and we don't have the authority to shut it down if there are any problems' (Lett 2008: 987). When a woman died in a Toronto clinic during a liposuction procedure performed by a physician who was not a licensed plastic surgeon, the province of Ontario began developing a comprehensive licensing regime. The province of Nova Scotia does not as yet have legislation covering private medical facilities.

Is the use of private facilities to reduce waiting lists a valid utilization of health care resources? Certainly this strategy is common in several countries with public health care systems: in the United Kingdom, for example, the Departments of Health in England and Scotland have established an Independent Sector Treatment Centre (ISTC) program, in which private facilities provide elective surgery and other clinical services paid by the public National Health Service (Pollock and Kirkwood 2009). But one must keep an eye on the distortions produced by the waiting list reduction strategies. Ottawa has provided extra money to the provinces to reduce waiting lists in the following four priority areas (in addition to diagnostics): cancer care, hip and knee replacements, cardiac surgery, and cataract surgery. There is some concern that funds are directed to these categories away from non-targeted areas. Thus, while $250,000 of a regional health authority's fund may go directly to private sector profits in order to facilitate hip replacements, a surgeon who performs delicate ear surgery may find that he loses several days per month of operating room time so that the health region can keep its total costs down. This may not seem either efficient or fair, but to the extent that receiving extra federal funding depends on meeting waiting-time benchmarks in orthopaedic surgery, it is politically rational. In any case, it is simply not clear how much provinces depend on private facilities (and in what areas) as these data, if kept by provinces at all, are not publically accessible: 'the upshot is that no one knows the extent to which people are using private facilities or the number of such facilities' (Lett 2008: 986).

BRITISH COLUMBIA

More difficult examples of the role and status of private facilities can be found in British Columbia. There are at least sixteen of these facilities in British Columbia and, unlike the case of Nova Scotia, these clinics are designed to attract private-paying patients directly. There has consequently been a storm of controversy over the extent to which these clinics have resulted in a two-tier system in British Columbia. Unlike Ontario, British Columbia does not forbid its physicians from opting out of the public system. These doctors can charge patients directly for medically necessary services. Moreover, unlike Manitoba or Nova Scotia, opted-out physicians can charge their patients whatever they like. It is important to point out that the practice of considering private facility fees (where the physician is not reimbursed through public insurance) as *not* constituting user fees is a convention based on an interpretation of the CHA (or, more specifically, an interpretation of the 1995 'Marleau Letter,' itself written to clarify the federal government's position on private medical facilities). As Boychuk (2008b: 21) points out, 'should the federal government choose to interpret such fees as prohibited user fees, it would be free to do so under ministerial discretion (either under provisions relating to the reporting of user fees or the general accessibility criterion) although the federal government has never yet exercised these provisions.'

While private surgical facilities have operated in British Columbia for years, a new phenomenon appeared in November 2006: a private emergency centre. This facility, designed to treat minor medical emergencies like broken bones, provided urgent treatment in a sleek and luxurious environment without long waits. The catch? A $200 facility fee, in addition to fees for services ($150 for stitching up lacerations or $70 for casting a broken bone) and any extras required (such as X-rays or blood tests). The clinic originally employed twenty-four emergency doctors, all of whom intended to continue working in the public system (Howard 2006). A howl of public outrage ensued, and within a week the province took action, asking its Medical Services Commission to audit the facility and seek a court order to close it (Stueck 2006). The clinic agreed to change its procedures, billing the province according to its fee schedule, rather than billing patients higher fees directly. The clinic maintained that it had not violated the CHA, but did not wish to engage in lengthy legal proceedings. Nevertheless, the private clinic could not recoup its costs within the public fee structure and, within four months, the clinic had reopened with a new business plan. This time, it only employed physicians who had completely opted out of the public insurance plan: in this way, it did not violate the CHA. But British Columbia does not permit private health insurance: thus, all transactions at the private surgical and emergency facilities must be out-of-pocket transactions. This is why a coalition of private health facilities launched a Charter challenge against the British Columbia government in January 2009, arguing that the ban on private health insurance is unconstitutional (see Chapter 4).

Another instance of controversial funding practices is exemplified by a Vancouver-based chain of medical clinics that charged private membership fees, but provided both private and publicly insured services. Originally, the clinic charged $1,200 to join and $2,300 in annual fees; but when the B.C. health minister declared that this membership fee violated the CHA, the clinic changed its fee structure to a $3,500 'first-year fee' and $2,300 for each subsequent year (later raising fees to $3,900 and $2,900 respectively). Unlike the previous case, the clinic's doctors remain within the public insurance system; but clients who join the clinic have access to services such as psychological or nutritional counselling and physiotherapy (which are not generally insured under most public systems) offered by trained staff who do not receive compensation through public insurance. Because the physicians provided publicly funded services, the clinic faced much criticism that the membership fees contravened both the CHA's accessibility condition and the Marleau Letter's prohibition of user fees, and acted as an upper tier of health care that permitted those with money access to enhanced and expedited care.

The clinic has been able to operate within the boundaries of the CHA, although there has been much dispute over its terms of operation. Legally, the clinic cannot turn away anyone who wishes to be treated for medically insured services, even if they refuse to pay membership fees. But there are clear physical limits on how many patients any doctor can see, and it is not uncommon across Canada for patients to be turned away by GPs operating fully within the public system because their rosters are full. It is difficult to know, therefore, whether a patient who cannot get in to see a physician at a 'membership-based' facility is turned away because there is no room, or because the clinic does not wish to take a non-membership client. If such a clinic is operating at undercapacity, it is in the interests of both patients and doctors for the non-membership patient to receive publicly insured care in any case. But if the clinic were operating at close to full capacity (because of, say, a flu pandemic), would it be able to choose a paying member over a client who had not paid membership fees? And exactly what kind of mechanism could monitor potential queue-jumping for public services by those paying the membership fees?

Is There a Better Way to Fund Canada's Health Care System?

How well is Canada's health care system doing? It is useful to glance at some statistics here to get a sense of how robust the system is in quantitative terms. But first, a cautionary word or two about the use of statistics in discussions of health care. Like the use of Scriptural verse, health care statistics can be presented to support almost any position. Statistics are useless without the capacity to interpret them, and a large part of interpretation depends on the context within which statistics are embedded. For example, health care spending (hcs) is normally expressed as a ratio, usually as a proportion of gross domestic product (GDP, the amount of wealth produced by a country annually): thus, hcs/GDP. It is also presented as a single 'snapshot' in time. Health care spending (the numerator) changes over time, largely in response to economic circumstances and political choices. But the denominator changes, too: during a recession, for example, the denominator contracts, which would make the numerator (hcs) appear much larger, even if *actual* health care spending remained constant. In such a case it would not be accurate to say 'health care costs are getting out of control,' as health care costs themselves would not be changing; rather, the *ratio* of health care spending to available wealth was shifting. (What one might say is happening, with some justified anxiety, is that 'the economy is becoming less able to sustain current levels of health care spending.') The difference is important insofar as it would not be ever-expanding health care costs, but rather the performance of the economy, that would be responsible for the statistic in question; and thus the solutions would likely be different than if the economy had remained constant, but spending had exploded.

Moreover, the mere fact that health care spending does increase over time does not give us a good explanation of whether there is a 'crisis' in spending. A province may see its health expenditure increase from, say, 40 to 44 per cent of its budget; but if it makes the political choice to cut taxes (thereby lowering its revenue), then the fact that health care eats up *more* of its budget is no reflection on the real nature of trends in health care expenditure per se (for an extended discussion of this, see Boychuk 2002: 5–6) but rather is a consequence of the political choices made. Hypothetically, public health care expenditure could decrease in real terms, but if tax cuts were significant enough, health spending could appear to have *increased* (as it would be presented relative to a smaller denominator). The time period one chooses for one's statistics is also quite important. If one looks at Canada's total expenditure on health as a proportion of GDP between 2003 and 2008, for example, the average would be approximately 10 per cent. However, if one looks at the figures for the period between 1996 and 2001, the figure would be closer to 8.8 per cent (OECD 2008). By considering these different percentages within the political context of federal health transfer cuts during the late 1990s, the much higher figures on public spending following the 2003 Health Care Accord could be seen as 'catch up' spending (not to mention political bridge mending) rather than as uncontrollable costs inherent in the system. Thus a *Globe and Mail* piece on health care spending trends reporting 'year-over-year double-digit status since 2002' might be quite alarming if one did not consider that much of this spending was actually the result of pent-up demand because of much *lower* spending in the mid-to-late 1990s (Priest 2008).

The same is true for international comparisons: Canada's international ranking in health care expenditure in 2005 or 2006 was much higher (because federal spending programs announced in 2003 and 2004 were coming online) than it was a decade earlier; but this must be considered against the fact that Canada was much more successful internationally in holding health care spending down throughout the 1990s. One would also have to examine Canada's spending increases in the private sector (about 30% of total health care spending) with spending increases in the public sector (about 70% of total health care spending): here one would see that spending increases are much *higher* in the private sector than the public (Canada's share of private spending increased from 25.8% in 1992 to 30.0% in 2007). If spending increases are largely driven by the private sector (with stable public spending levels), then it suggests that the *overall* rising costs often reported in the media will not lead to immediate crises in provincial budgets. *Globe and Mail* columnist Jeffrey Simpson, for example, has written that 'health care consumed 7 per cent of the nation's economic output in the mid-1970s, shortly after it was up and running. Now, it consumes 10.7 per cent. That share will keep on rising as the population ages, technology becomes more expensive, and demand grows' (2008: A19). But economist Robert Evans (2002: 27) counters that 'the claim that public spending is absorbing a rising share of national income, or of public tax revenue, is simply false': 'Spending on the Medicare programs – physicians and hospitals – took up almost exactly the same percentage of Gross Domestic Product (GDP) in 2001 (4.22%) as in 1981 (4.11%). This ratio has been virtually constant for the last five years, a full percentage point below its 1992 peak of 5.28% and lower than in any year from 1982 to 1996.'

If total health care spending increases are predominantly driven by cost increases in the private sector, then, it might make one hesitate when looking at greater privatization as a strategy for controlling overall health care spending. Finally, the simple ratio of 'total health care expenditure as a percentage of GDP' that is commonly used (e.g., by the OECD) does not make the distinction between 'who has the GDP' and 'who is responsible for health care costs.' This issue (of 'vertical imbalance') is highly relevant for a federal country such as Canada in discussions of whether 'crises' exist in health care spending. Where the budget surpluses arise at the federal level, but health care is largely funded at the provincial level, it is not uncommon to hear anxiety about 'the sustainability of public health care' discussed even as national GDP rises.

Canada spends approximately 10 per cent of its GDP on total health care (public and private). In comparison, the United States spends 15.3 per cent; France, 11.1 per cent; and Germany, 10.6 per cent. But the overall OECD average is 8.9 per cent: Australia spends 8.8 per cent; the United Kingdom spends 8.4 per cent; and Japan spends 8.2 per cent. Canada also has one of the highest per capita expenditures on health care: at U.S.$3,678 (compared with the OECD average of U.S.$2,824), only the United States, Norway, Switzerland, and Luxembourg are higher (all statistics, OECD 2008). Given the level of expenditure, one of the most emphatic criticisms of the health care system is that

'Canadians are paying more for government health insurance and getting less in return' (Skinner and Rovere 2008). This is why so much discussion regarding health care reform has revolved around whether there should be more (or less) privatization of 'the system.'

Again, however, one should be wary of talking about private or public 'systems.' All health care systems are a mix of public and private elements; and many are structured on mechanisms (like social insurance schemes) that are neither fully public nor private. There are numerous private and public components that can be assembled together in a particular 'health policy wardrobe' designed to fit a particular polity at a given time. It is the specific mix of elements that can more usefully be debated. Most of these policy elements can generally be categorized as belonging to the 'public' or 'private' sectors, although the lines can get quite blurred. Highly regulated 'mandated' private insurance (where individuals are required by law to buy some form of private health insurance) is one example. Another example is an 'internal market,' where public providers (hospitals) must compete for the contracts given by 'purchasers' (publicly funded GPs seeking care for their patients).

Nonetheless, the broader discussion over health care does tend to focus on the 'public-private' spectrum of choices. Those advocating greater privatization generally ground their position on two points: first, they argue, a private market-based system is more efficient, as it effectively connects supply to demand; and second, it provides more choice. These arguments are not mutually exclusive (there is often the assumption that a market system provides more choice); but the demand for greater choice can arise irrespective of whether this leads to efficiencies or inefficiencies in providing health care. Those espousing *public* health care also make the case for efficiency, but on different grounds. They also argue that, in the provision of health care across a population, fair access ought to take primacy over choice.

The Debate over Efficiency

The call for greater privatization is based primarily on the credo that 'the management of anything by investor owned, private enterprise is by that very fact more efficient than management of the same activity by publicly owned enterprise' (Reinhardt 2007: 1193). The basis of this position is that the market provides motivation for individuals to behave in a certain way: specifically, to think about costs and minimize consumption. The metaphor often used is free access to groceries at a supermarket: who, given the chance to receive free groceries, would only select what they absolutely need (or what they would normally select) if they did not have to pay for their choices? The 'fundamental flaw' of a public health care system, as Gratzer succinctly states, 'is that patients bear no direct costs for the medical services they receive' (1999: 118). Gratzer outlines a number of examples: patients will seek treatment for trivial cases, or even merely for the attention; they will use emergency rooms, which are more expensive than GP visits, for non-emergency cases simply because they are open 24 hours; they will demand tests for the most minor complaints; they will solicit several medical opinions for the same ailment; and they will stay longer in hospital rather than recuperating at home because they bear the immediate cost for none of these options (ibid., 143–5). But these 'perverse incentives' do not only apply to the patients: because of retrospective global budgets, hospital administrators are motivated to increase costs rather than diminish them. Hospital budgets are often based on previous years' expenditures: thus the more a hospital spends, the more it is assumed that the hospital needs. There is no mechanism to check whether these expenditures are used efficiently. Even politicians, argues Gratzer, contribute to inefficiency: they have incentives to keep medically unnecessary hospitals and emergency wards open when small constituencies can be won or lost on the issue of hospital closures.

There is, unsurprisingly, the vigorous counterclaim that *private* systems are the more inefficient alternative; and that public systems provide much more cost-effective services. In the first place, private health systems like those in the United States are inefficient because of the fragmentation of health care provision. In an uncoordinated, commercialized system, individuals can choose to see an expensive specialist (or even several of them) rather than a cost-effective GP for a minor complaint if they can afford to. Many public systems use GPs as 'gatekeepers,' so that only the most demanding cases get seen by specialists. Because health care providers have to compete for clients, they must spend money on advertising and marketing schemes to attract customers. This can result in inefficient *overcapacity:* if a hospital wants to offer 'no waiting time' guarantees, then it must have staff and facilities available for services at all times, which means that there must be unused facilities. This is like an airline flying with empty seats in order to promise last-minute customers that there will always be seats available on their flights: it is very costly. Hospitals can also compete with each other by offering the latest in technologies; but if several hospitals have all the latest equipment, then there is a good chance that each one uses this equipment only occasionally. Again, the inefficiencies result from overcapacity.

Similar inefficiencies result from overtreatment. As technology develops, drugs, diagnostics, and treatments are being applied despite evidence that they are unnecessary and pointless. Especially where direct-to-consumer advertising is allowed, patients will demand drugs or treatments even if the cost-benefit advantages do not exist. Wealthy clients will demand computed tomography (CT) scans for headaches or magnetic resonance imaging (MRI) for backaches despite prelimi-nary assessments that they are unnecessary: yet patients want them for peace of mind (for more discussion of this phenomenon, see Cassels, van Wiltenburg, and Armstrong [2009] and Deber [2008]). In a highly litigious culture like that of the United States, physicians may order tests simply to protect themselves against lawsuits: Brownlee (2007), for example, argues that 20 to 30 per cent of the tests done in the United States are needless. The same is true for surgery: in 2004, 345 individ-uals sued Tenet Healthcare, along with eight cardiologists and surgeons, for performing unnecessary major surgery, including superfluous triple-bypass surgery (*Consumer Reports*, November 2007).

The problem here is that market forces themselves actually produce inefficiencies. Thus cost containment, 'which is essential to maintaining an efficient and effective public health care system, cannot be recon-ciled with the growth requirements imposed by capital markets' (Evans 2002: 5). The drive for profits can lead health care organizations to cut corners when engaged in competition with other providers: when the primary goal of activity is the maximization of profits rather than the achievement of better health, argue critics of privatization, firms that must provide profits to their shareholders will, unsurprisingly, place profits above good health. In a public system, funds that would have been skimmed off as 'profit' in a private system would go directly into services or infrastructure. Fifteen to 25 per cent of the premiums given to private health care firms in the United States go directly to admin-istrative costs, marketing, and profits (Angell 2005), none of which are necessary in a public system.

Inefficiencies result not only from private health care provision but also private health *funding*. Again, the fragmentation of payment systems results in higher administration costs: 'comparative analy-sis of health care systems has conclusively demonstrated that private insurance requires much higher administrative overheads, for both reimbursing agencies and providers, than do public systems ... public systems can raise financing, administer claims, and spread risk over the population more efficiently than private firms can ... These excessive administrative costs account for nearly half of the difference between Canada and the United States in the share of GDP spent on health care' (Evans 2002: 30, 31). Angell (2005) corroborates this: in 2005, she notes, health care expenditures in the United States (with a predominantly private system of health care funding) were U.S.$6,697 per person; in Canada, the figure was U.S.$3,326 per person. Publicly funded systems are also better at overall cost control: the rate of public spending in health care systems such as that of the United Kingdom or Canada are consistently lower than those with a much higher level of private funding. Thus, it makes no sense to address issues of 'sustainability' by privatizing health care, as we have good evidence to show that higher levels of private health care would only drive costs higher.

Why, then, is there such insistence that publicly provided goods are inefficient because they lead to overconsumption? A few words about the RAND study on health insurance and 'moral hazard' are useful here. The administration of George W. Bush in the United States had for years based its private health care platform on this RAND study (Krugman and Wells, 2006); Gratzer (1999) also argues for greater private health care in Canada on the basis on RAND data. What was this study? During the late 1970s and early 1980s, the RAND Corporation in the United States conducted a health insurance experiment (HIE) to ascertain the role of moral hazard in health funding systems. 'Moral hazard' refers to the way in which behaviour changes when an individual is insured. Say I have serious food allergies: if I must pay $100 for each epinephrine injector, I may calculate that it is efficient to buy one injector, and keep it on me at all times. If my insurance plan covers all my costs, with only a $5 co-payment, then I may decide to buy six injectors: one for home, one for work, one for the car, one for my gym locker, one at my friend Meg's, and one at my in-laws'. The final cost to me with such good insurance is only $30. Because I pay less, I can consume more, even though this costs my insurer more, thereby raising overall health care insurance costs. But if I have more restrictive, or no, insurance, overall costs will be kept down (in this case, I would probably choose to buy one injector, and total costs would be $100, rather than $600).

But is the diminution, or even lack, of insurance *efficient*? If I have to pay for one epinephrine injector out of pocket ($100), and I am desperately short of funds, then I may forgo the injector altogether and just hope for the best, even though one shot may save my life. If I do buy one, but forget that I left it in my gym locker, then my risk of hospitalization or even death increases. Economists have suggested that the optimal insurance point can in theory be determined by a simple thought experiment: if I were given $100 in cash, would I buy an epinephrine injector, or some other consumer goods? (All things being equal, I'd probably opt for the injector.) If I were given $600 in cash, to use as I desired, how many injectors would I then purchase? ('Gee, for $600 I could buy an injector *and* an iPhone: hmmm, maybe I really don't need all those pens after all, given how organized I am ...')

The RAND study was designed to test these insights about moral hazard and health insurance. Under the study, participants were divided among those who paid a fee-for-service (FFS) with either no co-insurance or 25 per cent, 50 per cent, or 95 per cent co-insurance; others were assigned to an individual deductible plan with 95 per cent co-insurance. The lessons of the study, writes Nyman (2007: 761), were: (1) participants consumed less health care in plans with cost-sharing than in the free FFS plan, but (2) this reduction in health care consumption 'had little or no measurable effect on the health status of the average adult.' The lesson for health policy, as Gratzer (1999) indicates, would seem to be that user fees keep costs down without affecting the health of the population.

The RAND study has had considerable effects on health policy formulation, especially in the United States. But recent analyses of the study call some of its conclusions into question. Nyman observes that a significant portion of the cost-sharing group dropped out of the study. He suggests that they likely dropped out because they had poor health, and returned to their old plans where they could be treated at less personal cost. If, he speculates, those who dropped out had stayed in the study, 'the cost-sharing group would likely have exhibited a marked decrease in many of the important measures of health' (Nyman 2007: 773). Had these individuals stayed in the study (or had their ill health been followed up and calculated in), then the results of the RAND HIE study would have been considerably different: the study likely would have concluded that forcing people to bear the costs of their treatment led to diminishing health. Supporters of the original analysis of the study have argued that the reasons why so many in the cost-sharing program dropped out are simply speculative, as their health was not tracked after their exit (Newhouse et al. 2008). But Nyman holds that such speculation is both plausible and important to consider; for if he is correct, the conventional interpretation of the RAND HIE is potentially quite harmful: 'If cost sharing is applied across the board, it does not discourage between care that is efficient and inefficient, and it discourages both types of care. Discouraging efficient care by applying across-the-board cost sharing could have serious health consequences' (2008: 316).

'Choice' versus 'Access'

The second major criticism of public health care systems is that private systems offer more selection of goods and services. 'On a comparable basis,' states a report by the Fraser Institute, 'Canadians have fewer doctors and less high-tech equipment than Americans. Canadians also have older hospitals and have access to fewer advanced medical treatments and technologies that are commonly available to Americans ... Canadian patients who want to escape the delays in the public system are also prohibited from paying privately for health care services (in addition to what they already pay in taxes for the public system). In practical terms, Canadian patients are unable to buy quicker access or better care than what the government health insurance program provides' (Skinner, Rovere, and Warrington 2008: 1, 2). The very ability of public systems to keep costs down also results in what Gratzer has called 'the ugly truth' about Canadian health care: 'dirty hospitals, long waiting lists, and substandard treatment' (2007).

Private, for-profit health facilities are, as we have seen, essentially legal in most of Canada. The real issue, then, is not private delivery as much as private funding. The argument for greater privatization is generally to force provinces to permit user fees and co-payments as well as private insurance for medically necessary treatment. This, according to proponents, would allow greater choice in health care services, while taking pressure off the public system (Skinner and Rovere 2008). Yet critics of privatization argue that attempts to push health care into the private sector if successful would favour the wealthy while disadvantaging the poor and ill. Moreover, they hold that the existence of a separate private 'tier' is not a positive-sum solution: rather, it is negative-sum, as the addition of privately funded care actually undermines the public system.

Both user fees (including co-payments) and private insurance, argue defenders of public health care, disproportionately favour the wealthy.

User fees, as Steven Lewis (1998) states, amount to 'taxes on the sick.' They are also highly regressive. Those who can easily afford $30 for a GP visit will do so whether they are critically ill or just attention-seeking (they may well feel that $30 for a good chat with a nice doctor is well worth the money). Those for whom $30 is a significant sum may well put off treatment, which could result in a much more serious condition requiring expensive emergency or tertiary care. Ill health is also concentrated, rather than distributed evenly throughout the population: Forget, Deber, and Roos (2002) examined expenditures in Manitoba in 1997–9, and found that 26 per cent of expenditures were incurred by only 1 per cent of the population. This would mean a very high out-of-pocket or co-payment expenditure by a very small number of very sick people. At the same time, 50 per cent of the population incurred only 4 per cent of the expenditure. In other words, the vast majority of health expenditure is used by those who are very sick: in these cases, the imposition of user fees would not dissuade them from using services (nor would we want them to). This small number of very sick people is also less likely to be able to afford large sums of money for the required medical treatments. Conversely, a large majority of healthy individuals incur very few costs: thus user fees would not mean a significant reduction in an already-low rate of utilization among this group.

As Evans argues, cost pressures do not arise from people seeking inappropriate care. There may be lonely people seeking companionship from GPs, but they are not the cost drivers: 'The major pressures for cost escalation arise not from individuals' decisions to seek care, but from the therapies offered once the doctor's office has been reached, from the recommendations for various diagnostic and therapeutic procedures and prescription drugs that are under physician control. If inappropriate care is a concern – and it should be – then focusing on patient behaviour amounts to looking (perhaps deliberately) in the wrong direction' (2002: 39). Thus the 'supermarket' analogy is specious: people do not seek the *expensive* drivers of health care cost (dialysis, heart bypass surgery, cancer care) merely because they do not have to pay directly for it. Most healthy people probably would not opt for free dialysis simply because it was free.

But what of private health insurance? Greater use of private health insurance, according to the Fraser Institute, will relieve cost pressures facing the public health insurance system (Skinner and Rovere 2008). The difference in public and private health insurance is primarily how premiums are determined: in public systems, where the risk is widely pooled, contributions are based on income (health care systems funded through general revenues receive the funds through income taxes, which are generally progressive). With private health insurance, premiums are related to the expectation of illness, rather than income levels. To the extent that very ill people are generally less wealthy (especially if because of their illnesses they cannot hold employment), the poor and ill face much higher premiums for health insurance than do people in higher income brackets. The problem is compounded by risk selection. As private health insurers lose money on ill people, there is an incentive for them to court the healthy and ignore the sick. Woolhandler and Himmelstein (2007) document how private firms in the United States have attempted to cherry-pick healthier individuals through selective recruitment schemes, including the use of free fitness club memberships, recruitment dinners at 'times and places inaccessible to frail elderly people,' and advertisements placed in sports facilities. This is why the United States has had such a poor record of health insurance coverage, with so many individuals without adequate health insurance (or without insurance at all). Private health insurance systems tend to divide populations into 'insiders and outsiders': those who can afford comprehensive health insurance have a wide choice of sophisticated goods and services at their disposal; and those who cannot, face bankruptcy and refusal of treatment.

In Canada, the debate is less about *replacing* the public system with a private one and more about *supplementing* the current system with more private options. Those who want to use their wealth to secure better or faster health care should be allowed to do so, according to this account; and those who do not should still have access to a public system. (There are also discussions about replacing or supplementing the public system with one based on social insurance: see Flood, Stabile, and Tuohy 2008). Is this not the best of both worlds? It is not uncommon outside of Canada: Britain, Sweden, Australia, and New Zealand, for example, have private insurance systems operating concurrently with public ones. Critics point out, however, that countries with parallel public-private systems have problems with waiting times similar to the situation in Canada. Rather than alleviating pressure on waiting times, private systems seem to *increase* them (Flood, Stabile, and Tuohy 2008). There are a number of hypotheses for this: the private sector attracts qualified staff from the public sector, thereby leading to shortages in the public system; private facilities only select the easiest cases, 'thereby increasing the average complexity and dependency of patients continuing to use the public system' (ibid., 22); and providers 'have an incentive to maintain lengthy lists for publicly financed services in order to increase demand for privately financed services' (18). To this one might add the argument about political dynamics: the more that the well-off can afford private health care, the less they will also want to fund the public system through their taxes. This leads to a further undermining of the quality and scope of the public system.

Markets and Market Failure

For several decades now the debate over health care reform has been a debate about the role of the market. Especially where health care is based on a 'Beveridge,' or command-and-control, model, issues of information asymmetry (does the top know what those at the bottom really need?) and efficiency (is there any motivation to provide goods and services as effectively as possible?) are often addressed with reference to the beneficial tonic provided by market mechanisms. Many of these arguments are premised on the natural superiority of markets in determining the allocation of resources: if market mechanisms are always optimal, then any results that occur from the application of market mechanisms must also logically be the best possible outcomes. But there is no reason to accept this as anything other than a declaration of faith. The empirical record of market-based health reforms is mixed at best, and the discipline of economics has long seen a debate between those who believe in the natural salubrity of market mechanisms in health care and those who see health care as an outstanding example of market failure.

Chapter 3 examines in more detail the way in which market-based health care reforms grew in popularity from the early 1980s. However, there have been those who, over the same time period, have assiduously documented the failures of the market when applied to the provision of health care services (e.g., Evans 1984). Some of these have been discussed above, and more will be addressed in the comparative surveys presented in chapters 9 to 11. Here is a very brief summary of some of the ways in which market mechanisms impair, rather than improve, health care systems:

1. *Excessive bureaucratic and administrative requirements.* In a market-based health system, health care providers must field a massive number of various payment sources, and they must track payment

from each individual private or public insurance company (or patient, for out-of-pocket payment) for each service performed. Add to this the need for each health care provider to advertise for business, to collect bad debts, to address high legal liabilities, and accommodate much state regulation minimizing negative externalities (e.g., obliging private insurance companies not to refuse to cover sick people), and a very large amount of time and resources are spent on administrative work rather than on the provision of health care.

2. *Overcapacity.* In a competitive system, quick service, technological sophistication, and a variety of choices are the tools used to attract customers. But immediate treatment can only exist if there are beds or physicians on standby ready to treat any patient who may suddenly appear (medical treatments are not like aesthetic services; no one plans to get ill). If every hospital needs a positron emission tomography (PET) scanner to attract customers, then many of these machines will not be used as efficiently as they would be in a system where planning services tracked usage. Combine these with 'Wildavsky's Law,' which says that almost any available bed tends to get filled, and one can understand how the massive expansion of health care spending in market-based systems does not correlate to better health-care outcomes.

3. *Overtreatment.* In a contractual system in which profits depend on the volume of services performed or on the complexity of the treatment provided, there will always be motivation for providers to see as many patients in as short a time as possible, to provide expensive services when cheaper ones work just as well, or even to provide services that are completely unnecessary.

4. *Undertreatment.* In a market-based system, the provision of services is based on ability to pay rather than the need for treatment. The two may coincide, but do not have to. To the extent that health and wealth tend, like poverty and sickness, to coexist, a market-based system can be seen as regressive, unfair, and (given that illness is not in and of itself a criterion for treatment) inefficient. The problem is exacerbated by profit-based insurance. The point of private insurance is to make a profit, and *that* is best achieved by refusing to insure bad risks (i.e., sick people, or people likely to become ill), or to require sick people to pay higher premiums for fewer services. Again, this means that those who require health care the most are the least likely to receive it. Economists often use the principle of

'Pareto optimality' (the point at which no one's condition could be improved without making someone else's condition worse off) as the gold standard in health reform. But the use of Pareto optimality itself confers a value judgment in discussions about fair distributions. For, if the *starting* point is one of severe inequalities, then a 'Pareto optimal' outcome would conceivably reinforce existing inequalities rather than questioning whether they were fair in the first place (for a more detailed discussion, see Rice 1997).

5. *Information asymmetry.* Efficient markets depend on consumers being informed about choices. But the reason that individuals go to doctors in the first place is that they do not have the knowledge they need to make choices about expensive treatments. And it is the decisions of physicians, not patients, that are responsible for some 80 per cent of health care expenditures (Roemer 1982: 421). This is why user fees are so pernicious: they do not have any effect on the main cost driver (physician choices) but they do have a dampening effect on the cheapest, most efficient use of health care resources: primary care. User fees place a higher obligation on individuals to make decisions about 'important' or 'frivolous' conditions that they cannot be expected to make. Individuals often cannot know whether symptoms they experience (a chest pain) is evidence of a benign condition (a strained pectoral muscle) rather than a more severe one (a heart attack). Moreover, when given the choice, individuals are more likely to forego preventive services in favour of acute care, even though high utilization of preventive services significantly lowers the need for acute care. As Rice (1997: 415) summarizes, 'consumers do not seem to be able to evaluate the usefulness of medical services and to make the type of decisions that economic theory calls upon them to make.' Does the Internet provide enough information to allow modern consumers to make such decisions? Not really; for while individuals now have considerably more medical information at their fingertips, the sheer volume of information available requires them to have the ability to *evaluate* all the conflicting facts and claims. As Kenneth Arrow pointed out almost half a century ago, if a health care consumer 'knew enough to measure the value of the information, he would know the information itself' (1963: 946).

6. *Absence of economies of scale.* Market-based theories assume that competition is the key driver keeping prices low. As discussed above, competition in health care can have the opposite effect. But what

can keep costs low are economies of scale. This is especially true for the provision of goods like pharmaceuticals, where government formularies buying large quantities in bulk can demand considerably lower prices from manufacturers (this is the logic behind a national pharmacare system like Australia's). When economies of scale trump competition in the private sector, however, oligopolistic or monopolistic behaviour tends to increase rather than decrease prices.

How well markets tend to work in health care, in sum, largely depends on what one sees as the primary role of a health care system. If it is to produce profits, invigorate the economy, or meet the demands of those with ways to finance their demands, then a market-based system works quite well. From a consumer's perspective, the more resources one has, the better a market-oriented health care system tends to work. That is why wealthier demographic groups will generally tend to support private health care options. But if the role of a health care system is primarily to prevent illness and cure the sick, then market mechanisms can conflict with this fundamental objective in significant ways. That is why the debate over health care will always be a political one: different groups in society have conflicting opinions regarding whether health care ought to be a commodity (to be bought and sold according to ability to pay) or a public good (that is provided according to need). No one economic model can incorporate both of these positions. Thus the standards used to determine whether a health care system does what it ought to do will always be determined through some form of political tussle. It is worth reiterating that the debate between 'fully public' and 'fully private' systems occurs largely within the political realm; for policy makers, the more interesting discussion is how to combine the insights provided by advocates of public and private models in order to inch closer to the 'golden mean.' Britain, for example, introduced competition between payers and providers within their public system in order to avoid the inefficiencies in funding caused by global budgets. European states with social insurance systems have for years attempted to facilitate competition between payers. The energy and the ingenuity of the private sector, suggests Reinhardt (2007), must be constrained 'by appropriate laws, rules, and payment systems' in order to achieve optimal distributive objectives. But, argues Evans, 'the notion that some sort of automatic, self-regulating marketlike structure can be established that will *substitute* for public management and yet achieve public objectives is a fantasy: powdered unicorn horn' (1997: 462).

If the most politicized aspect of Canadian health care is the way in which it is funded, running close second is the way in which influence over health policy is distributed between levels of government. Canada is not unique in this respect. Many Western health care systems – including those in the United States, Australia, Germany, and Spain – are based on a federal model. Even Britain's National Health Service (NHS) has become fragmented into four separate political jurisdictions (England, Scotland, Wales, and Northern Ireland) since devolution. The particular nature of intergovernmental relationships depends on the constellation of several different kinds of variables, including the formal political institutions of each state, the traditional patterns of power, and other sources of influence (such as the relative economic strength and administrative sophistication of governments). Conceptually, federalism raises two kinds of questions for health care in Canada: first, does a health care system function better when it is governed at a national or at a regional level? Second, given the set of political and institutional constraints particular to Canada, what is the best way in which to facilitate an efficient working relationship between levels of government in the field of health care?

Health Care in Federal versus Unitary Systems

What, in general, can be said about the nature of health care in federal systems? Does comparative evidence show the superiority of federal (or unitary) systems? Any sweeping conclusions are difficult to find. This is because there are many different kinds of federal systems, as well as unitary systems. Good health care indicators (including cost containment, efficiency, equity, and choice) are strongly affected by numerous factors (such as the way in which health care is funded or the overall level of economic and social disparity in a country), and so it is difficult to say conclusively that the presence or absence of a federal structure has a strong impact on the nature of health care. One might assume, for example, that centralized systems would be more effective at containing costs. Yet France, a unitary state, does not perform as well on cost containment as does Canada, a federal state. Nonetheless, there are clear trends in the experiences of federal states that have led researchers to draw certain conclusions about the advantages and disadvantages of federal and unitary systems. How important each of these is usually depends on the diverse characteristics and qualities of each state.

The virtues of centralism seem especially pronounced to those living in federal systems. Certainly, when modern health care systems were developed in the wake of the Second World War, federalism was initially seen as an impediment. Britain's National Health Service, modelled on the provision of wartime health care, was very much a product of central planning. Unitary systems like Great Britain tended to facilitate much better coordination of service provision across the nation: lines of communication and accountability were clear, regional political resistance was less forceful, and resources could be targeted efficiently across geographical locations. Even today, federal systems often have slower reaction times to medical crises than unitary systems do: one example of this was Ottawa's inability to discuss the 2003 SARS (severe acute respiratory syndrome) epidemic in detail with the World Health Organization simply because the outbreak was under the jurisdiction of the province of Ontario, and the lines of communication between federal and provincial governments were not effectively structured.

At the same time, national-level governments have generally had much more economic and administrative capacity to establish expansive and complicated health care services. Where responsibility for health care fell to smaller jurisdictions with less revenue and expertise, the establishment of sophisticated modern health care systems has tended to take somewhat longer. While larger provinces in Canada such as Ontario had much of the fiscal ability and technocratic expertise to design and implement many postwar welfare programs, smaller and poorer provinces often struggled to maintain the status quo. The same kind of dynamic informs contemporary health system planning across Canada, as the larger and wealthier provinces are better able to take advantage of the advances in information technology (such as electronic health records) that require heavy capital investment.

Another disadvantage of federal systems is that severe regional disparities can lead to significant inequities in health and health care between citizens and, to the extent that access to health services is viewed as an aspect of citizenship, severe political resentment can lead to regional tensions. Most federal systems attempt to deal with geographical health care inequalities by implementing some form of intergovernmental transfers in order to allow for comparable health care between regions. This solution, however, does present its own problems: substantial federal transfers are often politically contentious and lead to resentment by those regions which bear most of the economic burden. Depending on the way in which transfers are structured, the unpredictability of transfer payments over time can lead to difficulties for regional governments in attempting to establish long-term health care strategies.

Much literature on federalism also notes the ability of unitary states better to resist powerful interests. While decision making in unitary states can be highly centralized, 'federalism multiplies the number of veto points at which action can be delayed, diluted, or defeated' (Banting and Corbett 2002: 5). It also increases the number of pressure points for interests lobbying for greater spending. Thus unitary systems, all things being equal, may be more effective at cost control. These issues are tremendously important for health reform. In the United States, for example, powerful private insurance companies or health care providers can play state representatives off against Washington (or even their own parties), thus undermining significant reforms. Likewise, the attempt to achieve a national pharmacare program in Canada (where a single national formulary could exert considerable pressure on drug companies to keep prices low) has been impeded by Canada's federal structure, as governments resist ceding power and jurisdiction even for reasonably advantageous policy objectives.

An increase in the number of jurisdictions responsible for health care also means a diffusion of responsibility. One of the administrative advantages of centralized systems is that there are clear pathways of accountability: one knows where the buck stops. One of the reasons that federal-provincial relations in health care became so acrimonious in Canada is the cost-shifting that occurred throughout the 1990s. The federal government may have reduced transfer payments to the provinces, but it was the provinces themselves that had to decide how to implement the cutbacks; and the resulting hospital closures were political liabilities for the provinces, not Ottawa. The problem was exacerbated by the way in which transfer payments were negotiated. By giving up tax points in exchange for lower cash transfers, it became unclear exactly what Ottawa's contributions to the provinces were (how do you measure foregone revenue over time?) and, because Ottawa delivered its transfer payments in a lump sum (including social welfare and education), it was impossible to measure how much federal money was spent in each province on health care alone.

But if federal systems have such a range of disadvantages, why are so many health care systems based on federal models? First, and primarily, the effects of federal structures on the provision of health care were generally not at the top of the list of important considerations when federal political systems were implemented. Most federal states came into being well before modern health care existed; and even federal states recently formed were based on more pressing political exigencies than the efficient delivery of social services. Second, the decentralization of service provision has become theoretically fashionable in the past few decades (see Chapter 3). The rethinking of service delivery based on principles of the 'new public management' has espoused ideas that federal systems have always articulated: that regional governments are more responsive to local populations, and that smaller governments in smaller jurisdictions have the capacity to be more flexible and innovative.

Provincial governments steadfastly make the claim that they, and not federal governments, are more accountable to their populations for a number of reasons. According to this position, provincial governments better understand the local political culture of a province (Alberta's political culture is dramatically different from Saskatchewan's, for example, despite the provinces' geographical similarities). They better comprehend the needs and limitations of the territory under their control. Moreover, they are not bound by the regional majorities in other parts of the country that the federal government would have to acknowledge. (This, however, works both ways: as those living in smaller provinces know quite well, a federal government can impose necessary but unpopular reforms in many areas with no fear of significant reprisal if its political base in other provinces remains stable.)

The capacity for responsiveness is important, but it is difficult to measure (even a local government is, arguably, only truly responsive to the majority that elects it). What has stood out in Canada's experiment with health care federalism is the dynamic flexibility built into federal systems. Different federal systems, of course, have varying degrees of autonomy for regional governments (the provinces of Canada and the cantons of Switzerland, for example, have a great deal more autonomy in health policy making than the Australian states or the German Länder). It is notable that it was Saskatchewan, with limited financial and administrative resources, and not Ontario, with a much larger fiscal and technocratic capacity, that was able successfully to develop a model of universal public health insurance. Even today, as health care becomes more complex and more dependent on expensive technological systems and processes, the ability to test new ideas and experiment with emerging technologies is facilitated by Canada's federal structure. It may be a valid criticism that we have become a 'nation of pilot programs' with little ability to establish overarching policies that reinforce and support each other from sea to sea (it makes little sense that there is, for example, no integration of vaccination programs for children across provinces). At the very least, however, a process of dynamic learning is taking place: the question is whether we can mitigate the worst of the disadvantages of federalism in order to take advantage of it.

Health Care Federalism in Canada

The discussion of the particular set of social, economic, and political forces that converged at a particular point in time to create a sense of collective solidarity on the issue of health care in Canada is a fascinating but intricate narrative; those who wish to delve into this discussion in more detail should consult Taylor (1978), Gray (1991), Naylor (1992), Maioni (1998), Tuohy (1999), or Boychuk (2008a). The political dynamics of federalism in Canadian health policy in the twenty-first century, however, are based on the simple fact that effective health care is complex, expensive, and wide-ranging, requiring collaboration, coordination, and communication. At the same time, the political framework of Canadian federalism is based on the creaky model of 'watertight compartments' of political responsibility. The two concepts are increasingly ill-suited for each other, and yet both are realities that have to be accommodated.

The Constitutional Framework for Health Care Federalism

When the Canadian Constitution was negotiated in 1867, health care was understood to be a private matter, to be provided by the family for those who could afford it, or by charitable organizations, for those who could not. The first instance of social health insurance did not arise until 1883, when it was introduced in Germany by Chancellor Otto von Bismarck for very specific political purposes. Thus health care, as a small matter of little public interest, was clearly seen as a good fit for provincial regulation, and was included in the list of provincial responsibilities under section 92 of the Constitution Act of 1867 (originally the British North America Act). Nonetheless, health care in Canada has been shaped by important documents and key pieces of legislation at both the provincial and federal levels (see Table 2.1).

Table 2.1. Key Dates in the Development of Canadian Health Care

1919 – First articulation of federal support for national health insurance
1919 – B.C. Royal Commission on Public Health Insurance
1933 – Canadian Commonwealth Federation (CCF) calls for socialized medicine in its
     Regina Manifesto
1936 – Public health insurance legislation passed in British Columbia (not implemented)
1937 – Public health insurance legislation passed in Alberta (not implemented)
1937 – Rowell-Sirois Royal Commission on Dominion-Provincial Relations
     (reported 1940)
1942 – Heagerty Report on health insurance (published 1943)
1947 – Saskatchewan implements universal hospital insurance
1957 – Federal Hospital Insurance and Diagnostic Services Act
1961 – Saskatchewan introduces public insurance for primary care
1964 – First Hall Report: *Royal Commission on Health Services in Canada*
     (published 1966)
1966 – Federal Medical Care Act
1974 – Lalonde report: *A New Perspective on the Health of Canadians*
1977 – Established Program Financing (EPF)
1980 – Second Hall Report: *Canada's National-Provincial Health Program for the 1980s*
1984 – Canada Health Act (CHA)
1996 – Canada Health and Social Transfer (CHST)
1999 – Social Union Framework Agreement
1999 – Kirby Report: *Standing Senate Committee on Social Affairs, Science and
     Technology Study on the State of the Health Care System in Canada* (reported
     2002)
2001 – Romanow Report: *Royal Commission on the Future of Health Care in Canada*
     (published 2002)
2003 – Accord on Health Care Renewal
2003 – Establishment of the Health Council of Canada (HCC)
2004 – 10-Year Plan to Strengthen Health Care
2005 – Establishment of the Public Health Agency of Canada (PHAC)
2006 – Kirby Report on Mental Health: *Out of the Shadows at Last*
2007 – Establishment of the Mental Health Council of Canada (MHCC)

Thus health care falls squarely under the regulatory authority of the provinces, which have in section 92(7) of the Constitution clear jurisdiction over 'the Establishment, Maintenance, and Management of Hospitals, Asylums, Charities and Eleemosynary Institutions.' Why, then, is there such a tension between levels of government in the area of health care? Primarily this is because the nature of health care has changed considerably, from a simple, private matter to a sophisticated and expensive system that is difficult for small jurisdictions to provide autonomously. In practice, the federal role in health care has become essential in a number of areas. As the Kirby Report (2002) points out, Ottawa now has at least five different functions in the health care arena. The first, obviously, is the *financing* role, which has been fundamental in allowing provinces to establish public insurance systems for their respective populations, but which has been important recently in allowing provinces to update their diagnostic and information technology (IT) systems. The second is the federal *research and evaluation role*, including the funding of bodies such as the Canadian Institute for Health Information (CIHI), the Canadian Institutes of Health Research (CIHR), and the Canadian Health Services Research Foundation (CHSRF). The third is the provision and monitoring of health *infrastructure*, including health human resources and health technologies. The fourth role, *population health*, has become increasingly important (see Chapter 5). As the public becomes more aware of the spread of pathogens throughout Canada (BSE, SARS, *e coli*, and *listeriosis* contamination, avian flu, West Nile virus, Lyme disease, and H1N1 influenza, to note the most visible concerns) there is a need to coordinate approaches to disease surveillance and prevention. The fifth role, *service delivery*, involves the direct provision of health services to specific groups (military personnel, Native populations on reserves). While this has not been a role of much public contention, the health conditions of Aboriginal people on and off reserves is becoming much more prominent.

What is the constitutional basis for the federal role in health care? The provinces manifestly claim the *regulatory* powers, but the federal government has substantial *expenditure* powers. Both the federal and provincial governments enjoy *taxation* powers that allow them to run public programs. The federal government also enjoys some influence through its residual powers ('Peace, Order, and Good Government,' which are relevant in discussions over public health issues) and through its regulation of 'noxious substances' (especially in regulating pharmaceuticals and the blood supply). The division of taxation powers is especially important for health care, as it has been the basis of much political controversy.

While federal involvement in health care has been premised on the position that the provinces cannot afford to run such programs without federal funding, Telford argues that this is largely because Ottawa 'commandeered' much of the tax room for itself during the Second World War: 'The provinces forfeited their fiscal autonomy with the understanding that the war-time tax agreement would be temporary. After the war, however, the federal government was anxious to renew the agreement' (2003: 33). By 1952 all provinces except Quebec agreed to permit Ottawa to collect their taxes, with the distribution of these funds becoming a matter of negotiation. Ottawa, observes Telford, 'is in the peculiar position of dominating the most lucrative source of provincial revenue only to transfer money to finance provincial programs' (ibid.). Thus there is little surprise that provinces became resentful of asking for money that they saw as rightfully theirs in the first place. To this, however, the federal government can rightfully respond that provinces have full ability to raise their own taxes any time they wish (they simply cannot demand that Ottawa lower its own share).

In 1977 the federal government became concerned with the tendency for health care costs to increase so rapidly, and decided to end the 50–50 cost-sharing system that it had established with the provinces on hospital and physician care. In its place, Ottawa developed 'Established Program Financing' (EPF), a system of block grants that permitted the federal government to place clear and predictable limits on the amount of funding directed to the provinces. As part of EPF, Ottawa ceded 'tax room' to the provinces: in other words, Ottawa lowered federal taxes, permitting provinces to increase their own taxes, over which they would have complete control. (As no government wishes to be seen to be increasing taxes, this was euphemistically referred to as 'a transfer of tax points.') This was not a major issue until the introduction of the Canada Health and Social Transfer (CHST) in 1995, when the federal government lumped both health and social transfers together while reducing overall funding levels. Then the provinces made much of the fact that Ottawa was only providing between 14 and 20 per cent of all health care funds, considerably down from its original bargain with the provinces to cost share these programs equally. But, as McIntosh (2004: 32) points out, 'if the tax points are provincial revenue and not a federal transfer, then provinces have to acknowledge that in accepting the tax transfer they accepted a new formula for calculating the appropriate federal cash transfer. From 1977 on, the "medicare bargain" agreed to was, to put it simply, fifty per cent paid by the provinces, twenty-five per cent paid in cash by the federal government, and twenty-five per cent paid by tax points transferred (which are now, of course, provincial own-source revenue).'

The third set of powers is even more contentious. These are the federal government's 'expenditure powers,' which have been the basis of Ottawa's nation-building exercises throughout the twentieth century. The problem is that this 'spending power' is not explicitly stated in the Constitution, but rather is inferred from the following sections: 91, the residual power based upon the principle of 'Peace, Order, and Good Government'; 91(1a), the power to make laws vis-à-vis public property; 91(3), the power to levy taxes; and 106, the power to appropriate federal funds. Others have advanced the position that the expenditure power has its basis in common law rather than in the formal Constitution (Scott 1977). The question, of course, is the extent to which Ottawa should be allowed to *spend* this money in areas outside its jurisdiction, where the Constitution forbids it from taking any regulatory or legislative action. Early judicial decisions on the extent of the federal government's spending power limited attempts by Ottawa to expand its reach, but this trend began to be reversed mid-century and, as Petter (1989) argues, despite the tentative legal status of the spending power, programs and institutions have been designed on the assumption of its legitimacy for over five decades. Any clear court ruling refuting the federal spending power would severely undermine a significant proportion of contemporary social infrastructure.

But federal nation building in Canada has two specific objectives: one is to develop a national set of social programs to enable its citizens to enjoy a comfortable range of modern services; the other is to limit the support for Quebec separation. In Canada's history, the two are closely intertwined. The federal spending power has been a source of perpetual resentment for Quebec. It is used most extensively in order to persuade individual Quebecois that Canada has provided a stable and commodious society for them, yet Quebec has never acknowledged the constitutional legitimacy of the spending power. Indeed, Quebec has in many cases negotiated separate agreements on numerous social programs, but this autonomy is largely symbolic to the extent that opting-out arrangements often limit the ability of Quebec significantly to change the nature of the programs themselves.

In sum, the constitutional institutions on which Canadian health care programs are based are themselves complex and contentious. Not only is Canada's federal structure not an ideal framework on which to build modern health care policies, but health care policies in Canada are often used to achieve political objectives that have little to do with health care itself. Health policy makers, therefore, must understand the wider political context within which intergovernmental relations exist.

The Dynamics of Health Care Federalism in Canada

The structure of federalism has both stymied and facilitated public health care in Canada, although not necessarily for the reasons we have come to believe. Boychuk (2008a), for example, argues that the 'incuba- tor of innovation' argument often presented by defenders of federal- ism is ill-conceived, as Saskatchewan's establishment of public medical insurance was in essence a 'strategic miscalculation' which took place only because provincial officials believed that a federal health insurance program was imminent. Moreover, he argues, Saskatchewan's success had the effect of crystallizing political interests *against* similar pub- lic health insurance programs across Canada, thereby weakening the capacity of other governments to implement robust public programs. However, at the same time, because 'support for the federal medicare program in Quebec proved to be higher than in any other region in Canada by a considerable margin,' Ottawa committed itself to a strong public health insurance agenda for the determined purpose of keep- ing Quebec in the federation (ibid., 134). More recently, interprovincial relations on health care were restructured for the primary purpose of federal fiscal retrenchment, with severe consequences both for health care and for interprovincial relations.

Most calls for health care reform in Canada have been very good at identifying the ways in which health care ought to be restructured, and very bad at identifying the entrenched interprovincial dynamics that tend to stymie them. Thus *Rekindling Reform*, the 2008 Health Council of Canada evaluation of health reform in Canada, noted that some of the most pressing policies (a national pharmaceutical strategy, a national human health resources strategy, and the Pan-Canada Healthy Living Strategy), all of which required much greater intergovernmental col- laboration, have been shelved or (like the Advisory Committee on Governance and Accessibility) disbanded. The problem, at least from the view from the street, is that the governments just can't get along. The reason they do not get along is not simply a matter of ideology or personality (although these can exacerbate existing tensions). It is rather that the logic of intergovernmental relations allows each level of government to provide perfectly rational and ethical reasons for its positions on various health care debates. To this must be added the normal political exigencies for democratic states to maximize autonomy while minimizing liabilities. Every elected government is ultimately answerable to its electorate; and an electorate that expects different things from two separate levels of government (make Canada more internationally competitive! lower taxes! just don't close our hospitals or scare our doctors away) does not facilitate intergovernmental cooperation.

Consider the federal perspective: We saw how provinces were struggling with the establishment of a public health care system, so we offered open-ended funding opportunities for the provinces to develop their own health caresystems through the 1957 Hospital Insurance and Diagnostic Services Act and the 1966 Medical Care Act. These pieces of legislation put Canada on the map in their establishment of a truly Canadian health care system that clearly distinguished us from Americans. It prevented severe regional disparities while developing modern, sophisticated health care in Canada. Unfortunately, we were a victim of our own success. The health care system grew and evolved at such a tremendous rate that, combined with the unforeseeable global recession of the early 1970s, it threatened to push our country into bankruptcy. In order to save our health care system – and our country – we were obliged to shift our shared-cost programs into a block-funding program in 1977. This allowed us to control costs, while at the same time the tax points we gave to the provinces allowed them both fiscal freedom and greater political autonomy. Now they don't have to endure the protracted yearly negotiations over eligibility issues, nor can they complain that their form of funding distorts their resource allocation process. Of course, we didn't realize then that, two decades later, the provinces would complain about the reduced cash transfers even while pocketing the tax transfers. No, they complained about how poor they were. Of course they were! They used the tax room we gave them to cut their own taxes – that was their choice. They could still have higher health funding if they wanted to. It's true that we had to cut back in the mid-1990s, and that the provinces found the CHST very upsetting. But what else could we do? The country was in dire straits. Federal public debt far exceeded the level of debt at the provincial level. And we made it up to them, didn't we? The 2003 First Ministers' Accord on Health Care Renewal injected $36 *billion* in federal money in addition to our regular health care spending and the following year's *10-Year Plan to Strengthen Health Care* added a further $41 billion to the health care pot, along with a 6 per cent increase in the regular health care transfers. How generous is that? In addition to that, we signed the 1999 Social Union Framework Agreement and promised that we'd never, ever make any sudden moves in health care without giving the provinces a clear indication of our intentions – even consulting them first, in some cases. Though, you have to understand, we really shouldn't have to, as it's our money. And yet they're still complaining that it's not enough! What a bunch of whiners.

The provincial perspective is slightly different: The provinces are the ones who took the initiative to establish public health care systems after decades of foot-dragging by the federal government. After seeing how well it worked, Ottawa decided to get involved and then started dictating terms and conditions to us, even though we're the ones who have the responsibility for running the health care programs, and we're the ones holding the can when things go wrong. There's a clear fiscal imbalance between federal and provincial levels of government: they're the ones who normally get the big budgetary surpluses, not the provinces. Our expenditures are growing more rapidly than theirs. Yet Ottawa makes us beg for money for operating a system for which they take credit – how many times have you heard them talk about the 'Canadian' health care system? They impose all sorts of rules and restrictions on us that limit our flexibility and distort our spending priorities, and they have no respect for local needs or political culture. Even though they only contribute a fraction of the total costs, they want to call the shots. Take the Canada Health Act: not only do they get to interpret it, but they get to enforce it – in other words, they're both prosecutor and judge! Sometimes we don't know year to year what the transfers will be – how is it possible to develop long-term policy plans when Ottawa makes unilateral decisions like the CHST out of the blue? Really, at times we're tempted to tell them to take their pennies and go for a hike. We could do this by ourselves – we do most of it in any case (with apologies to Lazar et al. 2002).

Where Are Intergovernmental Relations Taking Health Care? (And Where Is Health Care Taking Intergovernmental Relations?)

Federal systems are notoriously difficult to change. One reason is that federal systems contain multiple sites for veto options, so that many political actors can resist new policy directions. Any policy proposal, to be palatable to all, is generally stripped down to a point where little real change occurs. This is the phenomenon of the 'joint decision trap.' Each government guards its jurisdiction very carefully, and is loath to give up any advantage or basis of power that it enjoys. This is rational behaviour in any area such as health care, where these governments are ultimately accountable for whatever happens. If governments must bear the responsibility for a particular policy area, it is hardly surprising they should want as much control as possible in that field.

In Canada, the intergovernmental tussle over health care is structured on a (not always clear) constitutional framework, and is superimposed with (even more opaque) competing political dynamics. Provinces have good reason to pay close attention to their health care systems, as health care consumes the vast majority of provincial budgets (normally between 40% and 50%). Their electorates also hold them responsible for providing 'good health care' for each constituency. Poor policies can in this way get reinforced rather than eliminated: good democracy can mean bad health policy. This explains why so many rural emergency wards stay open, for example, when a 24-hour primary care clinic combined with an effective emergency transfer system may be superior from an epidemiological perspective. This also explains why so many provinces are so frequently tempted towards greater privatization of their health care systems: while the evidence linking greater privatization to higher costs is quite extensive, the costs are shifted from governments to the private sphere, leading (at least in the short term) to lower *government* expenditure.

The federal government, for its part, has for three decades been aware of the political pay-offs of promoting a public health care system with a national dimension. Polls consistently indicate that the Canadian public supports an accessible, universal, and equitable health care system, and no federal (or even provincial) government has been willing to take a strong stance against public opinion on this issue. To the extent that public health care has come to define 'Canadian values,' it has served as a powerful nation-building instrument, and any federal party – even those strongly sympathetic to market principles – will want to keep its hand at the helm of the 'Canadian health care system' by maintaining the ability of the Canada Health Act (CHA) to keep provinces rowing to the same beat.

How will these federal dynamics play out in Canada? Putting aside the status quo, there are three possible scenarios: greater federal involvement, greater provincial autonomy, and greater collaboration between governments.

Greater Federal Involvement

Given that the constitutional basis for health care in Canada gives clear jurisdiction in health care to the provinces, one might well assume that there is little capacity for greater federal activity in health policy making. It is an unlikely scenario, but not an impossible one. This scenario depends on the intersection of two variables: first, Ottawa's ability to capitalize on the golden rule (as in, 'he who has the gold, makes the rules') and second, the public appetite for (or tolerance of) an expansion of federal involvement into areas such as pharmacare and long-term care. The exclusion of such programs is a major weakness of Canadian health care (while most provinces have variations on these programs, they are usually offered on a needs-based or age-based allocation). To the extent that Canadian health care needs a major overhaul, it is in these areas. If Ottawa did decide to bankroll such programs, it could potentially buy its way into a more expanded political role in health care.

The federal government could use different instruments to expand its role in the provision of health care. The most contentious (by provincial standards) would be the direct delivery of insurance (e.g., for pharmacare or long-term care) at the federal level, by-passing the provinces completely. There would, in this scenario, likely be a constitutional challenge, but it could potentially survive such a judicial challenge (Lazar et al. 2002: 10). More probable would be a cost-shared system tacked onto the existing CHA. Another method of federal involvement in health care provision could include the transfer of health-related funds directly to citizens (e.g., through refundable tax credits or medical savings accounts). Given the nature of provincial territoriality in health care, any federal government would have to consider carefully whether the public support for such unilateral action would outweigh the provincial animosity such a program would likely provoke.

Greater Provincial Autonomy

A slightly more probable scenario is a more confederal system of health care. Provinces' participation in the Canada Health Act is completely voluntary; they can choose at any time to disassociate themselves from the CHA and manage their health care systems on their own terms. There was a great deal of discussion over this possibility in the late 1990s, after the unilateral introduction of the Canada Health and Social

Transfer by the federal government. In 1996 the Premiers' Council on Social Policy Renewal was established in order to determine how provinces could coordinate the management of interprovincial relations and bypass federal involvement as much as possible. One model of confederation in social policy was presented by Thomas Courchene (1996), who designed 'A Convention on the Canadian Economic and Social Systems' (ACCESS). Courchene's proposal included both an interim and a 'full ACCESS' model. The former retained a commitment by all provinces to the five CHA principles, but established a federal-provincial body for monitoring and adjudicating disputes over CHA transfers. The latter would remove the CHA entirely, and allow provinces themselves to determine which operational principles would underlie their respective systems. Federal health transfers would be converted into tax points, allowing the provinces to raise health care funds as they saw fit. There would be little binding provinces to any common standards, although it would theoretically be prudent for them to negotiate a system of portability for individuals moving between provinces (Maioni 1999).

There are problems with this scenario. The first, of course, is a deepening of asymmetry in the provision of health care across the country (although some argue that this in itself is not necessarily a bad thing: see Richards [1999]). The second is that Ottawa might be recalcitrant in handing over its tax points (although some of the wealthier provinces might decide that, given the small percentage of total health funding coming from Ottawa in any case, full autonomy was worth the price). But the third, and most formidable obstacle to a more confederal model is the electorate itself. Any federal government would be loath to walk away from such a powerful instrument of nation building as the Canada Health Act (Boychuk 2008a), and no provincial government has been successful in persuading its electorate to dismantle the public health care system (Maioni 1999).

In any case, the move by provinces to greater autonomy in health care was effectively checked by the vast infusion of health care cash offered by Ottawa to the provinces in 2003 and 2004, which is projected to continue until 2014. The only glue holding together the CHA to give Canada's health care system a national structure is cash and public opinion, both of which are nebulous and unpredictable variables. The provinces themselves have done little to organize a more collaborative confederal health care system. In 2003 the provinces set up the Council of the Federation, which was designed as a means of coordinating provincial and territorial activity independently of Ottawa. But there has been little development within the area of health care, except for a webpage posting a set of links to provinces' independent initiatives in health promotion. Thus the move towards greater provincial autonomy has been arrested, if only temporarily.

Greater Collaboration between Governments

The two scenarios noted above are premised on the rather pessimistic assumption that the relationship between levels of government will remain wary and acrimonious. There is certainly good historical evidence to entertain this possibility. But there is also the more optimistic view that governments have learned enough from the past to try to work towards more collaborative solutions. In this scenario, political actors increasingly understand the negative-sum consequences of competitive federalism, and they make an effort to develop health policy through a commitment to respectful negotiation, communication, and flexibility.

Despite the cynics' view that this development is as likely as international peace and good will, Cameron and Simeon document a number of factors that suggest that Canadian federalism is moving towards a more collaborative model. They point to the fact that most meetings and councils are now co-chaired by federal and provincial ministers; that territories are increasingly recognized as autonomous jurisdictions rather than as 'constitutional offspring of the federal government'; that governments articulate a respect for existing powers and a willingness to exercise them cooperatively; that efforts are taken to minimize duplication and overlap between jurisdictions; that a desire exists to share best practices, develop performance indicators, and monitor outcomes; that most agreements are formalized through individual bilateral agreements; that all parties express a concern for transparency and accountability; and that all governments acknowledge the need to collaborate more widely with non-governmental institutions and stakeholders (2002: 64).

The evidence in health policy is mixed. While collaborative processes have in some cases been increasingly formalized (as in public health), there is painfully little to show for it. Outcomes in planning, reporting, programming, and operation have been spotty at best. Despite agreement among first ministers in the 2003 Accord on Health Care Renewal to collaborate on a national health human resources strategy, for example, 'the reality is that planning remains fragmented. Except for some valuable efforts in regional collaboration, each province and territory does its own planning, without the benefit of pan-Canadian information needed for reliable decision making. The result is burn-out in the workforce and continued competition between jurisdictions for health care providers – and continued public frustration with wait times, uncoordinated care, and finding appropriate providers' (Health Council of Canada 2008: 28). The same problem exists in reporting on the state of health care, which remains fragmented between jurisdictions: 'too much of current reporting takes place in isolation, and most governments do not use or report the standardized data to which they committed' (ibid., 25). National-level collaborative programs articulated in 2003 and 2004 (such as the Integrated Pan-Canadian Healthy Living Strategy, the Pan-Canadian Public Health Network's strategy on control of communicable diseases, or the national pharmaceutical strategy) have quietly faded away. Nevertheless, where collaborative mechanisms have been established (as in public health), problems with communication and coordination still exist (Auditor General Canada 2008).

There is, of course, the response that not all overlap between governments is evidence of dysfunction. Having two jurisdictions involved independently in the same area can also contribute to the reliability of a system (in terms of ability to avoid or respond to error) and to innovation (by increasing the number of creative solutions available); see Lindquist (1999: 389). But in health care the most intergovernmental acrimony has not been caused by duplication of health services as much as by off-loading of the responsibility for funding – what Cameron and Simeon call the 'dis-spending power' or the 'exercise of the federal spending power in reverse' (2002: 54). The failure to coordinate programs or standardize reporting also presents problems in making services more effective. One possible strategy for achieving greater intergovernmental collaboration is a model that the European Union has been employing to facilitate policy making between autonomous member states. This model, termed 'New Modes of Governance' (or 'New Governance'), is based on a shift away from command-and-control systems towards approaches that are 'less rigid, less prescriptive, less committed to uniform approaches, and less hierarchical in nature' (de Búrka and Scott 2006: 2). Such approaches include deliberative decision making, multilevel networks, regulatory agencies, and peer review. The utility of such mechanisms is still being evaluated by

European policy makers and analysts, but because such procedures have been formalized and concretized over a period of years in the European Union, they may provide a rich source of ideas in fostering a greater capacity for intergovernmental collaboration in Canada.

There is, in sum, little reason to believe that intergovernmental relations will change considerably in the area of health care; but neither can the possibly for change be discounted. Currently, interprovincial relations are mediated by the 1999 Social Union Framework Agreement, a fairly general accord that articulates a commitment by the parties involved (Quebec is not a signatory) to greater communication, consultation, and public scrutiny. The agreement symbolized a mitigation of the rancorous intergovernmental relationship of the 1990s, but it has not substantially changed any of the underlying tensions between governments. In some ways the tensions are even more pronounced, with provincial governments publishing reports for radical reform (the Mazankowski and Castonguay reports) and Ottawa engaging in a potentially unilateral expansion of federal influence based on its strategy of infrastructure funding. As has been the case throughout Canada's past, health care in the future will be bound up with larger political strategies.

3   Health Care Administration and Governance

For a brief decade, the world experienced an exhilarating explosion of democratic reform. The fall of the Berlin Wall in 1989 and the end of South African apartheid in 1990 suggested that 'rule by the people' had finally become a global phenomenon. At the same time, Western states examined their own systems of governance, and program reforms were built around values of accountability, transparency, the dissemination of power, and democratic participation. All provincial health care systems experienced some kind of reform and reorganization throughout the 1990s, and most were influenced by these ideas to a greater or lesser extent. More recently, however, they have been moving away from organizational principles like 'regionalization' or 'citizen engagement.' What explains these shifts in the governance of provincial health care systems? What worked, and what did not? And in what direction is the governance of health care moving now?

The Rise of New Public Management

Historically, the major transformation of the way health care in Canada was organized was linked to the shift from private to public health insurance under key federal and provincial legislation. But another revolution in health care organization occurred throughout the 1990s. This transformation, however, was not driven by simple political objectives as the earlier reforms had been ('provide accessible health care for everyone') but by a rethinking of how public services ought to be administered.

The modern welfare state, and especially the modern health care system, rose from the ashes of the Second World War. It was, in fact, largely through the medical inspection of new recruits for the two world wars that most developed countries became aware of the poor state of health of their populations. During the Second World War, Britain's Labour Party became part of a coalition government from 1940 to 1945. Despite the restrictions of wartime governance, the Labour Party gained considerable ability to shape policy direction. Perhaps the most significant input was the development of the Beveridge Report of 1942, a document that outlined a series of social programs that would support Britons 'from cradle to grave.' Following the election of a Labour government in 1945, Britain's National Health Service (NHS) was established in 1948.

In Canada, research on postwar social reconstruction was directed by Leonard Marsh, who had conducted research for Sir William Beveridge in the United Kingdom before the war. Most of these social welfare reforms, including public health care, were implemented by the end of the 1960s. But the sheer size and complexity of such programs meant an expanding bureaucracy; and the best way of administering such a large organization was seen to be through a highly centralized and tightly controlled system (Aucoin 2008). By the 1980s the limitations of such a command-and-control system became apparent: a hierarchical and rule-bound organizational structure meant that flexibility and discretion were restricted and information flows were asymmetrical. Two sets of problems arose from these limitations. The first was *economic inefficiency:* those closest to the provision of services, and most knowledgeable about what was required, had too little or even no say in allocation decisions; while those making the funding decisions often had too little or no information about where the resources were most needed. The second problem was *poor service:* as those providing the services were responsible and responsive only to their superiors, and thus not to those receiving the services, there was often little incentive to treat recipients well, or to provide the best quality service.

The imperative of 'rolling back the frontiers of the welfare state' became the battle cry of Margaret Thatcher and other supporters of the 'new right' by the 1980s. One of the first politicians to systematically restructure the administration of public services, Thatcher based her reforms on ideas that had largely been developed within American academe and think-tanks. Despite the outcry and opposition to these reforms, Thatcher (and other proponents of the new right) also had considerable public support for them. Taxpayers were concerned about the high cost and huge inefficiencies experienced by the public sector, while many recipients of the services resented the shoddy treatment they experienced when using them.

The political traction of the 'new public management' (NPM) reforms was thus grounded in the rise of the new right. Nonetheless, the structural weaknesses of the old bureaucratic model were endemic to all developed welfare states, as evidenced in New Zealand and Australia where Labour governments led the way in implementing NPM. Not simply a 'handmaiden of neo-liberalism,' NPM is a tool that governments of various political inclinations have employed in order to improve the capacity of the state to provide services (Tupper 2001). While the new right as a political movement has become less strident, NPM has become the new orthodoxy for public administration (Aucoin 2008). What *is* NPM? Definitions are varying and overlapping, but at its heart NPM is a set of *goals* for the provision of public services, combined with sets of *processes and structures* to achieve them. The goals, broadly stated, are *cost control* and *individual empowerment* (both for those receiving services and those providing them). Generally speaking, it has not been the goals themselves but rather the means used to achieve them that have led to sustained criticism.

The first major structural reform informed by NPM was the detachment of policy making from service delivery. This account of the proper role of government ('steering, not rowing') argues that elected officials should develop policies and set priorities; but that services can be provided more efficiently by actors who do not enjoy monopolies. This 'alternative service delivery' takes many forms: privatization, contracting out, the use of private not-for-profit agencies, public-private partnerships, and so on. But it can also involve the restructuring of government services so that different public agencies have to compete with each other. The existence of competition, be it in the private or public sector (or between the two), would make those distributing the resources more responsible for doing so efficiently. It would reward innovation and risk taking, which would not only result in economic efficiencies but also in improvements to the services provided.

For those services that are not contracted out or subject to competition, business models were endorsed by NPM theorists as ways to measure performance and ensure accountability. These included clearly defined business plans, performance indicators, benchmarks, and framework documents. In this way, 'employee empowerment' was counterbalanced by administrative transparency: bureaucrats had more freedom of action, but they had to account publicly for both their successes and their failures in meeting targets. 'Citizen empowerment,' in contrast, was a much more nebulous concept. On the one hand, individuals as 'clients' or 'customers' had the freedom to reject an unsatisfactory provider for a better one. On the other hand, however, individuals who were actively engaged in determining what services were to be provided, and how to distribute them, would arguably be more 'empowered' than passive consumers.

New Public Management in Canadian Health Care Governance

Many of the characteristics of NPM were implemented (or articulated in vision documents) by provincial governments from the late 1980s to the early 2000s. The success of these reforms has been mixed at best. It would seem at first glance that health care would be an excellent subject for reform according to the NPM principles, as much of the decision making was already quite decentralized. Because of the nature of health care provision, which involves information gaps, the need for evaluative expertise, and a high error cost, both individuals and governments historically were willing to trust health care providers with decision-making authority on their behalf (Tuohy 2003). This 'agency' model of health care governance has been reinforced in Canada through the legal recognition of professional self-regulation by physicians. Self-regulation was negotiated by doctors in Saskatchewan after a bitter strike following the introduction of public health insurance, and it set a precedent for physicians in other provinces.

But the orthodox agency model of health care governance was problematic for three reasons. First, it was too expensive. Independent physicians with a direct line to government funding for 'all medically necessary treatment' in an era of skyrocketing treatment options meant that the only form of cost control was overarching funding limits. This resulted in waiting lists for surgeries, overcrowding in emergency departments, and shortages of family doctor in many areas. Second, it was poorly coordinated. Surgical care was stymied by bottlenecks in pre-operative consultations or postoperative therapy; patients with concurrent conditions were treated inefficiently; and there was little communication between the different fields of health care. Third, it was too one-sided. The information asymmetry underlying the agency model did not permit patients themselves any autonomous activity. The question for health policy makers, then, was whether NPM offered solutions to these specific problems.

Provincial health care reforms over the past decades have been significantly influenced by NPM. Interestingly, despite the different physical realities and ideological outlooks of the provinces, these reforms have been quite similar in their successes and limitations. With some hindsight, it is possible to say that some of the reforms (such as regionalization and citizen engagement) were based largely on a combination of faith and political opportunism. Other aspects of NPM theory (such as the use of performance indicators) have become more prominent.

The 'agency' model of health care governance ties into NPM theory quite well to the extent that both are based on the principle of autonomous, self-regulating players. However, the very factors that make health care governance well suited to the agency model – especially information asymmetry – also make it particularly unsuitable for market-based reforms. A clear commitment to more market-oriented reform was expressed in only two provinces: Alberta (in the 2002 Mazankowski Report) and Quebec (in the 2008 Castonguay Report). In both cases, proposals to privatize health care were quickly shelved because of public opposition. This is similar to the experience of many Western European countries; for,'unlike other sectors that were privatized (e.g., transportation), competition in the health sector is harder to trigger. This explains that while New Public Management theory has been around since the 1980s, it was only applied to the health care sector much later in the mid-1990s, the exceptions being the U.K., and with limited depth' (Simonet 2008; see also Chapter 9 below). In Canada there was an increased level of contracting out, greater spending reductions, and even, in some cases, the elimination of services altogether, especially during the late 1990s; but this had little to do with the principle of competition, and much to do with the cutbacks in federal transfers. But if clear market-based reforms were not prevalent in Canada, there were other manifestations of NPM ideas. Three themes which were much more prominent across provinces were *results-based* practices, *citizen engagement*, and *regionalization*.

Results-Based Management

While open competition in health care was not apparent in provincial reforms, business sector practices were nonetheless influential in a different way. This was in the overall shift from process-based to *results-based* management. This meant, first, that departments of health were required to post 'business plans' explaining what their objectives were for the year and how they intended to implement them, as well as an accounting of the previous year's business plan. Facilitated by the development of Internet technology, the articulation of clearly defined organizational objectives obliged departments of health to be accountable not only to the political executive, but also to the population at large. More profound was the development of benchmarking and performance indicators, which not only forced governments to meet their own objectives, but allowed for comparisons between provinces. This was not simply a result of NPM approaches, however: it was also a condition imposed on the provinces by Ottawa in 2004 for receiving extra funding. It was also the result of an increased capacity for data gathering that was facilitated by the establishment of several health research and data collection organizations, including the Canadian Institute for Health Information (CIHI) in 1994, the Canadian Health Services Research Foundation (CHSRF) in 1996, the Canadian Institutes of Health Research (CIHR) in 2000, and the Canada Health Infoway in 2001.

Results-based management has had considerable impact on the ability of health care systems to run more efficiently, but it has not been without problems. There has, for example, been some difficulty in getting provinces to agree on benchmarks. This is not surprising, given the diversity of capacity between provinces (whether a hospital can perform a hip replacement within a certain number of weeks depends on how well funded hospitals are, how successful the region is in recruiting necessary health personnel, how well coordinated its waiting-list management system is, and so on). Provinces that have limited capacity may also be less willing to 'sign on' to standard benchmarks because of the political pressures that can arise if they compare poorly with other provinces. Benchmarking and performance indicators in targeted areas also have the tendency to shift spending priorities away from local needs to national standards, which runs against NPM's push to decentralization. Targeted performance indicators in specific areas (e.g., hip replacements) can also drain funding away from areas *without* targeted performance indicators (e.g., the length of time it takes to see a psychiatrist after being referred by a GP), as there is less public accountability for decreased funding for low-profile services. There is even some concern that the success in establishing performance indicators and publicizing comparative ratings has actually led to *greater* conformity between regions (Hood and Peters 2004: 270). Another unintended consequence of the process imposed on public bureaucracies in order to secure public accountability has been an increase of 'formality and regulation' that, in some cases, is even more rule bound than the traditional form of bureaucratic management (ibid., 271).

Citizen Engagement

Like results-based management, *citizen engagement* was another ill-defined reform goal that had much rhetorical prevalence throughout the 1990s. By the early 2000s, however, the few experiments in citizen participation that had been implemented were quietly shelved, and the idea itself had lost its political traction. The role of citizens as active participants in health policy making had two very contradictory versions, neither of which ultimately gained a foothold in policy making. The first version was based on the concept of 'citizen as consumers,' and attempted to provide more choice to health care consumers, to give some guarantee of quality service, and to make health care recipients more responsible for their own health. This model was much more prevalent in both the United States and the United Kingdom, where the NPM ideas of 'new managerialism' suggested that money ought to follow patients, thereby forcing health care providers to make themselves attractive to potential 'customers.' While some economic efficiencies were gained through these 'client-based' reforms, there was little real citizen engagement, as the decision making regarding the choice of specialist was firmly lodged with individuals' GPs (in the United Kingdom) or employers and insurance companies (in the United States).

The only real acknowledgment of the role of individuals in health care was in the development of 'patients' charters.' The earliest version emerged from the Thatcher administration in 1991, but was revised in 1995 and then abandoned in favour of clearly articulated 'wait-time guarantees' under the Blair government. Tomblin and others have identified a number of reasons why the early attempts at a patients' charter were less than successful: 'it was a top-down creation; people and stakeholders did not identify with it and were threatened by it; the charter was designed to promote a consumerist culture or approach rather than a needs-based one; it encouraged competition and not the sharing of best-practices across health units; the emphasis was more on process, rather than outcomes; the focus was more national than community-based; it "encouraged people to cheat"; reinforced a "blame culture"; and "it muddled the concept of rights and aspirations giving patients rights but no effective redress when these rights were not delivered"'(Tomblin 2002: 20). More recent attempts at patients' charters have emerged in Scotland's devolved NHS in 2005, Germany's 2007 *Sozialgesetzbuch*, and West Virginia's 2006 Medicaid Redesign, although in all these cases the charters also include a series of 'patient responsibilities' that raise a number of ethical issues (Schmidt 2007). To the extent that individuals are held responsible for 'living well,' there are problems with ambiguity (e.g., is skiing a good means to keep fit or does it present an unacceptable risk of concussion and broken bones?), paternalism (who determines appropriate lifestyle choices?), and responsibility (how does one factor in illnesses due to genetic inheritance, poverty, or poor education?) And to what extent are prescriptions against 'unnecessary use' of the health care system unreasonable when only trained health care professionals can make the distinction between benign symptoms and symptoms of serious underlying health disorders?

Beyond the recent establishment of general waiting-time benchmarks, there has been relatively little evidence of this first model of citizen engagement ('patient as consumer') in Canada. The second version of citizen engagement widely discussed in provincial health care reforms throughout the 1990s focused more on a political or policy-oriented role for individuals. This, to a large extent, occurred concurrently with the phenomenon of 'regionalization' that began in the early 1990s: and, in many cases, it served as a justification for regionalization. Both Ontario and Quebec had experimented with some citizen governance of health boards in the 1970s, but the rhetoric of civic engagement in health care became a national phenomenon two decades later. In British Columbia, for example, the New Democratic government's 1993 document *New Directions for a Healthy British Columbia* articulated a commitment to devolved power from the provincial Department of Health to elected citizen boards in order to facilitate local accountability, community empowerment, and a reorientation towards preventive health care (Davidson 1999). Similarly, the Nova Scotia Liberal government employed the rhetoric of citizen participation in its 1994 regionalization reforms (Black and Fierlbeck 2006). Many other provinces, including Saskatchewan, Alberta, New Brunswick, and Prince Edward Island, also declared their support for elected regional health boards. Nevertheless, by the early 2000s, all provinces had backed away from commitments to engage a wide selection of lay individuals in health policy formulation and governance. Some governments, like Saskatchewan, couched their move towards more formal managerial systems as responses to electors' demands for more efficient management and greater accountability (Dickinson 2002: 21).

There are a number of reasons for this disillusionment in civic engagement within the health care arena. The first was simply bad timing: by the time representative bodies were established, the federal cutbacks to the provinces in the mid-1990s meant that the principal role of such bodies became the allotment of cutbacks. This worked to the advantage of provincial governments, who could pass on responsibility for hospital closures to 'the community,' but it certainly did little to facilitate a move towards population health models or an engaged citizenry. On the contrary, it led community activists to become even more cynical and alienated from the policy-making process. The second problem arose from the normal dynamics of democratic systems. Much of the rhetoric underlying citizen engagement rested on principles of democratic legitimacy; yet the turnout for the election of health board members rarely went above 10 per cent. This, in turn, raised serious problems for the 'capture' of health authorities by special interest groups, such as anti-abortionists (Davidson 1999; Lewis 2001; Tomblin 2002; Abelson and Eyles 2002). A third problem rested in the assumption (driven by the popular 'civil society' literature of the period) that public participation contributed to a more educated and engaged populace, in which collaborative problem solving led to tolerance, trust, and a commitment to the common good. In practice, it proved much easier to mobilize community involvement at a local level (especially when it came to saving or expanding local services) than to rationalize services more efficiently across larger areas (particularly when it came to closing small local hospitals or emergency wards: see Abelson 2001). By the end of the 1990s, the few experiments that evolved from policy rhetoric demonstrated that 'health board elections are costly, cumbersome and produce low voter turnout and have failed to foster a more active, engaged citizenry committed to collectivist goals' (Abelson and Eyles 2002: 12).

What the 'citizen engagement' reforms *were* able to do was not to hand power to individuals, but rather to wrest it further away from medical professionals. By eliminating hospital boards, where local physicians had more influence both formally and informally, and placing policy-making power in the hands of professional bureaucrats, the 'agency' model of health care governance was effectively undermined in most jurisdictions. It was by no means eliminated – the corporatist relationship between provincial colleges of physicians and the provincial governments that was established decades ago is firmly institutionalized – but it did restrict the input of physicians at a more local level. The traditional power of physicians – medical knowledge – is also being weakened by the large-scale data collection facilitated by technology. By analysing the statistical analyses presented by health data collection agencies (such as CIHI), governments are more able to make decisions about effective or efficient treatment options without relying heavily on medical experience. While governments are formally accountable to their electorate, however, this shift in power clearly falls short of what could reasonably be called 'citizen engagement.'

Regionalization

By far the most prevalent manifestation of governance reform in health care throughout the 1990s was regionalization. The principle of regionalization was based on the argument, explicit in NPM, that centralized control over management and the delivery of services was both unresponsive and inefficient. This was, from the late 1980s, an international trend (Saltman, Bankauskaite, and Vrangback 2007). While the decentralization of authority in many countries took the form of privatization and deregulation, in Canada the phenomenon of decentralization was clearly based on territorial jurisdiction. Decentralization as 'regionalization' has been, in Canada, 'an organizational arrangement involving the creation of an intermediary administrative and governance structure to carry out functions or exercise authority previously assigned to either central or local structures' (Church and Barker 1998: 468). In other words, while decision-making power was diffused *downwards* from the provincial departments of health to regional health authorities (also known as district health authorities), it was also consolidated *upwards* from several local hospital boards to single regional health authorities (see Figures 3.1 and 3.2). In Ontario and Quebec, the regional bodies are much larger and have therefore allowed local health services networks to have more organizational responsibility.

This intermediary form of decentralization is distinct from *devolution* insofar as the regional units had little if any ability to collect and spend their own funds. Fiscal authority remained at the provincial level, while managerial responsibility rested with the regions. Policy-making authority could be made at either level, depending on the type of policy involved. At least initially, this was a matter of some dispute, as critics argued that 'severing the link between health service provision and local taxation was tantamount to converting the health boards into agents of the government' (Davidson 1999: S38). Yet as regionalized institutions

Figure 3.1. Basic governance structure before regionalization

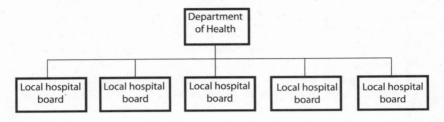

Figure 3.2. Basic governance structure after regionalization

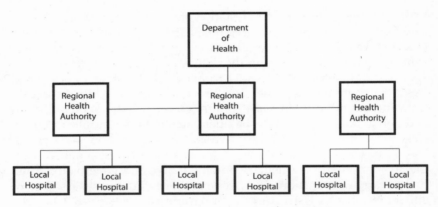

were being designed it became apparent that the devolution of fiscal authority could lead to intractable problems. The most apparent was the potentially inequitable distribution of health services within provinces. Given that the tax base of each region varied enormously (especially between urban and rural/northern areas), there was much concern that provinces would transform into a patchwork of health care regions, some being of much higher quality than others. This would also present the problem of 'bargain shopping' by health care users outside of their own regions, which would then require some form of administrative system to monitor this kind of usage and possibly provide for compensation. The second problem was liability: if regions themselves became responsible for raising their own funds, who would be responsible for cost overruns? Simply forcing regions to bear the costs of administrative miscalculations by eliminating essential health care services would be politically untenable. Given that the provincial governments would ultimately have to bear the costs of rescuing profligate regions in the last instance, provincial executives determined that being able to control costs systematically would, in the long run, prove to be more economically effective and politically uncomplicated.

How successful has the two-decade experiment with regionalization been? There is certainly no dearth of criticism regarding the implementation of regionalization but, as Lewis and Kouri (2004) point out, neither has it been shown to be drastically *ineffective*. To a large extent, the biggest fault with regionalization has been the failure to live up to the goals and expectations imputed to it. Regionalization may well have been implemented so widely precisely because so many disparate interests saw it as a means of achieving their own set of objectives: those on the left saw it as a means of establishing a system of citizen empowerment; those on the right saw organizational rationalization as a means of achieving economic efficiency; health promotion advocates saw it as a way of shifting a medical model of health care to one supporting preventive health care; governments saw it as a means of deflecting direct accountability for cutbacks, and so on. Many of these objectives were blatantly contradictory, and some of them were simply not feasible given the complexity of modern health care provision. Provinces themselves have passed widely disparate judgments on the utility of regionalization: some (such as Alberta and Prince Edward Island) have eliminated regional health boards altogether; while others (Ontario) have more recently established them. What can be said with more certainty (and some optimism) is that the relative strengths and limitations of regionalization have become much clearer. Given the solid experience Canada, and other countries, have had with the regionalization experiment, there is now more focus on achieving and refining the aspects of regionalization that work well, and on jettisoning those that were ill-conceived or overly optimistic. While the theoretical perspective on health care governance has been tempered by experience, however, competing political interests still have the capacity to impede further managerial reforms.

Beyond New Public Management: Lessons Learned for Health Care Governance

As a way of approaching the governance of public institutions, NPM has not been refuted or transcended as much as it has been refined into a much more circumscribed set of ideas for achieving much more limited goals. There has also been a clearer realization that the political and policy-making environment has changed radically – both for the better and the worse – since NPM was articulated in the 1980s. Moreover, as parties with quite different political values have had to grapple with the same sets of intransigent obstacles over the past few decades, many of the strident ideological overtones of NPM have been discarded even as some of its basic premises have become the new orthodoxy in public management.

Much, too, has depended on the particular sector of public administration. In the area of health care, for example, the siren call of 'competition' (which was one of the most fundamental aspects of early NPM theory) has remained muted. This has been so for a number of reasons. The nature of health care itself makes it a difficult commodity for the marketplace (see Chapter 1); public support for 'market solutions' in health care in Canada has been quite limited; and the bureaucratic fragmentation of health care administration in Canada was seen to require greater collaboration, not competition, between actors. The 'consultation, cooperation, and coordination' needed to integrate health care sectors within and across regions was not something that could be facilitated through a market-driven system. The three aspects of NPM that characterized administrative reforms in health care – results-based management, citizen engagement, and regionalization – still exist, but they have morphed into different manifestations based on the lessons learned in the past two decades. These lessons are: first, facts are your friends, but only if they're used the right way; second, accountability is easier to achieve than empowerment; and third, it's not really about regionalization, but about 'integration.'

'Facts Are Your Friends'

One of the most discernible improvements in health care administration has been the advance in data collection and analysis. This has been an international trend. Since the 1990s, 'with new information storage capabilities, more powerful computers and relational database methodologies it has become feasible to collect, store, and analyze vast amounts of data. The challenge in the measurement of healthcare performance is rapidly changing from one of the availability of information to the identification and management of the specific data elements and the use of the information to assess performance and guide improvement' (Baker et al. 1998: 22). Canada, as a whole, has been much slower than other countries to utilize new technologies for managing the performance of health care. This is partly a reflection of its federal structure, as many of these systems are quite complex and costly to establish. Poor intergovernmental relations throughout the 1990s limited the systematic development of health performance measurement, but by 2004 Ottawa promised financial support for the development of infrastructure to facilitate data collection and interpretation as part of its program of political bridge building with the provinces after a decade of acrimony.

All provinces now have units for the collection and evaluation of health care data. These are used for the development of patient safety and quality improvement; the monitoring of waiting times and access to services; the evaluation of resource use and outcomes (such as the effectiveness of specific health procedures), patient satisfaction surveys; comparative financial measurements; and the development of electronic health records. Most provinces even post some of these data – especially on waiting times – on websites for public information. The primary utility of such measurement instruments is that it gives a much clearer account of what works, what does not, and what the problems are. Where such information is publicly accessible, it also holds officials to account for the achievement of policy objectives.

Problems remain in the way in which such information is interpreted and applied. Although the Canadian Institute for Health Information collects a great deal of raw data on health care, it is the provinces that are ultimately responsible for the how information is collected and for the areas in which information is to be collected. Provinces do not always agree on comparative indicators. Often data are collected but not analysed, or they are analysed but not reported. As the Health Council of Canada's report states, 'data systems have been expanded and refined. However, these efforts have not led definitively to the "enhanced accountability" and "improved performance reporting" that the accord promised. Too much of the current reporting takes place in isolation, and most governments do not use or report the standardized data to which they committed' (2008: 25). The collection and reporting of data has also been hobbled by the implementation of new privacy laws in Canada. Moreover, there is little oversight to ensure that data are reported (and interpreted) correctly. In some areas – such as 'democratic accountability' – the ambiguous nature of the term makes performance measurement difficult to ascertain. Nonetheless, the growth of information technology in the health care sector has been nothing less than revolutionary. While the explosion of electronic capacity-building is not a consequence of NPM itself, the school's insistence on measurement and performance has fit well with the ability of technology to provide such information.

'Focus on Accountability, Not Participation'

The emphasis of NPM on a 'citizen-centred' and participatory management culture reflected the wider interest throughout the 1980s and 1990s in the nature of democratic governance. The size and unwieldiness of the modern welfare state had raised concerns about the responsiveness of those providing services to those for whom such services were designed. Those on the right argued that the utilization of market mechanisms would oblige health service providers to become more attuned to the demands of health care consumers; while those on the left held that the involvement of individuals in the planning and allocation of resources would give citizens a much better sense of ownership of, and connection to, public services. The ideological line between the two groups was usually sharply drawn: those on the right worried that public participation in health policy making would place unfair burdens on citizens as taxpayers; while those on the left argued that the uneven distribution of wealth in society would mean inequitable influence in a market-oriented health care system.

In the end, neither approach proved successful. In Canada there was some movement towards the contracting out of non-medical services (such as housekeeping and food services) and public-private partnerships, with mixed results (see, e.g., Vining and Boardman, 2008). But there was little appetite politically for large-scale privatization and no persuasive evidence internationally that out-sourcing or contracting out would lead to improved outcomes (Simonet 2008: 628). But if the model of 'citizen as consumer' conflicted too sharply with the entrenched view of health care as a social good, not a market commodity, the model of the 'engaged citizen' proved equally problematic.

Theoretically, the idea of citizens as 'involved stakeholders' is premised on the assumption that 'empowering people to provide input in decisions that affect their lives encourages support for those decisions, which in turn improves the public's trust and confidence in the health care system' (Bruni, Laupacis, and Martin, 2008: 15). Some provinces, such as British Columbia and Nova Scotia, attempted to formalize public participation through the establishment of community health councils (or boards), which were designed to provide a conduit for public opinion at the local level (see Figure 3.3).

The role for community health councils (CHCs) envisaged in British Columbia's 1993 document *New Directions* was quite extensive. Under this model, 'inter-sectoral collaboration would be achieved through the

Figure 3.3. Community health councils

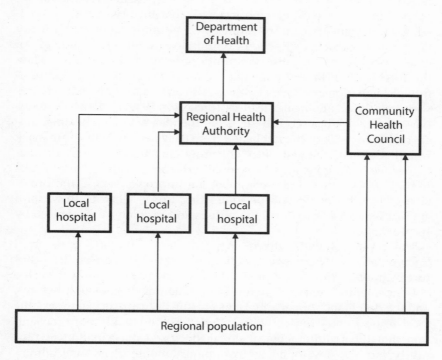

integration of a broad range of services at the community level under the control of the CHC; intercommunity collaboration by requiring community plans and expenditures to be vetted by representatives of all the communities within the region (RHB [regional health board]). Local governments were mandated partners through legislated representation on CHCs' (Davidson 1999: 35–6). These plans, however, were dramatically curtailed by 1996.

Nova Scotia's model of community health councils was clearly influenced by British Columbia's discussion of community engagement (Bickerton 1999). While Nova Scotia's 1994 *Blueprint for Health System Reform* saw the community health boards (CHBs) playing an important role in the administration of health policy, problems with the development of regional health boards throughout the 1990s meant that the role of CHBs became marginalized. By the time CHBs were formally recognized in legislation in 2001, their role was strictly limited to an advisory capacity (Black and Fierlbeck 2006). Despite the fact that recessionary politics were partly responsible for the failure of the CHBs to live up to expectations, the difficulty of institutionalizing citizen engagement in health policy administration had already been noted in Quebec's Rochon Commission Report. An evaluation of Quebec's experiment with community participation a decade earlier, the 1988 Rochon Report concluded that the mechanisms of community participation employed by the health and community care centres were 'paralyzed and nearly useless' (Bickerton 1999: 164). Interestingly, New Brunswick has recently revisited the idea of citizen health councils: in March 2008, it established a sixteen-person New Brunswick Health Council, charged with 'engaging citizens in meaningful dialogue,' evaluating health service quality, communicating these results to the wider public, and recommending improvements in the provision of health care. It will be interesting to see whether this health council will be able to avoid the pitfalls and problems experienced by its precursors.

The problems with citizen engagement are by now quite well known: lack of expertise in complicated technical areas; political capture by interest groups; shifting and unclear paths of accountability; the entrenchment of local hierarchies within new institutional structures; and the dominance of parochial concerns or, as theorists like to say, 'the local resource attachment phenomenon.' There is now more recognition that the requirements of engaged citizen participation involve much 'capacity development,' 'community mobilization,' and administrative supports which, in turn, means 'a slow, messy process that requires enormous amounts of time and resources' (Bickerton 1999: 182). Others have argued that citizens still have a role to play in 'setting overall directions for the health care system' and 'ensuring the system reflects public values and principles' by focusing on the contributions of individuals' 'lived experiences' and 'value-based deliberations' (Bruni, Laupacis, and Martin, 2008: 16; see also Dickinson 2002).

But the fear that individuals are marginalized and powerless in opposition to a monolithic bureaucratic entity may itself be an obsolete view of the modern citizen-state relationship. Contemporary reality is both more complicated and more dynamic. Democratic governments have, in the past two decades, been confronting the political pressures of the 'new public governance.' According to this account, modern democracies are facing unprecedented demands for openness and disclosure fed not only by the theoretical debates over 'good governance' but also by recent phenomena including the following:

- The transparency resulting from the modern communications technology revolution
- The emergence of greater assertiveness and aggressiveness by mass media
- The openness that comes with the advent of a public right to access government information
- The establishment of a host of more intrusive and independent audit and review agencies
- The public exposure of public servants as witnesses before parliamentary committees as well as in public engagement or consultation exercises
- A less deferential citizenry that demands great public accountability by both ministers and public servants. (Aucoin 2006: 303–4)

This has had both negative and positive consequences for health care governance. On the one hand, governments have had to reconfigure the way that they govern in order to maintain stable bases of political support. As discussed below, this has resulted in a greater tendency to micromanage governance from the top. But it has also allowed policy makers to distinguish between kinds of 'democratic governance,' and, specifically, to clarify the distinctions between the *representation* of interests, the *accountability* of individuals and agencies for decisions made, and *advocacy* for those with grievances against the system. 'Citizen empowerment' was seen as a means of accomplishing all three of these goals; but it may be that they are more usefully addressed in separate ways. The experiment with community health councils showed that attempting to achieve too much tended to paralyze the bodies and to diminish public support for them. For those community health boards in Nova Scotia or citizen advisory boards in Saskatchewan that have been seen as constructive and innovative participants in health care systems, the roles have been strictly limited to a consultative capacity rather than one responsible for raising funds, allocating resources, and/or managing programs. Whether such bodies are appointed or elected seems to be less important than whether they are constituted by well-informed and fair-minded individuals; and the formal powers they have are less important than the informal willingness of political officials to listen and to act on good advice. Given the complexity of health care management and the heterogeneity of the populations that health care managers are expected to serve, it is useful to have a clear channel for communication between administrators and client populations. This is a stripped-down version of 'citizen participation' as it was originally envisaged, but it may well be no less effective. The Rousseauean imperative of developing a mature citizenry through direct involvement in the political process will likely remain too unwieldy to be institutionalized in health care governance, but the recognition that individuals' voices must be *represented* for effective policy development remains. In the United Kingdom, for example, there is some evidence that individuals desire not direct participation but rather the opportunity to express their views 'with a guarantee that their contributions will be heard and an explanation of the rationale for the decision ultimately made' (Abelson and Eyles 2002: 15; Litva et al. 2002).

What citizens seem to want is not responsibility for decision making, but rather the ability to express their views and to hold decision makers accountable for their actions. This does not require ongoing participation but rather a clearly defined and transparent set of rules and processes that permit citizens to judge the quality of stewardship of their public services. To a certain extent, this goal has been increasingly facilitated by the development of performance indicators, as noted above, as well as by the culture of openness and accountability that has arguably been a residual effect of NPM. The development of advocacy mechanisms for those experiencing problems is less common, but is receiving more attention (Abelson and Eyles 2002). Often individuals have no interest in general policy directions, but they care very much about specific aspects of a system that may not be working well. This is another aspect of business management that has been effectively adopted in public governance (e.g., in the establishment of 'ombudsman' offices). Complaints that are dealt with effectively and respectfully can establish a strong sense of satisfaction with the way in which health care is provided. In sum, the idea of 'accountability' (that one's voice has been heard, that one knows why decisions have been made and who has made them, that the decision makers can be held to account, and that there is direct recourse for problems that arise) may well be more powerful in establishing a sense of 'empowerment' in health care than a model of 'direct participation' could ever hope to do.

A secondary legacy of the quest for citizen engagement has been the more circumscribed practice of *patient* engagement. This approach facilitates the active participation of patients in managing their conditions. It can, for example, take the form of 'patient decision aids,' which educate patients in order for them to make reasoned decisions about treatment options; or peer support groups, which present a perspective on illness and treatment that is more experientially based. The goals of patient engagement are more limited than those of citizen engagement, but because they are better defined and more closely monitored, they may well have a much better likelihood of becoming institutionalized as standard treatment practices.

A third, and more recent, development has been the phenomenon of organized non-governmental groups acting as 'policy watchdogs' through their willingness to measure and evaluate the performance of government bodies and report back to the general public. The problem of citizen accountability, as some observers note, is that such bodies are expected to assume governments' responsibility for ensuring accountability to the public, rather than merely supplementing it. They are rarely given the resources to be able to do so efficiently and rigorously, and their role as forensic auditor increasingly precludes their ability to engage in policy development (Findlay and Anderson 2010).

'It's about Integration'

Since 1992 all provinces have experienced some form of regionalization in health care; however, the counter-trend of *deregionalization* has also become apparent. This has not been limited to Canada: across Europe, various countries have reversed the practice of decentralization and have increasingly been taking more responsibility for policy making and financial control in the health care sector. There have been a number of reasons for this. Several countries have become concerned with increased disparities across regions where regional authorities have been responsible for raising their own health care funds. Others have become aware that expensive technologies and services are provided more efficiently at a central level where there is less duplication. The deregulation of health care markets in the European Union has led some member states to worry that there is need to wrest control back from the marketplace. Some countries have found that the lines of accountability are not clearly drawn, leading citizens to hold their national government responsible for shortcomings in regional systems. Further, advances in technology have allowed states to monitor and manage health care systems more closely from a distance, diminishing the need for administrative bodies to be 'close to the people' (Saltman 2008).

It is useful to point out that recentralization has not only been occurring in the health care sector, but across the public service more widely. As noted above, the pressures imparted by the 'new public governance' have led to the concentration of power at the centre. These pressures – sophisticated communications technology, more right of access to government information, more intrusive media, new external audit and review agencies, aggressive parliamentary committees, more public polling, and a less deferential citizenry – have, paradoxically, all been instrumental in the trend towards the concentration of power. But the trend to regionalization exacerbated the problem. The more power is diffused, the more discretion managers have, and the less direct control government has over problems that arise. Especially in the wake of the Gomery Commission, governments have been more circumspect about micromanaging administrative decisions, which itself leads to greater centralization. 'By trying to ensure that the necessary controls are in place to prevent the abuse of government resources by managers who manage resources with some discretion, the government response risks the adoption of centralized management systems that cannot but impede the achievement of economy and efficiency, staff commitment and engagement, or citizen-centred service delivery' (see, e.g., Aucoin 2008: 18). But regionalization has also evolved in different directions across provinces for different reasons. To an extent, this is because different jurisdictions had varying reasons for implementing systems of regionalization in the first place. The goals of regionalization that were articulated in various documents presented by provincial governments throughout the 1990s and early 2000s included the following:

• The rationalization of services to address excessive fragmentation and discontinuity
• The amalgamation of jurisdictions to achieve economies of scale in management and procurement
• The establishment of administrative bodies more responsive to local populations
• The facilitation of wider public participation
• The development of a focus on promoting population health.

A political objective that was rarely articulated but usually implicit was the limitation of the ability of the medical profession directly to influence the way in which health services were provided, both at an individual and at a systemwide level.

The results of these experiments in regionalization were mixed. Smaller communities which had elected local residents to municipal hospital boards perceived themselves to be more disconnected from the health care administration of their immediate area, as 'the pluralistic nature of local decision making was replaced by more concentrated and centrally directed regional decision making involving numerically fewer community representatives in the process' (Church and Smith 2008: 234). The fact that representatives on regional health boards often had more power than elected hospital board officials had enjoyed did not, in the eyes of many small town inhabitants, make up for the fact that their municipality was not represented at all in the new administrative structures. This was especially true in provinces like Alberta, where close to 200 local boards were amalgamated into seventeen (and then nine, and then one), or Saskatchewan, where 435 boards were whittled down to thirty-two (and then twelve). This perceived lack of representation was exacerbated by the cutbacks of the late 1990s. As noted above, most experiments with elected representation in place of political appointments were unsuccessful over time. The administrative reorganization of governance structures was also insufficient to achieve any major health promotion goals. The attainment of a system that actively embraces preventive health care was limited by a range of political, economic, cultural, and institutional barriers (see Chapter 5); and the hope that regionalization by itself could facilitate significant health promotion goals proved to be unrealistic. Economically, the move to regionalization was more successful in closing smaller or redundant hospitals and in allocating regional services more efficiently, although there was little evidence that 'scale economies' were achieved by regional health authorities (especially in provinces where even the regions themselves were too small to effect real economies of scale). Interestingly, Alberta's move in 2009 to recentralize into one single 'superboard' was done on the grounds that this rationalization would cut administrative costs.

Where regionalization has been more successful has been in the reduction of fragmentation within the health care system. By reducing duplication, eliminating barriers, and coordinating programs across sectors, regional health authorities have been able more effectively to connect resources to needs. In some cases, discrete units with more autonomy have been able and willing to act as 'more active incubators of innovation' (Lewis and Kouri 2004: 26), and they can 'respond quickly and strategically to challenges where there are fewer autonomous agencies and affiliations' agreements to deal with' (ibid.: 28; see also Casebeer 2004). In other words, the main success of regionalization has been its ability to facilitate greater integration between health sectors, agencies, and services. A major criticism of the provinces' experiments with regionalization is that they have not been integrative *enough*. Most regional health authorities have focused on the coordination of primary care and hospital care with some reorganization of public health. Provinces differed in their willingness to include cancer care, mental health, long-term care, and alcohol and drug addiction programs in their regional health authorities; very little was done anywhere in thinking about the integration of physicians or the development of a comprehensive prescription drug policy.

Thus, even under a system of regionalized health care, gaps in timing and treatments remained, as well as unnecessary duplication, lack of communication, and poor access to services at all levels. The focus on health administration has shifted from 'regionalization' (where integration was only one objective) to 'integration' itself. While the two concepts are closely linked, there is some debate about whether geographical regionalization is useful or even necessary to achieve the integration of services (Forest et al. 1999; Lewis and Kouri 2004). 'Integration,' by definition, is more about the *organization* of services than about the governance of management systems. Originally developed in the early 1990s, integrated health care shared with NPM the concept of organizing health delivery around the needs of consumers rather than the convenience of providers, and focused on the following: greater choice in treatment and in providers; efficient and timely treatment, including quick access and 'one-stop shopping'; and high quality services. The 'organized delivery systems' on which integrated health care must be structured have been defined as 'networks of organization that provide or arrange to provide a coordinated continuum of services to a defined population and who are willing to be held clinically and fiscally accountable for the outcomes and the health status of the population being served' (Shortell et al. 1993: 447).

Integrated health systems mean in practice (ideally): seamless communication between patients and all health care providers, including case histories, test results, and appointment schedules; the elimination of gaps between treatment, including pre- and post-operative care; quick access to primary care, usually through team-based primary health care practices; effective management of chronic care conditions or multiple concurrent medical conditions; accessible and comprehensive information about medical treatments and administrative processes; and the merger of preventive and medical care (Leatt, Pink, and Guerriere, 2000; Rachlis 2004). The point is to eliminate the rigid barriers between health care 'silos' so that the different components of a health care system mesh together like the gears of a well-oiled clock to provide 'seamless care.'

Despite its failings, regionalization has in most cases been a firm step towards greater integration of services. What has emerged from the experiments with regionalization is that innovative attempts at integration (such as Edmonton's Capital Health District) have been relatively successful (Decter 2006; Lewis and Kouri 2004). Unfortunately, there is no clear model or working template for integrated health care per se: each attempt at establishing an integrated system is based on evaluations of what has worked in different jurisdictions. Ontario's implementation of fourteen local health integration networks (LHINs) in 2007, for example, was more clearly designed to facilitate integration than other provinces' attempts at regionalization in earlier years. It is, in part, easier to inch towards integration now because of the extent and quality of technology (especially electronic health records), the growth of team-based primary health clinics, and coordination on communicable disease surveillance systems. But there is no panacea. Integrated systems will have to work out relationships of collaboration and accountability just as painfully as regionalized systems did. To the extent that shared governance tends to disperse responsibility, the structures of authority and accountability will have to be carefully negotiated and monitored as formerly discrete 'silos' become more closely integrated. In short, the traditional patterns of political influence that made it difficult to integrate physicians, establish a clear policy on pharmaceuticals, diminish health disparities, or focus on the promotion of health still remain in place.

In conclusion, the way in which health care is administered is very much influenced by larger trends in governance. Each public sector has its own distinct characteristics, and health care is quite unique for a number of reasons, including the highly technical nature of medical knowledge, the entrenched power of the medical profession, the size and complexity of the sector, the high 'life or death' stakes involved in much decision making, and so on. New public management has had a clear influence shifting health care from a provider-centred to a more patient-centred focus, although the original market orientation of the approach was never substantial. The use of performance indicators, business plans, benchmarks, and feedback mechanisms – themselves borrowed from the business sector – became the preferred method of establishing more responsiveness in the health care sector.

The attempt to 'empower' patients, and even administrators, was much less successful. The institutionalization of citizen engagement proved difficult to formalize effectively. While it is important for those who design and administer health care systems to have a good sense of what is desired at a local level, as well as of what works and what does not (and why), the mass mobilization of grassroots involvement was too unwieldy and problematic in practice. The election of local representatives had its own difficulties, and did not prove to be significantly better than appointed bodies. Allowing civil servants more latitude for decision making at the regional level was useful in many instances, but was limited by lack of financial control. Pressures on governments to micromanage bureaucratic decisions also impeded the flexibility that regionalization was expected to facilitate, while local interests remained sceptical that regional bodies were as representative of local concerns as the old structure of local hospital boards had been.

The experiment with NPM was both disadvantaged and assisted by the financial difficulties of the 1990s. The attempt to construct a new system based on an engaged public, a fully integrated system, and a more preventive focus was clearly hamstrung by the need for governments to make cutbacks an immediate priority. It also made very clear the need for a more rationalized health care system, and the larger political focus on fiscal restraint facilitated the reduction of many health services and the closure of numerous hospitals and wards. By the time additional cash was pumped back into the system ten years later, advances in information technology allowed provinces to capitalize on their emphasis on greater efficiencies.

The lessons learned from almost two decades of NPM have had a profound impact on the political debate over health care reform in Canada. Where the debate two decades ago was whether to 'make it private' or 'keep it public,' the discussion has shifted to the extent to which internal system reforms (such as integration and the effective utilization of information technology) are sufficient to save the Canadian health care system (Rachlis 2004). The two questions that now dominate management of the health care system are how we can use technology to remove inefficiencies (e.g., waiting-list management systems), and how we can facilitate greater integration between discrete units in the health care system. There is certainly reason to be optimistic; many success stories are emerging across Canada and elsewhere (Baker et al. 2008). What will become more challenging, however, is the nature of account-ability in health care. One reason that free-standing silos remain in health care systems is that they are based on hierarchical, clearly delin-eated patterns of accountability. The push towards greater collabora-tion between units means that responsibility for policies and funds becomes more diffuse and therefore more difficult to identify (Bakvis and Juillet 2004). Further, integration raises questions about how to ensure that bureaucrats not only remain accountable to those at the top, but also responsive to those whom they serve. How can integrated sys-tems stay responsive to those using services without being tempted to 'pass the buck'? Given the popular insistence that health care remains a public good accessible to all, there is also a political expectation that health care systems must remain responsive to all *equally*. Attempts at integration will require a great deal of concentration on developing clear structures of management and accountability between and across units (primary care, acute care, long-term care, mental health care, and so on) and a great deal of thought about how to manage competing pathways of accountability (to managers, to politicians, to taxpayers, and to patients). Integration is a required direction for reform, but it should not be seen as an easy one.

4   Health Care and the Courts

Do Canadians have a *right* to health care? Yes and no. Canadians like to think that the 'right to health care' is one thing that has distinguished them from Americans. But there is no explicit statement in the Charter of Rights and Freedoms that guarantees a 'right' to health care. Europeans, in contrast, arguably do have such a right: Article 35 of the European Union's Charter of Fundamental Rights stipulates that 'everyone has the right of access to preventative health care and rights to benefit from medical treatment under the conditions established by national laws and practices. A high level of human health protection shall be ensured by the definition and implementation of all Union policies and activities.' The situation in Canada is much more complicated. To the extent that universal access to health care is guaranteed at all, it is articulated by a federal statute – the Canada Health Act (CHA) – while health care itself is provided by the provinces, which are not legally bound by the CHA. Simply put, our 'right' to health care in the first instance is not enforced by law, but secured through a process that some would simply call bribery. Nevertheless, courts have become increasingly active in determining health policy in Canada. What impact do the courts have on the nature of health care in Canada?

The Limits of Politics and the Role of the Courts

While the Canada Health Act is a legal statute, it should be viewed more as a political document than as a legal one. To an extent, it is like a gentlemen's agreement that defines the rules of the game played by both levels of government rather than a document by which citizens hold their governments accountable. Thus there is little room for the courts. Traditionally, judges have shown deference to policy makers in the area of health care: unless criminal activities, Charter breaches (such as refusing treatment on the basis of race or gender), a violation of the constitutional division of laws, or breaches of administrative principles are involved, courts have chosen to respect the judgment of legislators. The problem is that the laws governing access to health care generally do not facilitate the input of individuals (as patients or citizens), and the only form of recourse available to Canadians who dispute the way in which the CHA is applied is through the courts.

What are the limitations of the Canada Health Act? As noted in Chapter 1, there is an expectation that the CHA covers all 'medically necessary' health services: in fact, the CHA only covers 'medically necessary' physician and hospital services (including diagnostics ordered by physicians). In practice, the CHA only covers the medically necessary hospital and physician services that the provinces perceive they can afford. The requirement of 'medically necessary' is itself a very flexible stipulation. Although the CHA requires the provinces to provide medically necessary services to all their citizens, it is the provinces themselves who determine what is to count as medically necessary. Likewise, the requirement established by the CHA that all services must be 'comprehensive' is highly circular: it simply means that all insured services must be insured (Flood and Choudhry 2002: 18). The stipulation of 'accessibility,' rather than being too broad, is arguably too narrow: it refers only to the lack of barriers due to income, as opposed to the time one must wait to receive the service. This is one reason there is such fragmentation across Canada regarding the kinds of services provided and the length of time it takes to receive treatment.

Another issue surrounding the CHA is the enforcement process. 'Despite the existence of a dispute resolution mechanism,' writes Boychuk (2008b: 5), 'the interpretation and enforcement of the CHA remains primarily a prerogative of the federal minister.' Political groups supporting public health care in Canada have decried Ottawa's lack of action regarding such perceived violations; but there are a number of reasons why the federal government is very conservative in exercising its right to impose penalties under the CHA. In the first place, Ottawa has attempted to resolve such issues through negotiation with the provinces, leaving financial penalties as a last resort. Second, the funding system of health transfers (conditional grants) is viewed by provinces as a contractual undertaking, and any unilateral reduction of this undertaking as akin to defaulting on established contracts. That cash transfers from Ottawa have decreased to less than 20 per cent of provinces' health care revenue means that the threat of such penalties is not a particularly menacing sanction, at least for the wealthier provinces. Finally, the federal government tends to defer to the provinces' right to determine what their particular needs and capacities are, and to their ability to employ health care funds to these ends (Flood and Choudhry 2002: 20).

In sum, the courts have played but a very small role in interpreting the CHA or in resolving disputes regarding its interpretation. One exception to this is a provision in administrative law that allows for the judicial review of policy decisions. Under this process, individuals can challenge administrative decisions (such as interpretations of what is covered by the CHA) on the grounds of 'unreasonableness.' Nonetheless, in practice, the courts have remained very deferential to the decisions of health policy administrators, and have only used the determination of 'patent unreasonableness' in the most egregious cases. There has only been one successful judicial review claim before the courts with regard to waiting times, and that is *Stein v. Québec/Régie de l'Assurance-maladie* (Flood, Stabile, and Tuohy 2006: 27). A much more radical path available to those who wish to contest the way in which the CHA is interpreted is through a Charter challenge. Despite the length of time it took for Charter cases to gain traction in the field of health care, there is some indication that the nature of Canadian health care could be radically altered by the Supreme Court. This, in turn, has led to much political polarization regarding the role of the courts in health care policy making.

The Canadian Charter of Rights and Freedoms

Since the establishment of the Charter in 1982, there have been very few successful challenges in the area of health care. Between 1985 and 2002, for example, only eleven out of thirty-three cases succeeded (Flood, Stabile, and Tuohy 2006: 28). It was clear, however, that the establishment of constitutionally entrenched rights had nonetheless widened the range of policy issues subject to 'judicial policy-making,' allowing the courts to establish policy in areas that were formerly under the sole jurisdiction of legislative bodies (Manfredi and Maioni 2002: 216).

Health care challenges under the Charter have focused on three specific rights: equality rights (section 15), mobility rights (section 6), and rights to 'life, liberty, and security' (section 7). Cases launched under section 15 have generally involved the attempt to increase the scope of health care coverage for particular conditions. 'With escalating drug costs and increasing reliance on life-saving drugs,' comments Greschner, 'it is surprising that major exclusions from Medicare, such as most prescription drugs and home care, have not been subject to more Charter challenges' (2002: 9). But given the lack of success of most section 15 challenges, it is perhaps understandable why there is little momentum in this area. The Supreme Court has ruled that the Charter does not support the expansion of health care coverage in the area of prescription drugs (*Brown,* in a 1990 decision), fertility treatments (*Cameron,* in 1999), and intensive treatment sessions for autistic children (*Auton,* in 2004). The only significant health care case to be successfully argued under section 15 was *Eldridge,* in 1997, which required that health authorities provide sign-language interpretation for the deaf in hospitals. *Eldridge,* however, was quite distinct from the other attempts given that 'the plaintiffs were not asking for a specific medical treatment that the government had decided not to fund,' but rather that 'they wanted equal access to all the services, and no more than those services that were available to the hearing public' (Greschner 2002: 7). Because deafness constituted a disability under section 15, the claimants were successful.

In contrast to section 15, which has been generally employed by health care *consumers,* section 6 challenges have been utilized by health care *providers* in response to physician-supply mechanisms used by provinces to entice physicians to underserviced regions. Under such a policy, only new physicians working in an underserviced area would receive full compensation for services provided. Doctors employed in 'adequately serviced' areas could claim 75 per cent of the full compensation rate, and those in 'overserviced' regions would receive only half of the full amount. In a case launched before the British Columbia Supreme Court (*Waldman,* in 1997), physicians argued that this policy violated their right to practise freely where they chose. What is striking in this is that the court chose to disregard specific empirical findings (that the policy was necessary in order to provide accessible health care to citizens in all regions of the province) and articulated their decision 'on the basis of reason and logic' (Manfredi and Maioni 2002: 225, 228). This approach was troublesome for many commentators. 'Judges,' writes Greschner, 'are not well equipped to deal with the enormous ramifications of changing elements of the health care system ... assessing health care policy is a quintessentially interdisciplinary undertaking.

Yet judges will be wading into these thorny areas without expertise'
(2002: 12). Echoing this sentiment, Manfredi and Maioni point out that
judges rarely concern themselves with the wider policy context within
which specific measures are enacted. The articulation of human rights,
under this account, is so important that it cannot be qualified or cor-
rupted by considerations of financial costs or logistical consequences.
'Given this predisposition of judicial policy-making,' they conclude, 'it
is hardly surprising that the Supreme Court of Canada has explicitly
excluded administrative efficiency and cost from the list of "pressing
and substantial" objectives that might justify limiting a protected right'
(2002: 218).

These perceptive observations proved to be extremely well grounded.
When the Supreme Court of Canada released its decision on the *Chaoulli*
case in June 2005, precisely the same criticisms were levied against the
court; but the political consequences of this decision were even more
profound. *Chaoulli* was launched in 1997 as a section 7 challenge against
Article 15 of the Quebec Health Insurance Act, which forbids private
health insurance of services that are covered by public insurance, and
Article 11 of the Quebec Hospital Insurance Act, which prevents opted-
out physicians from participating in publicly funded hospitals. Jacques
Chaoulli, a physician who had opted out of Quebec's public health
insurance plan, launched the challenge with George Zeliotis, who
had had to wait eleven months for his left hip replacement, and seven
months for his right. Together, they argued that these excessive waiting
times were a result of Quebec's ban on private health insurance and that
such a ban therefore amounted to a violation of 'life, liberty, and security' under section 7 of the Canadian Charter of Rights and Freedoms,
as well as section 1 of the Quebec Charter of Rights and Freedoms.

Both the trial judge in 2000 and the appeal court judge in 2002 agreed
with expert witnesses who argued that permitting private insurance
threatened to undermine the integrity of the public health care system. Zeliotis was quite clear that he was 'arguing for the right for more
affluent people to have access to parallel health services' (*Chaoulli* 2000,
cited in Flood, Roach, and Sossin 2005: 532.) The trial court judge found
that there was no infringement on the Charter's section 7 provisions
on life, liberty, and security. Even if there had been, there was a further
question of whether such an infringement was, in fact, justifiable. In
this case, stated the trial judge, 'an analysis under s. 1 [of the Canadian
Charter] would show that the impugned provisions in the case at bar
are a reasonable limit in a free and democratic society.' Moreover, she

added, 'it is entirely understandable that a government with the best interests of the public at heart should adopt a solution that will benefit the largest number of individuals' (quoted in ibid., 557). On appeal, the trial judge's decision was unanimously upheld. One of the appellate judges even added the observation that the rights for which Chaoulli and Zeliotis desired protection were, in fact, not fundamental rights to life, liberty, and security, but merely 'economic' rights. At neither level was legislation discussed with reference to the Quebec Charter of Rights and Freedoms.

The case was appealed to the Supreme Court. By this time, the political nature of the case had become quite apparent. Numerous parties asked for intervenor status, including five other provinces, activist groups supporting public health care, and commercial health clinics supporting private health care. Even the senators involved in the Kirby health reform document were allowed to appear as intervenors. As two of the Supreme Court seats were waiting to be filled, the case was heard by only seven judges, rather than nine. Ultimately, the judgment overturned the two lower court decisions; but the judgment was contradictory, fragmented, and confusing. Three justices (Binnie, LeBel, and Fish) agreed with the lower courts that Quebec's legislation did not violate the Canadian Charter of Rights and Freedoms (nor, they added, did it violate the Quebec Charter of Rights and Freedoms). Three justices (McLachlin, Major, and Bastarache) found that the legislation violated both the Canadian and Quebec Charters, and that this violation could not be deemed to be justifiable under section 1 of the Canadian Charter. A final justice (Deschamps) agreed that the legislation did violate the Quebec Charter, but refused to rule on the status of the legislation with reference to the Canadian Charter.

There were at least three separate kinds of criticisms made of the decision. The first addressed the lack of clarity: despite the fact that the lower courts' rulings had been overturned, there was some perplexity in attempting to determine what the decision actually meant for the purposes of policy making. This was partly because of the conditional nature of the decision of the majority: 'where the public system fails to deliver adequate care, the denial of private insurance subjects people to long waiting lists and negatively affects their health and security of the person' (*Chaoulli* 2005, para. 152; cited in Flood, Roach, and Sossin 2005: 596). It was not clear whether private insurance could therefore be denied where the public system was deemed to deliver adequate care; nor was it clear exactly what constituted 'adequate care' in any quantifiable form. Moreover, as Peter Russell points out, provincial legislators could simply re-enact the legislation banning private insurance 'with a statement that it stands notwithstanding s. 1 of the Quebec Charter' (2005: 9). Had four, rather than just three, of the justices held that the legislation unreasonably violated the Canadian Charter as well as the Quebec Charter, adds Russell, the Quebec National Assembly could simply have enacted the notwithstanding clause of the Canadian Charter of Rights and Freedoms.

The second set of criticisms is based on the argument that the court was engaging in judicial activism, imposing its belief that negative individual rights were simply more important than positive collective rights. As the trial judge and appeal court judges had recognized, the question of whether a violation of rights occurred was separate from the question of whether such violations may be considered *justifiable*. In the case of health care, if a private parallel system provided superior care for the wealthy while undermining the quality of public care, then the rights of a wealthy minority would be protected at the expense of a larger number of individuals who would be unable to access private services. In this way, individual rights would be protected at the expense of the collective right of a society to provide universal access to good quality care. Moreover, there is the issue of the kind of right being protected: is the right to purchase private care really a fundamental right to life and security? (And, if so, then is it significant if all individuals cannot enjoy this right equally?) Or is it, as appellate justice Delisle suggests, merely an economic right? Choudhry (2005: 87–8) argues that the majority of justices on the Supreme Court have interpreted the right to 'life, liberty and security of the person' to encompass 'liberty of contract,' thereby turning an economic right into a 'fundamental' one. In this way, critics maintain, the court has exhibited a form of judicial activism biased in favour of the protection of market principles over those of redistribution (see, e.g., Petter 2005; Sossin 2005; and Roach 2005).

One of the most remarkable characteristics of the *Chaoulli* case was the way in which evidence was selected and interpreted by the Supreme Court. This led to a sustained barrage of criticism by health policy analysts. One commented that 'one of the most unsettling aspects of the *Chaoulli* decision was the misuse, and ignorance, of the data' (Barer 2005: 217), while another called the court 'jurisdictionally arrogant, substantively ignorant, and politically irresponsible' (Evans 2005a: 20). What provoked this response?

At issue was the kind of evidence the court chose to consider, and the way in which an 'expert witness' was understood. On the one hand, the appellants (Chaoulli aand Zeliotis) depended on practising physicians, who gave anecdotal evidence of the effects of long waiting times on their own patients. On the other hand, social scientists presented comparative analyses explaining why private health insurance did not decrease waiting times and had, in some cases, even increased them (Wright 2005: 221–2). The majority decision, however, called these studies 'common sense' assumptions based on 'apparent logic' (*Chaoulli*, 2005, para. 136). Because these were not randomized, controlled studies (the gold standard in scientific research), the social scientific evidence was, in the end, given less weight than the daily experiences of two physicians, neither of whom claimed expertise in waiting-time management. To the disbelief of academics who had presented comparative research on the relationship between waiting times and private health insurance, the majority decision (written by Justices McLachlin and Major) stated that the government of Quebec did not 'present economic studies or rely on the experience of other countries' (*Chaoulli* 2005, para. 136). The Supreme Court decision also notes that no study was presented in the Quebec Superior Court showing private health insurance to be problematic (ibid., para. 64). This, writes one health policy analyst, is 'utterly inexplicable' and 'the most bizarre comment in the entire judgment,' given that the 'published results of specific studies, statements from respected leaders in medicine, and research in prestigious medical journals' were what ultimately had convinced the Superior Court to rule against Chaoulli and Zeliotis (Wright 2005: 223). It should be mentioned that the minority decision of the Supreme Court (comprised of Justices Binnie, LeBel, and Fish) did find this evidence persuasive. So what accounts for the decision of the majority, which overturned two lower court judgments?

It may be, as McIntosh speculates, that 'because the anecdotes related to the Court in this particular case fit so well with a long-standing public view that wait times continue to grow across the country, the Court felt no need to probe these claims in any depth' (2006: 3). But Roach (2005) offers another explanation: because Chaoulli and Zeliotis were granted 'public interest' standing in the Supreme Court, the case was discussed at a much more abstract policy level (what is best for Canadians?) rather than according to the simple facts of the case, as it was in the two lower courts. This may have influenced the case considerably, as the delay Mr Zeliotis experienced was to some degree self-inflicted given his indecision, his other underlying medical conditions, and his history of 'unfounded medical complaints' (also cited by the dissenting minority in *Chaoulli* 2005, para. 211). Because of the 'public interest' standing granted to so many parties on both sides of the case once it reached the Supreme Court, the kind of arguments considered by the judges shifted slightly. What became relevant were not the actual facts of what happened, but the counterfactual nature of the arguments presented ('if we don't do *this*, then *that* will happen'). Thus, as Stewart (2005: 209, citing Hagan 1987: 215) explains, 'the crucial factual question was the effect of the availability and quality of health care under the public system. This is not a question about what happened in the past, but a question about what is likely to happen in the future if the statute in question is not invalidated. That is, the facts at issue in *Chaoulli* are not "adjudicative facts" but "legislative facts." They "involve the use of social and economic data to establish a more general context for policy-making."' The majority was unwilling, however, to examine this social scientific data closely, referring to them only as 'speculative' and 'common sense logic.' Consequently, the majority made a number of distinct errors in their interpretation of the public policy evidence (Flood, Stabile, and Kontic, 2005).

The first error is the assumption that a public insurance monopoly necessarily leads to lengthy waiting times. This conclusion was made despite clear evidence that countries with parallel public and private insurance systems (such as the United Kingdom, Australia, and New Zealand) also suffer from significant waiting times. The countries citied by the majority (such as Germany and the Netherlands) which did not have lengthy waiting times did not employ the public-private insurance mix that the appellants wanted, but rather were characterized by a mixed social insurance system (see Chapter 1). Thus the majority did not comprehend the different forms of health insurance that exist internationally, and drew the wrong conclusions from this comparative evidence (Flood and Lewis, 2005).

The second error is the assumption that the existence of a parallel private insurance system will alleviate the pressure on the public system. As noted in Chapter 1, there is evidence to show that the policy dynamics in such a public-private system can lead to the opposite effect, for a number of different reasons: qualified medical staff are drawn out of the public system; private systems are less cost-effective; and those working in private systems have an incentive to make the public system less efficient (Flood, Stabile, and Touhy 2004; Flood and Sullivan 2005).

The third error is the assumption that private health insurance would benefit 'many ordinary' Quebecers. However, private for-profit health insurance constitutes but very small proportion of health care coverage in most countries. Rather than 'many' Quebecers benefiting from private health insurance, there is solid comparative evidence to hold that only a *few* would benefit. Moreover, given the premiums involved in a parallel private system, the few that actually would benefit would not be 'ordinary,' but would be the wealthy individuals who could afford to carry these premiums (Evans 2005a). It is also worth noting that the purchase of private health *insurance* (as opposed to services) is generally only affordable to healthy individuals: thus Mr Zeliotis, with all his medical conditions, probably would himself not have qualified for any private health insurance. It is difficult, as McIntosh (2006) points out, to obtain private health insurance once you need it – just as it is difficult to purchase home insurance when your house is on fire. Finally, the right to purchase private health insurance is meaningless where a market in private health care *services* does not exist (especially relevant where provincial laws disallow physicians from practising in both public and private sectors).

Another explanation for the decision of the majority in *Chaoulli* is that the majority was simply playing to its own bias: the protection of the rights of the *individual*. This is, after all, generally the intent of most charters of rights in the first place. But there are exceptions: the collective rights of linguistic, religious, and cultural groups are recognized by the Canadian Charter. There is certainly room to argue that the overall well-being of Quebecers, as a society, overrides the economic rights of individuals to contract for future services. This was precisely the reasoning the trial court judge used in her decision: 'The only way of ensuring that all health resources will benefit all Quebeckers without discrimination is to prevent a parallel care system from being established. That is precisely what the disputed provisions in the case at bar do' (*Chaoulli* 2000). Given that the laws in question were upheld in two lower courts, one might assume that the burden of proof would have to be on the appellants to show that the health care system was not, in fact, 'benefit[ing] all Quebeckers.' The appellants would presumably have had to show that there was 'no reasoned basis' for the legislation. However, given the amount of evidence showing (at the very least) that there *was* good reason to suppose that preventing private insurance was benefiting Quebecers as a society, the case could hardly be made that there was *no* reasoned basis for the provision (Stewart

2005). Thus, while the burden of proof rested with the appellants to show that Quebec's legislation was not in accordance with the principles of fundamental justice, the majority shifted the burden of proof to the government of Quebec, requiring it to show that anyone in Quebec would *not* be denied access to medically required treatment because of its ban on private health insurance. This, writes Roach (2005: 187), 'meant that Quebec had to justify every possible waiting list and every possible counterfactual.' And because the majority held that health care is a private commodity rather than a public good, they refused to allow economic access to health care to fall under the rubric of 'principles of fundamental justice.'

The majority was certainly correct in a sense: there is no explicit right to public health care in the Charter of Rights and Freedoms. But the right to buy private health insurance is not explicitly mentioned either. These are matters of interpretation: and critics of the decision hold that where public values are precisely what are at issue, the courts should defer to the legislative bodies that represent the people. That the government of Quebec, as well as Quebec judges at two levels, held that health care in Quebec ought to be considered a public right was a clear expression of Quebec's social values that should have been respected by the Supreme Court. There was much concern in Quebec that a federal institution was attempting to impose market values on Quebec's more solidaristic society and that this attempt went well beyond its purview.

The Fallout from *Chaoulli*

Will the *Chaoulli* decision have a lasting and decisive impact on the Canadian health care system? Newspaper headlines following the decision suggested that the ruling could dramatically change the nature of health care in Canada. Commentators suggested that provinces would begin to change their laws immediately to comply with the ruling. The *Globe and Mail*, discussing the twenty-fifth anniversary of the Charter of Rights and Freedoms, listed *Chaoulli* as 'one of the most important and influential Charter cases since 1982' (10 April 2007: A7). But what is so remarkable about *Chaoulli*, in retrospect, is that so little radical action ensued. Why?

The first reason is the nature of the decision itself. The ruling did not strike down medicare. In fact, the Supreme Court decision did not make a conclusive determination on the Canadian Charter of Rights and Freedoms at all. The decision addressed only the status of Quebec's health legislation under the Quebec Charter of Rights: the Court was evenly split 3–3 on whether the laws violated the Canadian Charter. The case revolved around the legality of a public insurance monopoly, not the legality of public insurance per se. Moreover, the decision was couched in conditional terms, allowing Quebec (and other provinces) to focus upon one aspect of the ruling (*if* you don't do something about waiting times) rather than the other (*then* you will have to allow private insurance).

Actually, provinces had already been working on managing waiting lists. By December 2005 all provinces and territories had announced benchmarks for treatment times for a number of common procedures. This would have happened independently of the *Chaoulli* decision, as the establishment of benchmarks was a condition of receiving supplementary federal funding under the 2004 health care agreement. Many waiting-time management programs had by 2005 already been developed. The annual Taming of the Queue conferences, which permitted the dissemination and discussion of best practices from numerous regions in Canada as well as abroad, had already been established. The Wait Time Alliance, a group of medical practitioners, had also presented a discussion of benchmarks necessary to address waiting times. Within four years, all provinces had some form of waiting-list management strategy. Early waiting-time management strategies include the Western Canada Wait List Project and the Ontario Cardiac Care Network; the most recent development has been the Ontario Wait Time Information system (WTIS). By 2009, a report issued by the Canadian Institute for Health Information (CIHI) showed definite progress on waiting times, although the results differed province to province. These accomplishments most likely had less to do with the *Chaoulli* decision and more to do with a combination of public pressure and advances in information technology (including the capacity to gather data efficiently); but the ruling certainly ensured that political attention on the issue did not slip.

In response to the Supreme Court ruling, the government of Quebec asked for, and received, a twelve-month stay of judgment. It then released a health care consultation paper which reasserted a strong commitment to public health care and guaranteed waiting times for certain aspects of cardiac and cancer care, as well as hip, knee, and cataract surgery. It proposed the development of 'affiliated specialized clinics,' or private facilities that provided contractual services to the public system, and it removed the ban on private insurance for hip, knee, and cataract surgeries. Quebec's political strategy was quite savvy. It permitted private insurance, but only in areas where (given waiting-list management) there would be little incentive for patients to purchase it. The province also placed clear limits on fees paid to physicians opting out of the public system, and prevented physicians from practising in both public and private systems, thereby removing incentives for physicians to provide private services (as opposed to removing incentives for patients to buy them). None of these measures was particularly radical; all were practised in various provinces in Canada. When Claude Castonguay released a report in 2008 calling for more private health care, the provincial government repudiated the report immediately (Maioni 2008). Certainly Jacques Chaoulli himself has expressed 'surprise and disappointment' that the ruling, in retrospect, was not more transformative (Kondro 2006a).

Does this mean that the most radical effects of *Chaoulli* have effectively been prevented? Only for now: the courts may still have the potential to change the landscape of Canadian health care. At the very least, it takes time for the effects of a judgment to ripple throughout the legal system. By 2007 *Chaoulli* had been cited in thirty-one decisions, in almost every province (Solomon 2007). But the most dramatic challenge to be launched in the shadow of the *Chaoulli* decision was a 2009 writ filed in the British Columbia Supreme Court by a number of private clinics, most of whom, in fact, had been given intervenor status in the 2005 *Chaoulli* case. In the British Columbia Supreme Court case, the plaintiffs argue that the 2005 judgment should be applicable in British Columbia, and that the province's Medicare Protection Act violates the section 7 rights of those who wish to purchase private health insurance where health care is not provided in a timely manner. Similar cases exist in Alberta and Ontario. Whether these challenges will be successful likely depends on variables such as waiting times in these provinces and, perhaps ultimately, the constitution of the Supreme Court of Canada (of the current nine judges, only five participated in the *Chaoulli* ruling: two supported the majority decision, and three opposed).

Another Kind of Legal Challenge

It is important to remember that Canada is not only subject to its own laws, but to those it negotiates with other states. Two international legal agreements have the potential to affect the nature of health care in Canada. Canada is a member of the World Trade Organization's General

Agreement on Trade in Services (GATS) agreement, which facilitates the liberalization of trade in services. While there is some 'exceptional' recognition for the protection of national health care, there remains much debate regarding the level of protection such exceptional status affords (Sanger 2001; Ouellet 2002; Crawford 2005). The second document is the 1994 North American Free Trade Agreement (NAFTA), signed by Canada, the United States, and Mexico. This agreement attempts to promote trade liberalization through the reduction of economic barriers between the signatories. NAFTA's effects on health care in Canada are determined by chapters 11 and 12 of the treaty, dealing with investment and services. Specifically, the 'national treatment' and 'expropriation' provisions pose special challenges: the national treatment stipulation, for example, means that American and Mexican firms must be treated on par with Canadian ones. The expropriation clause means that once foreign firms are active within Canada, they cannot be removed without penalty. Two annexes to NAFTA were established with the intention of protecting the public nature of Canadian health care; but, again, debate exists over the effectiveness of these annexes. The first merely protects NAFTA-inconsistent practices in health care put in place before 1994; the second protects future health care services from NAFTA regulation only if they are 'maintained for a public purpose' (Epps and Schneiderman 2005). What this means is that services provided by the public sector for general social utilization are exempt from regulations governing fair trade. Thus government monopolies in, say, sewage treatment or electrical power are not normally subject to anti-competition laws.

But problems arise over health care, as some countries (such as the United States) consider it to be a private commodity to be bought and sold in the marketplace; while other countries (such as Canada) see it as a public service. What NAFTA specifies is that as long as Canadian health care stays firmly in the public sector, the rules of the marketplace will have no bearing on it. Once Canada begins to permit health care services (such as insurance) to be offered in the private sector, anti-competition rules can be applied. These rules limit the participation of actors (especially governments) who are seen to have an 'unfair advantage' over the private firms. At issue, then, is whether allowing greater privatization of health insurance in Canada will trigger an action by another country which will lead to a trade arbitration, which might then decide that the public insurance provider had an 'unfair advantage' in relation to private companies. This would mean restrictions on public health insurance providers which would, by definition, limit the effectiveness of public health insurance. 'It is thus quite possible,' writes one international law specialist, 'that some services that Canada sees as covered by a reservation or exception will not be considered in the same way by our trading partners, or by a panel arbitrating a dispute between Canada and another Party seeking access to our health care market for one of its nationals' (Ouellet 2002: 17).

This scenario is not simply speculation. It is the dynamic that has strongly shaped European health care since the late 1990s. The treaties signed by European Union member states since the early 1990s (Maastricht, 1993; Amsterdam, 1997; Nice, 2001; and Lisbon, 2009) have, like NAFTA, attempted to provide a more integrated market. Despite the implicit political understanding between member states that their health care systems were not to be subject to regulation by internal market laws, the European Court of Justice has, since 1998, systematically been ruling that health services should be considered 'economic transactions' rather than 'domestic social policy.' Thus the courts have upheld, often over the protests of national governments, the free movement of patients and health professionals between European Union countries. But they have also increasingly found that the utilization of market mechanisms and private sector components in the public health care system is to be subject to anti-competition law. There is thus widespread concern that 'European competition law will apply to any entity that participates in markets even if the purpose is a social one and even if the market is highly regulated' (Prosser 2009: 139). The best way to prevent national health care systems from being restricted in their functions by anti-competition laws, argue European health policy analysts, is to prevent the infiltration of private insurance and services in the first place. 'If policy-makers are genuinely concerned about access to health care,' warn Thomson and Mossialos, 'one strategy might be to make sure that statutory health coverage is universal, falls squarely within the boundaries of "social security" and covers a wide range of services, thus eliminating or lowering the need for private health insurance' (2008: 7).

What is most interesting about the experiences of both Canada and the European Union is that the courts, which had historically acted with deference to the policy makers in the area of health care, are increasingly playing an active role in determining the parameters of health policy (Fierlbeck 2011). Moreover, judicial involvement in health policy making has had a liberalizing effect on health care, notwithstanding the existence of charters of rights which specify protections for life, liberty, and the security of the person (in Canada) and a 'high level of health protection' (in the European Union). The idea that judicial power is expanding into sectors previously determined by legislative processes has been observed by political scientists for some time (e.g., Tate and Vallinder 1995), but it is notable that judicial activism has now begun to manifest itself in health policy. The effect of this is still too early to determine, but it will be worth the scrutiny.

5 Public Health and Population Health

'Public health' and 'public health care' are not synonymous. 'Public health care' generally refers to the way in which a health care system is funded, and it signifies that the provision of certain important health services are free or subsidized at the point of delivery for the general population (usually through a form of public insurance). 'Public health' is, at its simplest, just that: the health of the public. But it is rarely that simple. Formally, public health is an approach that focuses on 'population health' and attempts to address its determinants (Deber, McDougall, and Wilson, 2007). 'Population health,' according to Health Canada, is 'the health of a population as measured by health status indicators and as influenced by social, economic and physical environments, personal health practices, individual capacity and coping skills, human biology, early childhood development, and health services.' As an approach, population health focuses on the interrelated conditions and factors that influence the health of populations over the life course, identifies systematic variations in their patterns of occurrence, and applies the resulting knowledge to develop and implement policies and actions to improve the health and well-being of those populations' (Health Canada 2001). Thus a *population health approach* is 'a unifying force for the entire spectrum of health system interventions – from prevention and promotion to health protection, diagnosis, treatment and care – and integrates and balances action between them' (ibid.). In general, public health is divided between two primary functions: health protection and health promotion. On the surface, public health is a very straightforward branch of modern health care based on common sense and good policy. Dig any deeper, however, and the highly politicized nature of public health quickly becomes apparent.

The Structure of Public Health in Canada

That public health and political structures are indelibly linked was apparent as early as the fourteenth century, when a wave of bubonic plague swept the Italian city states. As these cities were the European gateways for traders from China and the Middle East, they were the first to succumb to the effects of the Black Death. Cities like Florence and Genoa, in which power was effectively held by merchant guilds, were hit the worst as the guilds refused to close the ports on which they depended so heavily. But cities like Milan and Mantua were governed by autocrats who were able to construct a cordon sanitaire around their cities and to enforce it with absolute sanctions; and in these cities the plague was much more effectively contained (Hawthorne 1991).

The political structure of public health has almost always been reactive. In Great Britain, the first milestone in public health infrastructure was the 1848 Public Health Act, designed to establish better public sanitation in an increasingly urbanized, industrial society. In Canada, formal institutions governing health at the national level began with the Spanish flu and, most recently, were reformed in the wake of the epidemic of severe acute respiratory syndrome (SARS) in 2003. The pre-eminent political institution underlying attempts at public health reform in all modern liberal states is the ideology of liberalism itself. Because liberalism stresses individual autonomy as a keystone of political organization, there is always a tension between those who view health as primarily an individual responsibility and those who see it as a consequence of social organization. Is nutrition, for example, a matter of getting people to take responsibility for eating more healthy food, or is it also firmly linked to patterns of work, the cost and availability of fresh food, the strength of the agrifood industry, urban design, socioeconomic disparity, and so on? The second political institution informing the character of public health in Canada is federalism. When the division of powers in Canada was established in 1867, health care was limited and basic, and it did not require much public infrastructure. What hospitals did exist were generally run by charitable (usually religious) institutions, which themselves fell under the jurisdiction of the provinces. Thus provinces were given the legal responsibility for the provision and management of health care within their respective jurisdictions (see Chapter 2).

There are a number of reasons that public health has become so politicized; and while they are not indigenous to any one country, each state has had a distinctive way of responding to them. The first is simply *the prevalence of modern pathogens*, including both the increase of new strains and the speed at which pathogens spread. While the occurrence of water-borne diseases such as cholera, dysentery, and typhoid fever was effectively controlled by the end of the nineteenth century through better sanitation and water management, air-borne illnesses such as diphtheria, tuberculosis, scarlet fever, measles, and whooping cough remained recurrent threats into the twentieth century. Modern disease, however, is built on a completely new trajectory. The unprecedented level of human travel, for example, has exposed us to the unpredictable risk of virulent pathogens. This realization became especially pronounced in Canada, which saw forty-four deaths due to a mystery virus that was transferred from rural Guangdong Province in China to Toronto in a matter of weeks. In February 2003 a doctor from the Chinese mainland flew to Hong Kong, where he infected a number of people including an elderly woman from Canada, whose son subsequently was treated at a Toronto hospital, leading to the rapid spread of SARS to staff and to those in the emergency department. Given the relationship between human migration and the spread of infection, Canadian epidemiologists have even developed a model predicting patterns of viral infection based on air travel patterns.

The spread of modern pathogens is also very much influenced by the way that the food supply is designed and managed. The prevalence of bovine spongiform encephalopathy (BSE) in British beef in the 1980s, for example, was due to the introduction of rendered meat byproducts into cattle meal; and the export of British beef and live cattle led to contamination of the food supply in numerous other countries, including Canada. The dependence on imported vegetables has led to numerous outbreaks of *Escherichia coli* and salmonella throughout North America; while the taste for highly processed foods has increased the risk of listeriosis, spread through contaminated meat-processing equipment. Pathogens are also spread through the importation of non-food products. West Nile disease, which was found only in Africa, Asia, and southern Europe prior to 1999, was likely spread through the export of materials such as scrap tires (the mosquitos that carry the disease tend to breed in water pools, e.g., those left inside used tires). Mosquito colonies in Canada were first found to have the West Nile virus in 2001; in 2007 alone – only half a dozen years later – over 2,000 cases of human infection in Canada were reported.

A second factor in the politicization of public health is the *complexity of the systems* needed to monitor and address the spread of modern pathogens. Fragmented regional institutions simply cannot effectively address the monitoring and surveillance of modern pathogens, let alone organize an effective response against them. Many of the surveillance systems in place, like the Global Influenza Surveillance Network established by the WHO, are part of an interconnected international reticulation. The WHO also requires governments to meet certain requirements as part of its International Health Regulations system. The response to mass infection must be carefully coordinated, as a single weak link can compromise the coordinated efforts of other jurisdictions. Thus all governments have, at a national level, implemented strategies for dealing not only with infectious diseases, but also chemical, biological, and radiological disasters. At the same time, individuals expect their governments to manage disease effectively, and administrations are judged critically by how well they respond to such incidents. The political dynamics underlying public oversight of disease control are especially unstable because governments are generally loath to expend considerable money on things that may, in fact, not occur. While public officials know that they will be held responsible for outbreaks that do occur, they will generally not be rewarded for preventing ones that did not.

Another issue politicizing the public health system is the *extensiveness of the scope of issues* that public health must address. This is especially true for the health promotion goals of public health systems. To the extent that public officials recognize that the 'social determinants of health' (income and social status, social support networks, education, employment, social and physical environments, personal health practices and coping skills, healthy child development, gender, culture, and access to health services, in addition to biological and genetic endowment) are relevant in establishing good health, there is little that does not fall under the rubric of 'health care.' This means active intervention by government departments overseeing employment, housing, social services, justice, education, and environment, among others. Some jurisdictions, such as the European Union, have actually attempted to implement a system in which all departments recognize the health consequences of their own activities. This is done through the establishment of 'health impact assessments' of all significant new policies, although this is a relatively new policy, and evaluations of its success have yet to be undertaken (it is notable that health impact assessments are also undertaken in the province of Quebec). But the involvement of numerous governmental and non-governmental organizations leads to disputes over responsibility: who is accountable for which outcomes? Whose budgets get spent? And who takes the blame for negative outcomes?

Issues of accountability in public health are not restricted to governmental jurisdictions but, as noted above, are also influenced by *ideological perspectives*. While there is less dispute over the necessity of a public role for an emergency response and risk prevention organization, the belief that governments should be held responsible for all manner of social indicators is a much more controversial position. The final source of political friction is the set of *institutional structures* on which public health must be administered. In Canada, of course, the most important of these is the system of federalism, which clearly gives the jurisdiction over public health to the provinces. Thus coordination between units must be negotiated rather than imposed, and disputes must be resolved in an ad hoc manner. To this must be added the need for interdepartmental collaboration, both across federal and provincial departments. Schematically, the organization of public health is remarkably complex (see Figure 5.1).

Prior to 2005, the public health system in Canada was very decentralized, with some formal coordination occurring through the Council of Chief Medical Officers of Health (comprising the provinces' top medical officials). This changed radically in 2003, with the sudden appearance of the SARS virus. But SARS was the culmination of a decade of high-profile outbreaks, including BSE in cattle, the Krever Inquiry's report on a tainted blood supply, the contamination of drinking water by *Escherichia coli* in Walkerton (Ontario) and by *Cryptosporidium* in North Battleford (Saskatchewan), West Nile virus, avian influenza, and H1N1 influenza. The perception of the Canadian public that governments were increasingly unable to manage such outbreaks was further punctuated by the publication of two reports by the auditor general that were critical of Canada's public health system. Most countries by this time were already reflecting on the effectiveness of their own public health systems. The United States, experiencing not only the terrorist attack of September 2001 but also the release of anthrax spores through the U.S. postal system and inept responses to major hurricanes, had already begun to examine the capacity of its own public health infrastructure.

For Canada the turning point was the report of the National Advisory Committee on SARS and Public Health (the Naylor Report) in 2003. This report highlighted the disadvantages of such a fragmented system, including problems in determining accountability, a lack of effective cross-jurisdictional communication, inadequate resources (especially factoring in the need for 'surge capacity' in times of crisis), and disparities in capacity within and between jurisdictions. The new public health system in Canada came into effect in April 2006 with the passage of Bill C-5. This legislation established the federal Public Health Agency of Canada (PHAC) as well as a national chief public health officer. This new body was to be a discrete agency separate from other branches of Health Canada, but still under the direct authority of the minister of health. The new agency was designed on the principle of *collaborative federalism*, which is characterized by the assumption of equality between federal and provincial governments (underscored by the co-chairing of major committees), the stipulation of the need for cooperation to minimize duplication and overlap, the intention to share 'best practices,' the negotiation of bilateral agreements based on framework agreements, the desire for greater accountability, and stakeholder participation (Cameron and Simeon 2002: 64).

The main locus for federal-provincial coordination in public health is now the Pan-Canadian Public Health Network, established concurrently with PHAC. The Pan-Canadian Public Health Network is governed by a council comprised of representatives (generally either assistant deputy ministers or medical health officers) from each province and territory, and is co-chaired by provincial and federal representatives (the federal official being the chief public health officer). The council reports to the federal, provincial, and territorial deputy ministers of health (who are, in turn, responsible to the Council of Ministers). The Pan-Canadian Public Health Network provides a body of expertise to the council in a number of ways: there is, in the first place, a set of six 'expert groups' specializing in communicable disease control, emergency preparedness and response, public health laboratories, surveillance and information, chronic disease and injury prevention, and health promotion. These expert groups are, in turn, supported by twenty-three standing and five temporary issue groups. The Council of Chief Medical Officers of Health still exists, and serves as a forum for advice for the Pan-Canadian Public Health Network (see Figure 5.1).

In addition to formal federal-provincial-territorial relations, there is a strong regional component to public health. The Public Health Agency of Canada itself maintains five regional centres which have informal connections with local academics, policy makers, stakeholders, and provincial governments. There are also six National Collaborating Centres that are regionally based. These were established, while the national public health system was being reformed, as a means of collecting information and

Figure 5.1. Horizontal and vertical links with the Public Health Agency of Canada (PHAC)

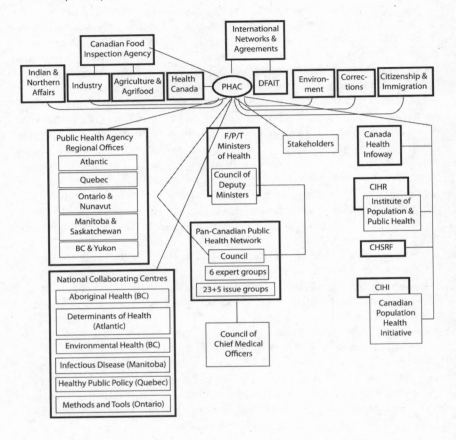

promoting evidence-based public health practice and policy development. They address six specific public health priorities set by the government, and they are funded by the federal government, but they formally remain at arm's-length from government. PHAC also maintains connections with Canada's data- and research-gathering institutions (CIHI, CIHR, CHSPF, and Canada Health Infoway), as well as with numerous stakeholder groups. PHAC must also maintain close ties with international groups such as the World Health Organization (e.g., as a member of surveillance networks and as a signatory of the International Health Regulations).

How does the Public Health Agency of Canada coordinate disease control during an epidemic? There are essentially two interrelated pathways. When an individual is diagnosed with a suspected infectious disease, the physician generally informs the regional health authority (RHA) or public health unit, which reports to the provincial Department of Health, which informs the Public Health Agency of Canada. At the same time, the physician sends a sample to a qualified testing laboratory, which is obliged to contact the RHA, which in turn, reports to the province and thence to PHAC (see Figure 5.2).

The Politics of Disease Prevention

The SARS outbreak of 2003 illustrated quite vividly the flaws in Canada's public health system. As a consequence of SARS, as well as other public health issues, the Public Health Agency of Canada was established in 2005 as a means of making the public health system more effective. Nevertheless, by 2008, two independent reports criticized the public health system for not making 'satisfactory progress' on strategic direction, data quality, results measurement, and information sharing (Auditor General Canada 2008; Canada Standing Committee on Health 2008). The public health community has become quite impatient with the political obstacles impeding better public health integration: public health advocates argue that the attempt to achieve federal-provincial cooperation through negotiation is simply ineffective, that 'Ottawa must now legislate to compel [the provinces] to share epidemiological information in times of emergency' (Attaran 2008: 9) and that 'Ottawa should use its conditional spending power' to improve innovation, cooperation, and reform in public health (Lewis 2002: 1421; see also Wilson, von Tigerstrom, and McDougall, 2008). An editorial in the *Canadian Medical Association Journal* the same year snapped that 'parliament's deference to the provinces [on disease surveillance] has reached a ridiculous, potentially tragic level. In a deadly epidemic, Ottawa's laws to protect Canadian poultry are stronger than its law to protect Canadian people' (1 July 2008). This observation proved percipient given the 2009 listeriosis outbreak, which killed twenty-two people. The report into the management of the outbreak underscored the absence of effective coordination, noting that 'the lack of a clear understanding about which organization or level of government was responsible for doing what – including which organization should lead the response to

Figure 5.2. How surveillance information gets to the Public Health Agency of Canada (PHAC)

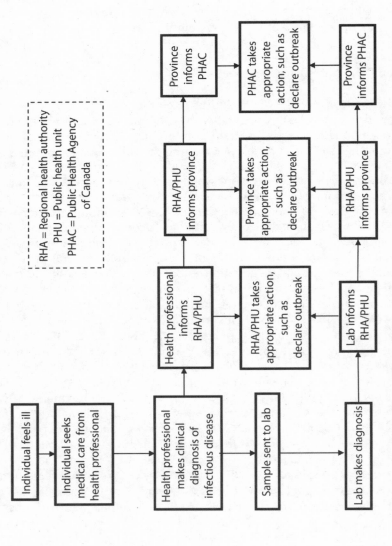

RHA = Regional health authority
PHU = Public health unit
PHAC = Public Health Agency of Canada

Source: Auditor General Canada, 2008.

the crisis – contributed to the inconsistent management of the outbreak'
(Weatherill 2009: xii).

Intergovernmental Cooperation

The reasons for this are, unsurprisingly, political. The main axis of dispute is (again unsurprisingly) the intergovernmental tension over jurisdiction on public health. As Chapter 2 explains, the provinces have clear
constitutional responsibility for health care within their respective jurisdictions; however, the federal government has some claim for authority
in this area as well. One of the earliest instances of federal involvement
was its responsibility under section 91(11) of the British North America
Act in determining regulations over the quarantine of immigrants
arriving in Canada (PHAC is still actively involved with Immigration
Canada in coordinating health regulations regarding incoming migration). Another federal power is that over criminal law under section
91(27) of the BNA Act, including section 245 of the Criminal Code of
Canada (which discusses the administration of noxious substances to
individuals), which became relevant during the investigation over the
blood supply in Canada.

Much more widely debated has been the 'residual power' of the federal government to legislate in order to maintain 'Peace, Order, and
Good Government.' Case law has provided a strong foundation for the
federal role in infectious disease control: the 1946 *Canada Temperance
Federation* case stated that 'it would seem to follow that if the Parliament
could legislate when there was an actual epidemic it could do so to
prevent one occurring and also to prevent it happening again' (cited in
Gammon 2006: 15). However, the utility of federal activity in infectious
disease control has been counterbalanced by the 'provincial inability
test,' which requires evidence that 'the failure by one province to adequately deal with the subject matter would lead to harm for the other
provinces that had taken steps to address the matter' (ibid., 19). Even
the 'emergency powers' of the federal government under the 'Peace,
Order, and Good Government' clause of the Constitution are limited
to periods of actual, as opposed to potential, crisis and therefore cannot be used to establish a unilateral federal framework for disease
surveillance.

The most prominent powers of the federal government in public
health have been exercised under its spending powers (section 36). As
Chapter 2 here notes, this is not a formal power per se but rather a

secondary power derived from the interpretation of sections 36, 91(1a), 91(3), and 106 of the Canadian Constitution, which address the commitment to equalization, the power to levy taxes, the ability to legislate in relation to private property, and the power to appropriate federal funds. Quebec, especially, holds that the spending power is an illegitimate exercise in 'nation-destroying' due to its trespass on Quebecers' 'sovereignty in their sphere of jurisdiction and on sufficient revenue to make that sovereignty meaningful' (Telford 2003: 41). There are thus two impediments for Ottawa in its exercise of constitutional powers to reinforce the public health system: first, a challenge by the provinces could result in a clear setback if the courts determine such action to be uncompromisingly ultra vires its constitutional authority. At present, federal powers to legislate in the area of public health are ambiguous, but they arguably do exist. Second, the federal government has in recent years established a policy of 'open federalism' in order to build bridges with Quebec. This policy is built on 'a recognition and a respect for the constitutional division of powers; a recognition that there exists a fiscal imbalance in the federation; a commitment to redress this vertical fiscal imbalance; a related commitment to rein in the federal spending power in areas of exclusive provincial jurisdiction; and, finally, a commitment to work with the Council of the Federation to improve the management and workings of the Canadian federation' (Courchene 2008: 20). Any unilateral federal push in public health – even in the relatively 'soft' area of spending – could exacerbate political tensions with the provinces (and especially Quebec).

Federal-provincial tensions are thus the main reason that so little progress beyond the 2005 reforms is being made in the area of public health: national coordination is most effectively attained at the national level, but the federal government is unable (and unwilling) to coerce such coordination. To the extent that such coercion is possible, the political price is very high. The provinces, for their part, are also unable and unwilling to cede authority to a national body despite the policy gains in such an approach. They are, for example, hobbled by recent privacy legislation, which obliges them to be very careful about the kinds of information about private individuals that they release (even to Ottawa). They are also loath to hand over authority for coordination to a body they see as having many coordination problems of its own. These are a separate kind of headache for public health systems. The problem here is not vertical (federal-provincial) but rather horizontal (federal interdepartmental) coordination.

Interdepartmental Collaboration

As illustrated in Figure 5.1, the Public Health Agency of Canada must communicate and coordinate different kinds of policy between quite different federal departments. There are even tensions between the two most similar federal bodies: PHAC and Health Canada. When PHAC was established, for example, many key areas of public health (such as tobacco and nutrition) remained within Health Canada. Both are well-funded areas. In addition, while one of PHAC's original strategic objectives was the development of 'a strong Aboriginal public health policy,' little has been accomplished because the First Nations and Inuit Health Branch also remains squarely within Health Canada. Other issues arise in the attempts by PHAC to coordinate policies with other federal departments. A 2008 report by the auditor general observed that the relationship between PHAC and the Canadian Food Inspection Agency has still not satisfactorily been sorted out in order to determine health risks and to establish surveillance roles. Disputes still arise regarding the respective responsibility that Immigration Canada and PHAC have in monitoring the health of immigrants. Despite PHAC's original intentions to focus on environmental health, there is little concerted effort between Environment Canada and PHAC to address this. Even more formal linkages between PHAC and various departments show signs of strain (where, e.g., the status of memorandums of understanding signed between Health Canada and other departments have been disputed when PHAC took over the function of various branches of Health Canada).

It would be a mistake to place the responsibility for such functional problems directly with PHAC. As a large agency that was established quickly in the wake of a serious crisis, many organizational issues have yet to be sorted out. More significant is the difficulty of reconciling a strategy of interdepartmental collaboration with a management structure based on hierarchy and vertical accountability. The push in public policy (and especially health policy) towards greater integration has been built on the recognition that effective service delivery depends on the development of seamless service between sectors (e.g., primary care, surgical care, postoperative care, rehabilitation, and follow-up care) but also potentially between departments (e.g., between health care, mental health care, social services, justice, and police services). But if 'horizontality' is the 'new reality,' there is less understanding of the obstacles to collaborative management. A different set of skills and values, for example, must be present to achieve the consensus necessary where hierarchical decision making is absent. Line departments will be uneasy about committing their resources to horizontal initiatives where funding is already stretched. The shared accountability required by horizontal management can be problematic: decision makers may have opposing views regarding how objectives ought to be pursued, and responsibility may be unfairly allocated when outcomes are less than positive (Bakvis and Juillet 2004). Moreover, while efficiency concerns may be the primary reason that such horizontal initiatives are pursued, effective collaboration can require a significant investment in time, planning, and resources including increased meeting time, more paper work, the development of shared performance indicators, and more complex reporting requirements (ibid., 2).

The Role of the Chief Public Health Officer

When the idea of PHAC was originally conceived, the intent was to give the chief public health officer (CPHO) in charge of it considerable autonomy vis-à-vis the federal government (Fierlbeck 2011). The limitations facing a CPHO who was directly accountable to, and served at the pleasure of, the minister of health were articulated in the 2003 SARS report. In the end, however, the CPHO was established at the level of a deputy minister, reporting directly to the minister of health. The advantage of this arrangement is that the CPHO is firmly ensconced in government and is always 'in the loop' regarding administrative and policy developments. This facilitates the communication of information, policy coordination and, ideally, interdepartmental collaboration.

But detractors have pointed out the costs of this model. Both the U.S. surgeon-general and the British chief medical officer have greater autonomy in their roles than has the Canadian CPHO, and they have used their respective positions to speak out against government policy on certain occasions. Canada's CPHO must be more circumspect. The ability of the CPHO to report directly to the public is a very powerful and effective public health tool, but this is precisely why political executives find it threatening. It is not surprising that the CPHO has not spoken out publicly on issues that the public health community itself has been quite verbal, including the use of safe injection sits, the *listeriosis* outbreak, or the evisceration of health promotion policies. Deputy minister status may seem to confer a great deal of authority on the CPHO (and it does vis-à-vis civil servants), but it also means that the CPHO cannot speak out against his employer (the federal government). The CPHO can be removed any time by the minister of health, for any reason, and he is not protected against unfair dismissal by the Public Service Employment Act, as are most other civil servants (Keelan and Wilson 2008). The theoretical distinction here is whether the CPHO should be directly accountable to government (like the minister of health is) or to the people (as is the auditor general).

This distinction makes a considerable difference for the particular function of the CPHO. In the former, the purpose of the CPHO is to direct and manage a sizeable bureaucracy, develop policy, negotiate connections within government (and between government and stakeholder groups), present government with specialized briefings, and coordinate strategy during public health crises. In the latter role, however, the purpose of the CPHO would be to represent the interests of the Canadian public: even against the immediate interests of the government, should this be necessary. This situation might arise if the CPHO determined that the government was withholding important public health information about which the public ought to be apprised (such as a viral outbreak or contamination of the food supply), that a current policy was misguided, that there was too much foot-dragging on policy formulation, or that any aspect of the public health service was receiving insufficient funding to protect the health of the population.

There has been some criticism that the CPHO does not have sufficient autonomy to do his job properly (Keelan and Wilson 2008), and that he is effectively muzzled by government. While the CPHO does, for example, have the ability under the Public Health Agency of Canada Act to 'communicate with the public' and to present reports to the public, there are concerns that the CPHO will engage in strategic self-censorship due to the insecurity in the terms of tenure regarding his or her position. The chief medical officer in the United Kingdom enjoys protection from dismissal without cause; and the position of the American surgeon-general, which traditionally enjoyed some autonomy, is being strengthened even further through amendments to the American Public Health Service Act. These reforms will also allow the surgeon-general to request public health funds independently (ibid.). Similarly, provincial chief public health officers in Canada are governed by a wide range of legislation. Some chief public health officers (such as those in British Columbia and Ontario) enjoy a significant degree of autonomy in relation to the provincial executive; others have very little.

There is ongoing debate about the degree of autonomy that the CPHO of Canada should be granted. Some see the restricted role of the CPHO as a manifestation of the federal government's propensity to micromanage public policy. Nonetheless, the decision to subsume the duties of the CPHO within the government, rather than place them in opposition to it, was a reasonable choice at the time. Given that the public health service was being built from the ground up, it was important to emphasize interdepartmental and intergovernmental collaboration, to coordinate policy and practices within and between units, and to establish communication between public health and other governmental officials. The particular context underlying the establishment of the federal public health service was not that federal officials did not act responsibly to the population, but rather that there was insufficient coordination of pandemic planning between units and regions. It follows that the best way to address such shortcomings would be the development of a well-organized administration under the direct control of a government official whose first responsibility would be the effective organization and coordination of various public health systems and related departments and agencies.

The question remains what the duties of the CPHO should be now that the organization, function, and duties of the public health service have been established. Should the primary duty of the CPHO be to keep an eye on his or her department (as a deputy minister) or to keep an eye on his or her government (as a watchdog)? The more established the Public Health Agency of Canada becomes, with a clear protocol and institutional memory, the more reason there is to shift the duties of the chief public health officer from administration to vigilance. To this end, it would make sense to change the legislation governing the position of the CPHO so that it is de-politicized (an appointment made by the Public Service Commission rather than a political appointment). This could allow the CPHO greater discretionary ability to request funds, stipulate the right of the CPHO to communicate directly to the citizens of Canada, and offer protection from arbitrary removal (e.g., through requiring Parliament to agree to the removal of the CPHO).

The Politics of Health Promotion and Population Health

The formal functions of a public health service are generally said to be population health assessment, health promotion, disease and injury control and prevention, health protection, surveillance, and emergency preparedness (Mowat and Butler-Jones 2007). In practice, however, the objectives of most public health systems have become bifurcated into functions related to infectious disease control and prevention (surveillance systems, data collection and research, emergency response systems) and those addressing health promotion and disease prevention (usually focusing on the social determinants of health). Most public health officials would agree that public health is marginalized in Canada, with only 2 per cent of total health spending being directed towards public health (Alikhan and Lozon 2007). Others would point out that, even within the public health system itself, more resources have been directed towards emergency response (outbreaks of disease) than towards improving the social (or 'non-medical') determinants of health (income, education, housing, etc.). The Kirby Report stated that 75 per cent of Canadians' health is determined by physical, social, and economic environments. Why, then, has the attempt to *prevent* poor health been so neglected?

That the health of a society could be addressed more effectively through changes in people's environments than through medical intervention was recognized as early as 1842, when Edwin Chadwick published his *Report on the Sanitary Conditions of the Labouring Population* in Britain. The diseases endemic within the working classes, he wrote, almost always 'point to one particular, namely, atmospheric impurity, occasioned by means within the control of legislation, as the main cause of the ravages of epidemic, endemic, and contagious diseases among the community, and as aggravating most other diseases.' Data on sanitation throughout the country, he wrote, 'show that the impurity and its evil consequences are greater or less in different places, according as there is more or less sufficient drainage of houses, streets, roads, and land, combined with more or less sufficient means of cleansing and removing solid refuse and impurities, by available supplies of water for the purpose.' This was compounded by 'the effects of overcrowding the places of work and dwellings, including the effects of the defective ventilation of dwelling-houses, and of places of work where there are fumes or dust produced.' Chadwick's quaint Victorian observation that 'the good or evil moral habits promoted by the nature of the residence' were also to blame for ill health seems strikingly modern when rearticulated as the observation that 'behavioural choices are influenced by social environment' (Chadwick 1842: 4).

The link between living standards and public health was brought more forcefully into a modern idiom by Thomas McKeown, who made the compelling argument that it was the improvement in living conditions (and especially better nutrition) rather than in medical care which accounted for the decrease in morbidity levels and the increase in age of mortality (McKeown 1976a, 1976b). The debate became sidelined over time by discussions of accuracy in historiographical technique, but it nonetheless resonated with those who were becoming concerned that modern medicine was increasingly enthralled with expensive technological and pharmaceutical treatments at the cost of neglecting poor health caused by widening social disparities.

At roughly the same time that McKeown's thesis was provoking debate over the allocation of health care resources, Canada produced the first major public policy paper addressing the social determinants of health. *A New Perspective on the Health of Canadians* (the Lalonde Report), published in 1974, challenged the primacy of the biomedical model in addressing the health of populations and stressed, instead, a set of factors encompassing environment, human biology, lifestyle, and the organization of health care. The timing of the report was not propitious. Canada was, along with the rest of the world, struggling to deal with a major recession provoked by the fuel crisis and the Organization of Petroleum Exporting Countries (OPEC); and there was little inclination to invest in a health policy focusing on improving broad social indicators.

Nonetheless, the WHO released a major position statement in 1986 entitled *The Ottawa Charter for Health Promotion*, and Canada capitalized on its publication by presenting its own policy paper, *Achieving Health for All: A Framework for Health Promotion* (the Epp Report) in 1986. This position became known as the 'population health' perspective – or 'social determinants of health' (SDOH) perspective – and differed slightly from the more traditional public health perspective in that the population health approach identified socioeconomic inequality (as opposed to levels of overall economic prosperity) as a critical factor in determining the health of individuals. While the field of public health has always been viewed as 'a grand social intervention' going far beyond orthodox health care (Sretzer 2002), the more recent population health strategy is highly political. The issue addresses the allocation and redistribution of resources throughout society: 'Are public health ends better served by narrow interventions focused at the level of the individual or the community, or by broad social, political, and economic resources that exert such a profound influence on health status at the population level?' (Colgrove 2002: 728).

Canada's record on this is mixed. Notwithstanding the great emphasis placed on the redistributive nature of Canada's health care system vis-à-vis its American neighbour, Canada's level of socioeconomic inequality has remained quite high. On the other hand, the institutionalization of population health advocacy has solidified in the past two decades. A population health group was created within the Canadian Institute for Advanced Research in 1989, and the Federal/Provincial/Territorial Advisory Committee on Population Health was created in 1992. In 1999 the Canadian Population Health Initiative (CPHI) was established under the auspices of the Canadian Institute for Health Information (CIHI) to produce an annual set of health indicators to gauge the health status of Canadians across jurisdictions, and to 'contribute to the development of policies that reduce inequities and improve the health and well-being of Canadians' (CPHI 2007). The Canadian Institutes of Health Research (CIHR) also established a discrete institute to address population health issues (the Institute of Population and Public Health) to analyse the impacts of physical and social environments on health and to develop policies aimed at reducing health disparities in Canada. In 2003 Canada's ministers of health established the Intersectoral Healthy Living Network, charged with designing policies that would improve health outcomes and reduce health disparities. This body, working in conjunction with the Federal/Provincial/Territorial Advisory Committee on Population Health and Health Security and the Federal/Provincial/Territorial Healthy Living Task Group, developed the 2005 Integrated Pan-Canadian Healthy Living Strategy, a conceptual framework for long-term public policy making based on the principle of 'healthy living.' Moreover, of the six National Collaborating Centres established in 2004, one addresses the social determinants of health directly; a second, focusing on risk assessment, places emphasis on the social determinants of health and the physical environment; and a third focuses on environmental health.

The institutionalization of population health in Canada coincided with population health policies launched by the European Union, including its 2005 program 'EU for Health and Wealth,' a politically astute strategy that focused on the capacity of a healthy population to produce greater wealth (as well as on the fact that healthy societies consume fewer social resources on health care). The EU's 2006 strategy of 'Health in All Policies' (HiAP) addressed the need of all sectors to understand the health consequences of policies enacted under their jurisdiction. The World Health Organization, too, launched its report on the social determinants of health, *Closing the Gap in a Generation: Health Equity through Action of the Social Determinants of Health* in 2008.

The sophisticated evidence produced by this most recent wave of public health practitioners has been impressive, provocative, and unsettling. Researchers at the Canadian Institute for Advanced Research, for example, produced a seminal book in 1994 entitled, simply, *Why Are Some People Healthy and Others Not?* This volume made the clear case that 'lower income and/or lower social status are associated with poorer health ... Whatever is going around, people in lower social positions tend to get more of it, and to die earlier – *even after adjustment for the effects of specific individual or environmental hazards*' (Evans and Stoddart 1994: 45, 46; emphasis added). Taking Chadwick and McKeown a step further, the contributors argued that it was not only the direct effect of poor housing, nutrition, or sanitation that contributed to the higher incidence of ill health among lower socioeconomic groups. Rather, stated Evans and Stoddart, 'the psychological dynamics of status and class may have even more powerful, if subtler, effects' (ibid., 50). Thus health becomes influenced by the quality of one's social relationships, sense of self-esteem, hierarchical position, and social status.

The point here is that targeted medical interventions may be cost-ineffective (at best), or futile (at worst) if the context within which they exist is defined by severe social inequalities. This is where comparative epidemiology presents some interesting statistics; and the social policy experiment that resulted from Canada's divergence from the U.S. model of health care funding provides a clear illustration of this hypothesis. Fifty years ago, as Hertzman and Siddiqi (2008) write, Canadian and American health indicators (such as life expectancy and infant mortality) were very similar. But by the end of the twentieth century, the severe health inequalities present in the United States were absent in Canada, where the *very poorest* 20 per cent of Canadians enjoyed the same life expectancy as *average-income* Americans. Likewise, a British study has noted that each 1 per cent rise in income inequality led to a 4 per cent increase in deaths for those at the lower end of the socioeconomic scale (Wolfson et al., 1999). This would seem to indicate that it is not the overall prosperity of a society that determines the health of its inhabitants, but rather how the wealth is utilized and distributed. Canada spends considerably less on health care as a society than does the United States, yet its overall health indicators are significantly better. Other authors have made similar observations among the member countries of the Organization for Economic Co-operation and Development (OECD): those countries with the smallest socioeconomic gradients (such as Japan and Sweden) have much better health indicators than those countries with large inequalities (see, e.g., Pickett and Wilkinson 2009). Evans (2008: 26) points out that the set of health indicators of even a very poor (but more egalitarian) country – Cuba – 'matches or exceeds, on average, that of the United States.'

The question that such observations naturally lead to is why, given the overwhelming evidence of the impact of the social determinants of health, so little change has occurred. As the Health Council of Canada states, 'despite considerable investments by all governments in activities to promote healthy living, the idea of an integrated pan-Canadian strategy that cuts across specific diseases (which health ministers agreed to in 2005) seems to have been shelved. Overall, public spending to foster healthy living still represents only a fraction of what we spend on treating preventable illness and injury' (2008: 30). A more positive interpretation would begin with the observation that a shift in policy focus from a biomedical model to a population health model requires considerable groundwork before any noticeable change of direction could occur. The development of such groundwork has been evident in the past decade. Conceptual frameworks, data gathering, policy formulation, and policy networking are crucial first steps in shifting course. When the institutional capacity is ready, actual policy implementation can be undertaken effectively.

However, the line from policy development to policy implementation is rarely a straight one, and the very nature of 'population health' itself complicates the process considerably. If the provision of orthodox health care services is highly political, the attempt to incorporate population health models is even more so. What are the political obstacles to a more preventive health approach?

Causality

The very dominance of the biomedical model of health care has its basis in the development of enlightenment rationality. 'Truth,' in this account, is based on the collection and evaluation of empirical evidence. If it can be shown persuasively that X (contaminated water) causes Y (cholera), then the solution is to ensure a sanitary water supply. The evidence rests on the identification of an organism (*Vibrio cholerae*) in the water, observation that those ingesting cholera bacteria will likely become ill with predictable symptoms, and an understanding of how, precisely, cholera affects human health. (*V. cholerae* can penetrate the mucus lining the intestine, producing toxic proteins that cause severe diarrhea, leading to intense dehydration and potential death.) When such causal links weaken and become less clear, the evidence of causality is less persuasive. Some low-income individuals working in stressful, highly controlled situations may have certain indicators of poor health, but others might have different sets of indicators. Some might not suffer significant ill health at all. Some individuals will manifest poor health early in life, others later. Where, then, is the evidence that poorly paid, strictly regimented employment leads to ill health?

What counts as evidence here is, to a large extent, indirect: epidemiologists use statistical data to show that individuals in highly regimented, low-income jobs tend to exhibit worse health indicators than those who are well paid and who have substantial control over their employment conditions. This was Edwin Chadwick's strategy: to show, statistically, that the health of the 'labouring classes' was clearly connected to their living conditions. But statistical analysis has, since Chadwick's day, become sophisticated enough that it is easier to adjust the analysis to eliminate all possible causal links except the one under investigation. For example, one can remove such factors as smoking, drinking, and poor nutrition from the data set and still be able to show a clear causal link between low-income, high-stress jobs and illness. A bigger problem is that it is difficult to explain the biological pathways that link certain kinds of stress and ill health: why does an office worker with an abusive manager suffer worse health than a chief executive who must produce profits for boards of directors and for shareholders? Both experience a great deal of work-related stress. Because such biological mechanisms are unclear, the statistical data alone remain unpersuasive for many. Population health advocates argue that this is similar to the debate over smoking several decades ago, where the statistical correlation of smoking and lung cancer was rejected (by smokers, tobacco companies, and some health officials) because it was not clear how, exactly, tobacco smoke led to lung cancer – why did some smokers *not* end up with lung cancer? The psychosocial dimension of the population health approach, however, does lead to additional problems. It is possible, for example, to determine how many cigarettes particular individuals smoke and to observe how much tar has collected in their lungs. It is not as simple to determine how much 'self-esteem' these individuals have, or how much control over their social environment they perceive they have, even if one can make the statistical correlation between self-esteem (or perceived lack of control) and ill health.

Thus epidemiologists tend to talk in terms of a 'web' of causality, in which there may not be a single cause for a particular disease, and in which the causes of disease may be interconnected. The issue is further complicated by the temporal nature of the presentation of disease. While the most problematic dimension of causality is the issue of competing causes – how do we know it is stress that leads to ill health, rather than the poor nutrition often practised by a person undergoing considerable stress? Another important dimension is the length of time it takes social determinants of health to become evident. The effects of low income (living in mouldy housing or violent neighbourhoods, suboptimal nutrition, unstable employment, low self-esteem, and so on) generally only become evident over longer periods of time. Obviously the provision of clean, verdant, socially integrated neighbourhoods is preferable to ones that are not. But when such programs must compete for funding with hospitals, which require staff and technology to treat patients with immediate medical needs (cardiac or cancer care), then illnesses resulting from long-term underlying causes will simply not be able to compete. This is exacerbated by the electoral cycles of democratic politics: 'policies with longer-term horizons are often neglected because they do not produce immediate political capital' (McMillan and Nagpal 2007: 62).

Diffusion and Fragmentation

Compounding the complexity of causal attribution for disease is the fact that jurisdiction governing both prevention and treatment is spread out both geographically and sectorally. As noted in the discussion over disease surveillance, the prevention of ill health (and the promotion of good health) is most effectively pursued through cooperation between regions and collaboration between line departments; however, such synergetic activity is often difficult to attain. The rationale for such collaboration is mutual gain: it is in the interests of each and every jurisdiction to cooperate in order to improve public health. Yet this condition also encourages 'free-rider' behaviour, in which actors can still benefit from others' collective actions even if they themselves do not contribute directly. Further, where results are diffuse rather than clearly evident, the political pay-offs diminish as any one political jurisdiction cannot take full credit for successful outcomes. Accountability for unsuccessful outcomes is also a source of political anxiety, as incompetence by one set of actors could compromise the integrity of other participants. The sheer effort involved in communicating with disparate units (including the meeting time needed to establish effective communication), the clash of bureaucratic cultures, and the expenditure of good will (e.g., to establish who will contribute what level of funding) are all costs that must be calculated in the attempt to achieve collaborative action.

This is especially true for disease prevention and health promotion, as the *social* determinants of health are quite disparate and fall under numerous separate jurisdictions. As McGinnis et al. (2002) explain, while medical treatments often focus on a single biological symptom, prevention requires intervention in a number of upstream areas; and 'when multiple factors need to be addressed to assure prevention, multiple funding streams need to be coordinated, and incentives for numerous actors need to be addressed through a broad health strategy.' Treatment strategies which involve a 'single decision node' (increasing federal funding to target cancer or cardiac care) are much simpler to implement than wide-ranging collaborative ones (establishing an intergovernmental strategy for community-wide programs aimed at improving nutrition, encouraging physical exercise, eliminating excessive stress, and limiting alcohol and tobacco use). This, in sum, is why the attempt in 2004 to target five high-priority areas – cancer and cardiac care, joint replacement, cataract surgery, and diagnostics – has been a qualified success, while the Pan-Canadian Healthy Living Strategy has simply vanished.

Competing Interests

Not all interests perceive that health promotion can result in positive-sum gains. On the one hand, unless a considerable amount of new monies are dedicated to the task, medical personnel involved in acute care may resist attempts to address non-medical determinants of health if they believe it will involve a redistribution of resources away from them. On the other hand, to the extent that provincial health care budgets are perceived to have cannibalized those in other areas (such as social services or education), promoting further involvement by non-health sectors in order to achieve health-related goals is viewed as 'health imperialism' and is the focus of deep resentment by those not directly involved in acute care (Collins and Hayes 2007; Lavis 2002; Glouberman 2001).

More intense is the influence from large commercial interests. Powerful, well-organized lobbyists representing sizeable agricultural groups (such as tobacco and corn in central Canada, beef in Alberta, or potatoes in Prince Edward Island) may be able to influence regional policy makers through their disproportionate economic status in certain geographical regions. The most powerful agricultural industries are rarely the ones that contribute most to good health: one rarely sees large glossy advertisements promoting the sale of fresh broccoli. As Michael Pollan (2003) argues, even corn is not promoted for its value as a vegetable, but as 'the building block of our fast food culture':

> For the food industry, the real money will never be in selling cheap corn (or soybeans or rice), but in using cheap raw materials to make the kind of snacks that consumers are willing to pay top dollar for. That's one reason why the number and variety of new snack foods at the supermarket have ballooned. The game is in figuring out how to transform a penny's worth of corn into a $3 bag of gourmet corn puffs, or a dime's worth of milk and sweeteners into Swerve, a sugary new 'milk based' soft drink to be sold in schools. As concern over obesity mounts, the focus of political pressure has settled on the food industry and its marketing strategies. Certainly Big Food bears some measure of responsibility for our national eating disorder – a reality that a growing number of food companies have accepted and are beginning to respond to. But the food industry is only playing by a set of rules written by our government (and maintained with the industry's political muscle).

In Canada, the agricultural lobby has been assisted by the historical organization of dairy producers through marketing boards. Milk is a staple of childhood development, but the cost of milk can be prohibitively high for many families (much higher than the price of soft drinks). This is because the dairy boards are able to negotiate base prices for milk and milk products in each province. Farmers' organizations argue that such policies are important in maintaining the family farm as a viable unit, and in maintaining the quality control of dairy products. Thus the public health objectives must be balanced against those of the agricultural interests.

The situation is even more complex when the problem of tobacco regulation is considered. Again, public health goals are constrained by the consideration of conflicting political objectives. When high cigarette taxes led to a sharp increase in the number of contraband cigarettes in Canada, the problem was addressed by lowering the price of cigarettes, even though evidence was clear that high cigarette prices were an effective means of dissuading people from smoking. However, because contraband tobacco involved the political minefield of Aboriginal autonomy (contraband cigarettes are often either smuggled through or produced in territory under Aboriginal jurisdiction), a simpler and less adversarial policy solution to contraband cigarettes was chosen even though it undermined public health goals. A similar dilemma is found within the gaming sector. Governments have enjoyed increasing revenues from a number of forms of gambling, including lotteries, casinos, racetracks, and slot machines, even though research has suggested that approximately one-third of this gambling revenue comes from problem gamblers (Priest 2009).

The same difficulty arises with any large corporate player whose interests are not served by the population health model: car companies and suburban developers do not benefit from strategies promoting pedestrian-friendly urban planning; chemical producers clash with environmental health advocates; and pharmaceutical companies do not profit from the message that good nutrition and physical exercise provide as many benefits as do some drugs. Then there is the tension between recipients of health care. The best-organized (and best-funded) health care lobby groups are those focused on single chronic diseases, such as cancer, diabetes, arthritis, and heart disease. 'In contrast,' note McGinnis, Williams-Russo, and Knickman, (2002), 'the millions of people who benefit from health promotion interventions each receive seemingly small benefits – usually sometime in the distant future.'

The outlook is not completely pessimistic. Clear successes focusing on non-medical factors have been achieved through political will, especially through organization, advertising, and lobbying. Past decades have seen results in statistics on drunk driving, smoking levels, the use of seat belts and, more recently, an effort to shape nutritional choices in schools. In a survey of numerous health regions in Canada, Frankish et al. (2007: 44) report a clear effort by most regional health authorities to address non-medical determinants of health in such areas as 'personal health practices' and 'child development' (areas that were 'less threatening to vested economic interests'). Health regions were much less likely to focus on other determinants of health, such as those related to social and income status, employment and working conditions, culture, and gender. But selective progress, one might optimistically state, is progress nonetheless. Whether such areas represent a beachhead from which further efforts might be expanded, or whether they are the extent to which population health successes will be limited, is unclear.

Values and Ideologies

Strategies based on the social determinants of health have themselves palpably changed over time. From the early 1970s to the early 1990s, the emphasis was on getting people to change their 'lifestyle choices.' Poor health, from this perspective, was almost a reflection of a weak character: one suffered high blood pressure or developed obesity because one was too indolent to get up off the couch to exercise, or too lazy to cook a nutritious meal rather than grab fast food. By the 1990s there was more interest in *why* people were making what, by that time, were clearly understood to be poor health choices. The reasons, again, are diffuse and wide-ranging: but often they are rational responses to a particular social and physical environment rather than merely character flaws. Certainly there are people who do not exercise because they can't be bothered to, even though they have every opportunity. But there are also those who do not exercise or eat well because they are working parents who spend off-work hours taking their own children to various activities; because they are the children of working parents and are expected to stay safely inside the home until their parents arrive home; because they cannot afford to live in safe neighbourhoods and thus remain indoors as much as possible; because they cannot afford the sports fees that would allow them to become involved in organized sports; because they must work irregular shifts; because they cannot afford the time to cook from scratch, or the money to buy large amounts of imported fresh food; and so on. In an ironical historical twist, this development reflects Edwin Chadwick's belief that 'good and evil habits' are 'promoted by the nature of the residence.'

But social attitudes do not always follow social research in lock-step. The 1980s and 1990s saw the efflorescence of neo-liberal values that stressed individual responsibility and self-reliance. It was difficult to square a strategy of population health with a philosophy of public administration based on individualism and market mechanisms. Social values can also be a barrier to regional collaboration on strategies to address the social determinants of health. Many regions have historically determined value patterns, which is why one can often find more generous social benefits in poorer provinces with a long-standing political culture of social integration (such as Newfoundland) or collective action (Saskatchewan) than in some wealthier provinces (such as Alberta) with their own political cultures of individual independence and self-reliance. The problems are compounded by the call for more extensive and organized government activity, as regions that are normally skittish about 'state intervention' at the best of times tend to balk at strategies that involve greater state involvement or expansion. Fears about the protection of privacy, for example, are only exacerbated by the call for better high-tech monitoring tools that could usefully identify links between social and environmental variables and chronic disease.

Public health, by its very nature, has rarely been able to compete effectively with acute health care services for public funding. Cross-jurisdictional administration, antithetical social values, ambiguous causal connections, and entrenched political influence have, in combination with each other, erected intransigent barriers to political reform. But there are also reasons to believe that a window of opportunity may be developing that could push public health issues more forcefully onto the political agenda. For the first time in forty-one years, for example, the World Health Organization in 2009 declared the existence of a global pandemic in the face of H1N1 and, compared with the sudden emergence of SARS, the institutional framework for addressing pandemic management was considerably different. Canada, like most developed countries, now has a system for disease surveillance and a strategy for rapid response to the spread of virulent pathogens. Public awareness (and fear) of global pandemics, the contamination of food and water supplies, and non-medical determinants of health have increased the political capital of public health advocates. Sophisticated data collection and analysis, as well the institutionalization of formal bodies charged with collecting evidence and developing policies, has fortified the institutional capacity to address public health issues not only in the prevention of disease but also in the promotion of health. While H1N1, among other potential pandemics, might have been ominous for public health, it was a good test of the development of a more seasoned and robust public health system.

Entrenched political interests that resist efforts to develop and expand public health strategies still remain. Jurisdictional disputes, as well as debates over the proper role of public health (and public health officials) continue to hamper attempts to streamline systems of disease surveillance and response. Even more diffuse and widespread forms of opposition manifest themselves against the development of a comprehensive, pan-Canadian approach to the promotion of good health. Notwithstanding the appearance of a possible 'window of opportunity,' any sustained political reform in public health will likely depend on the factors that successful policy making generally require: organization, support, resources, and possibly, luck.

6 Health Human Resources

The Debate over Doctors

Many Canadians say that the problem with the Canadian health care system is that we don't have enough doctors. Former Canadian Medical Association (CMA) president Brian Day has argued that Canada would need to add 26,000 doctors to its health system immediately to bring the country 'up to global standards' (Ubelacker 2008). This position makes sense to those who have difficulty finding a family doctor or GP, or to those who have to wait several months for surgery. But it raises the question of exactly *how many* doctors is the right number or whether gaps in health care service delivery are simply reducible to a shortage of doctors. Looking at comparative data, there is little direct correlation between the number of physicians and the health outcomes of a given country. According to the Organization for Economic Co-operation and Development (OECD), Canada has fewer practising physicians per 1,000 people (2.2) than most OECD member states (we come in 24th out of 30). Canada's mortality and morbidity indicators, however, consistently remain better than those for most OECD countries, and clearly meet or surpass those in OECD countries with the *most* doctors (Greece, Belgium, and Italy). This juxtaposition is even more pronounced with Japan, which has fewer doctors than Canada (2.0 per 1,000) but still better health indicators (OECD Health Data 2007).

So there is little statistical evidence that simply pushing more doctors into the system will improve health care. It is worthwhile to point out that more doctors *are* coming into the Canadian health care system: while Canada's population grew by 9 per cent between 1997 and 2006, the number of physicians practising in Canada grew by 12.9 per cent (of these, slightly more than half were family doctors, and slightly less were specialists). Moreover, between 2001 and 2006 (the last year for which data were available), the number of doctors leaving Canada declined by 56.9 per cent, resulting in a higher number of doctors *returning* to Canada than those leaving (CIHI 2008). The exodus of physicians from Canada peaked in the mid-1990s. This was due to the combination of several factors, including the migration of doctors disheartened by the considerable cuts to health care funding during this period (CMA 2009) and the expansion of the family practice residency to two years (from one) in 1993, which delayed entry of this cohort of physicians for an additional year (Evans and McGrail 2008).

The ratio of physicians relative to the Canadian population has actually *increased* noticeably over the past twenty years (CMA 2009). From 2004 to 2008 alone, the total ratio of physicians to 100,000 of the population increased from 189 to 195. This has been a combination of increased medical school enrolment (up by 6.6%) higher numbers of foreign-trained physicians (up by 10.4%), and favourable patterns of migration (the number of doctors returning to Canada outnumbers those who left); all statistics are from CIHI (2009). Why, then, is there a clear perception that Canada is experiencing a shortage of doctors? There is actually a confluence of factors. One is the way in which regional health associations choose to distribute their funding: they may, for example, cut back the number of days a surgeon is allowed to perform procedures in order to save money. Thus it is not the number of physicians per se but the number of procedures each is allowed to perform that contributes to the waiting times experienced by patients. Another contributing factor is the geographical distribution of physicians. The province with the most physicians per capita, for example, is Nova Scotia: but this fact would be met with scepticism in places like Digby County which, like other rural areas in Canada, has difficulty in attracting doctors. Administrative regions have considerable difficulty in directing physician supply to areas with the biggest need, as most physicians are 'free contractors,' and like most Canadians, they expect the freedom to work where they wish. In 1997 the *Waldman* case determined that provinces' attempts to withhold full billings from physicians who chose to locate in well-served areas was contrary to the mobility rights (section 6) of the Canadian Constitution (see Chapter 4). This meant that health officials were denied the sticks and left with the carrots in their physician supply strategies: but these carrots are expensive ones (recruitment and retention bonuses average around $10,000 per year for up to four or five years), further straining already limited health budgets for many regions.

Another reason is the nature of the changing physician cohort itself. Gender is one factor: female physicians have over time consistently worked fewer hours per week. CMA data show that in 1982 female physicians worked 44.0 hours per week compared with the 52.8 hours per week men worked; in 2007 the respective hours were 47.5 and 53.8; this is usually explained with reference to the greater domestic burden generally faced by women (see Gross 1998), but other factors – such as the type of specialization chosen – can also play a role. At the same time, women entering the practice of medicine are significantly outnumbering men: while the female-male physician ratio in Canada (total number of practising physicians) in 2009 was 22,753 to 44,239, the ratio for physicians 35 or under was 2,429 female to 1,921 male (CMA 2009).

Another variable explaining the perception of a physician shortage may be generational. For example, Watson et al. (2006) determined that there was a decline in average weekly hours worked by GPs of 8.5 per cent from 1993 to 2003; and Crossley et al. (2006) report a decline of 15.6 per cent from 1982 to 2003. This may be because of the desire of younger physicians to enjoy a more balanced personal and professional lifestyle. Interestingly, as Evans and McGrail (2008) point out, while physicians' overall hours may be declining, their average billings actually *increased* by 30 per cent. This, they explain, may be partly due to the noticeable rate of increase of billings by *specialists*, as opposed to GPs, as the increase in GPs' billings was only a third of that of specialists. The consequences of this trend, argue Evans and McGrail, have not been adequately recognized: given that a relatively constant number of doctors in the system have actually been costing us considerably more (a 71.6% cost increase between 1968 and 1989, with the share of GDP absorbed by physicians rising by more than 30%), what will it mean for us now that politicians have responded to the perception of 'physician shortages' by rapidly expanding the enrolment of medical schools to meet public pressure?

A related issue in physician employment is not simply 'how many' but also 'from where.' Throughout the 1990s there was much concern that Canada was not doing enough to facilitate the integration of foreign-trained physicians, who were relegated to driving cabs and working as dish-washers while physician positions went unfilled. Foreign-trained physicians from countries other than the United States must first pass written and clinical exams, at their own expense, and then find residency positions at hospitals. The problem is that residency positions are available to them only after Canadian-trained physicians have been placed. In 2003, only 67 out of 625 international graduates were given a residency position. This led to accusations of callousness (at best) and discrimination (at worst) against the Canadian government, as many foreign medical graduates are from a wide variety of ethnic groups. While the federal government is responsible for immigration, however, it is the provincial colleges of physicians and surgeons that set the standards for foreign-trained physicians. This is slowly changing. In 2006 Ontario required the provincial accreditation body to revise its procedures in order to speed up the certification and licensing of foreign-trained doctors; and in 2008 the province announced a system of transitional licences that would permit specialists to practise under the supervision of practising specialists, eliminating the need for residencies altogether. In 2010 federal and provincial governments jointly produced the Pan-Canadian Framework for the Assessment and Recognition of Foreign Qualifications, which stipulates that immigrants with professional qualifications (such as registered nurses, pharmacists, physiotherapists, occupational therapists, and doctors) should be informed within a year whether their credentials will be accepted in Canada. It also recommends the development of programs to inform professionals prior to immigration of all licensing requirements, to prepare them for competency exams once they have arrived, and to support them with linguistic and cultural training as needed.

But Canada has also been condemned for *encouraging* foreign-trained doctors to practise in this country. Like many countries (including the United States and Great Britain), Canada relies heavily on foreign-trained physicians. Approximately one-quarter of Canada's physicians come from abroad; of these, most come from the United Kingdom, Ireland, India, and South Africa. In the past ten years, the vast number of immigrant doctors came from South Africa, which has a strong medical program (and English-speaking graduates). There are 2,112 South African physicians in Canada; and in the western provinces the proportion is particularly high. Seventeen per cent of Saskatchewan's physician population is from South Africa (McIntosh et al. 2007). The figure in Alberta is approximately 8 per cent, although the number in rural areas is even higher: 'Without the South Africans,' declared one Alberta practitioner, 'there would be no rural medicine' (Lang 2008a).

The problem is that South Africa, like other developing countries, can ill-afford to lose its physicians. South Africa, with the highest rate of HIV in the world, is itself experiencing a critical physician shortage, with one in three medical positions in the public health sector remaining unfilled – although, as Lang (2008b) notes, South Africa's *private* health care system is able to maintain a 'reasonable supply' of physicians. Because of this, the active recruitment of physicians (as well as nurses and pharmacists) from countries like South Africa is often viewed as 'poaching.' There is increasing consensus that 'it is inappropriate for nations as relatively wealthy as Canada to solve their own domestic health human resources problems of undersupply and maldistribution by relying on the immigration of health professionals from developing countries' (McIntosh et al. 2007: 4), but there is less consensus on what 'ethical recruitment' should be.

For example, one could argue that an across-the-board policy of *not* hiring from third world countries is itself highly discriminatory. We do not make personal judgments against physicians who choose to come from Britain, for example, nor do we impose any moral expectations on them. Is it fair, then, to imply that South African doctors are opportunistic for leaving their country, or to hold that they have an obligation to serve the country that trained them? Surely they have, as individuals, a stronger moral claim to escape the violence and corruption that pervades their daily life than do individuals from European states. Finally, it particularly makes no sense to argue that Canada has a moral duty to *increase* its immigration quotas for individuals from developing countries, especially if they are highly qualified – but not if they are doctors.

An uneasy compromise has been developed in 'codes of conduct' for the ethical recruitment of foreign-trained physicians. This code of conduct differentiates between 'active' and 'passive' recruitment. The former, which is held to be 'ethically unacceptable,' includes bringing health providers to visit communities, sending out e-mails, setting up booths at job fairs in developing countries, and advertising in the professional journals of developing countries (McIntosh et al. 2007: 12). The latter form of recruitment, which is acceptable, includes listing job vacancies on Canadian-based web sites, advertising Canadian communities on Canadian-based web sites, and matching applicants with positions in Canada (ibid., 13). There are, however, many ethical problems with this position. In the first place, one might argue that if it is wrong to hire physicians from South Africa, then it is *wrong;* and any argument for gradations of attempt ('we just recruited a *little* bit') is a matter of degree rather than principle. Conversely, if some (probably well-connected) physicians from South Africa have learned about job opportunities in Canada, is it fair to make such opportunities more difficult to discover for physicians in remote rural areas of South Africa? Is the position that only foreign physicians 'in the know' should be hired in Canada simply rewarding South African elites at the expense of the less well-connected? Then there is the matter of moral hypocrisy: why should Canada hold that South African physicians should stay and work where they are trained (and where they are needed) when Canada does not do the same for its own medical graduates? Canada does not tell its own physicians that they must stay to work in underserviced rural areas or Aboriginal communities: what business does it have taking such a position against South African physicians?

Nevertheless, it is impossible to disregard the scope of disease and despair that so many South Africans face because of the lack of doctors. This is not a debate only facing Canada. Well before Canada was discussing this issue, the United Kingdom was a leader in establishing its own *Code of Practice for the International Recruitment of Healthcare Professionals.* Cynics, however, would note that the United Kingdom could well afford to take the high ground, given that European Union directives were at the same time confirming the rights of European physicians to practise anywhere within the European Union. Thus the United Kingdom has monitored its recruitment from South Africa much more carefully, but it has also increased its recruitment from other EU states such as Germany. The ethics of this seem unproblematic until one realizes that now Germany must recruit more doctors from countries such as Poland and Greece. The migration of European doctors to the 'old Western' EU states from the 'new Eastern' EU states is thus a concern for the poorer Eastern states which themselves spend more of their resources training physicians who consequently migrate in search of a better life. But, because the European Union has determined that these doctors have a clear legal right to do so, the ethical issues remain under the surface.

The 'Other' Health Care Professionals

A common indicator frequently used to compare the nature of health care across countries is the number of doctors relative to the size of the population, even though the link between numbers of physicians and the actual health of a population is rather tenuous. However, others argue that there is closer correlation between the number of *nurses* relative to the size of the population and the health outcomes of the patients (Tomblin Murphy and O'Pallas 2002:14). Physicians in Canada make up only 9 per cent of the health care workforce. Nurses constitute more than 40 per cent, while other health care professionals make up half of the health care workforce. Given that 91 per cent of health care workers are non-physicians, it is remarkable that so little attention is paid to them. Who are these 'other' health care professionals, and what influence do they (or can they) have on the Canadian health care system?

Nurses are the largest group of health care professionals, but they can themselves be divided into four distinct groups: registered nurses, licensed practical nurses, registered psychiatric nurses, and licensed nurse practitioners. The third-largest group is social workers (because some provinces – British Columbia, Alberta, and Ontario – regulate social workers as health care professionals), and the next-largest group is pharmacists. Beyond this (in descending order) there are medical laboratory technologists, dentists, dental hygienists, radiation technologists, physiotherapists, psychologists, occupational therapists, dieticians, respiratory therapists, chiropractors, speech pathologists, optometrists, health information management professionals, audiologists, midwives, and medical physicists (CIHI 2007a). One of the more positive aspects of Canada's health human resources landscape is that the Canadian Institute for Health Information is now able to track important information about many of these professions (such as demographics, education, and employment) through access to the Occupational Therapist Database, the Pharmacist Database, the Physiotherapist Database, the Medical Laboratory Database, and the Medical Radiation Technologist Database. Having clear factual information about the nature and scope of these professionals allows health policy planners a better basis from which to develop longer-term strategies.

Workforce issues must look at the interrelationships between these health care professions, rather than at each profession in isolation. Many problems with satisfaction and retention are related to the structure of work for the health care professions, and changes in this structure for any profession often have compound effects on several others. The structure of work is also tightly tied to larger social and cultural changes in the wider community within which health care professionals live and work. The most obvious example of this is rural medicine. As Canadian society becomes increasingly urbanized, fewer potential doctors see the attraction of rural life. Many have working spouses who cannot find suitable jobs in rural settings, and others are concerned about the educational opportunities (e.g., bilingual schools) for their children in rural settings. As medical technology becomes increasingly sophisticated, rural doctors are increasingly more divorced from specialist services and technological advances than their urban colleagues, especially in smaller hospitals with more limited facilities. Sheer geographical distances mean more difficulty in ensuring professional backup or collaborative practices, leading to longer working hours and greater burnout (Rourke 1993).

But the issue of rural medicine is not simply addressed by training more doctors, who are under no obligations to work in rural areas on completion of their training. Health policy planners are thus attempting two different kinds of strategies to address staffing shortages: reallocating work responsibilities among existing professions, and developing new health professions in order to redistribute the workload. These strategies are often employed first in desperately short-staffed rural areas, but they are becoming increasingly common throughout health care regions. The use of nurse practitioners, for example, has been established in northern communities for some time, but it is now becoming more prevalent in rural areas as well as underserviced urban settings. Nurse practitioners are registered nurses who have additional training to diagnose, evaluate, and treat common medical conditions, and well as to determine which conditions require further attention by specialist physicians. They can also order tests and help patients manage chronic medical conditions, although the exact duties and the degree of autonomy from supervising physicians is determined by legislation developed by each province.

Many other health care professionals are also gaining greater responsibility for meeting patients' health care needs. Several provinces (including Alberta, Ontario, British Columbia, Quebec, and Nova Scotia) allow pharmacists to write as well as fill certain prescriptions. On a province-by-province basis, midwives have been given increasing responsibility in delivering babies, dental hygienists can work independently, and physiotherapists can order X-rays and treat certain injuries. In some cases, remote communities depend on paramedics (supported by long-distance medical supervision) to offer basic and ongoing medical services. A parallel strategy has been to develop new professional categories: in Ontario, for example, five new professions have been formally recognized. These groups (physician assistant, nurse endoscopist, clinical radiation therapist, anaesthesia assistant, and surgical first assistant) were designed to address critical shortages in key areas (physicians, radiation therapists, anaesthesiologists, and registered nurses).

The strategy is increasingly common in most Western countries, and it is not difficult to see why. According to the Canadian Institute for Health Information (CIHI 2009) the average physician salary in Canada is $266,031 (up from $231,427 in 2003), which is considerably more than the average registered nurse's annual salary (although physicians generally spend a much higher proportion of their income on overhead). But the strategy of replacing higher-costing physicians with lower-costing health care professions faces objections from those who argue that effective cost-cutting measures are not necessarily good medicine (or even that effective at cost-cutting). There is the obvious fact that physicians have more intensive medical training than nurses, and that they therefore have a wider knowledge of possible conditions, and are less likely than nurses to miss unobtrusive clues about conditions. There is also the concern that the use of licensed nurse practitioners or other health care professionals to provide traditional medical services could be costly if mistakes resulted in litigation. Others argue that fear of litigation, simple uncertainty, or the lack of training to 'work autonomously' can lead non-physicians to order more (and more costly) tests to confirm their diagnoses, or to schedule more visits to specialists. One hospital consultant argues that 'there is a big difference in what nurses do if they see something. For example, if doctors see a stomach ulcer, they will decide on treatment and treat the patient. But nurse endoscopists will refer back to the consulting physician. Once you have the technical skills you have to apply them. Just sending patients back to the consultant is not helpful' (Coombes 2008: 661). Others would reply that the intensity of training that physicians experience is often more than balanced by the fact that most nurse practitioners have more overall professional experience than qualified but inexperienced GPs as they generally have a long service of clinical practice before upgrading from registered nurse to nurse practitioner. Moreover, many nurse practitioners have graduate nursing degrees (such as a doctorate of nursing), which involves a roughly similar number of years as a medical doctor (MD). But because the utilization of such professions to perform tasks traditionally performed by MDs is relatively new, there is little empirical data on either the clinical- or the cost-effectiveness of these roles.

A more subtle concern in the structure of work for medical professionals is the organization of the system itself and, in particular, the level of autonomy and flexibility that it provides commensurate with training and skill levels. 'One of the most frequently cited factors affecting job satisfaction,' write Rivet, Ryan, and Stewart, (2007: 92), 'is control of the job or being able to balance personal and professional commitments.' Thus health human resource planning must also examine how broad systemic changes affect the ability of the individual health professional to do his or her job. Physicians and nurses both experience stress and burnout because of long hours and unresponsive clinical conditions: doctors cannot find adequate services for patients, nurses are not given sufficient time to establish a humane care relationship with their patients, and so on. Why are these problems so intransigent?

The Politics of Human Health Resource Planning

The immediate response to crises in health human resource issues is often just 'let's hire more' (doctors, nurses, etc.). We have more than sufficient evidence to show that this is bad planning: physicians alone, for example, make up 13 per cent of total health care spending (and are only 9% of the health workforce). Increasing medical staff drives up health care costs, which in turn, leads to public outcry over the 'crisis of health care spending,' which leads to cutbacks (in medical school enrolment, or in hiring, or in operating room hours, and so on). This 'boom and bust' system of human resource planning seems manifestly inefficient and destabilizing. Nevertheless, it continues because it is so easy to get political mileage out of it. In the 2008 federal election campaign, for example, all three political parties called for 'more doctors!' even though numerous academic studies were written in the preceding decade arguing against such a simplistic approach.

The most nefarious example of the intractable politics of health human resource planning is perhaps the fate of the (now infamous) 1991 report by Barer and Stoddart, *Toward Integrated Medical Resource Policies for Canada*. The one recommendation in the 355-page report that is well known is the suggestion to cut medical school enrolments by 10 per cent. Yet 'the authors made 53 recommendations, in an integrated package, and emphasized that "cherry-picking" from this package could easily do more harm than good. Provincial governments promptly (and predictably) cherry-picked the easiest, in hopes of saving money' (Evans and McGrail 2008: 20). Why is it so difficult to design a model of efficient human resource allocation in health care? The first problem lies in the determination of who is responsible for making allocation decisions. In a fully private system, the market makes these decisions;

and in a fully publicly run system the government is required to do so. But in Canada, physicians are self-employed; most (but not all) are remunerated by government insurance plans. The majority (but not all) nurses are publicly employed; while most (but not all) other health care professionals are privately employed. Thus governments have a limited set of tools to use when attempting to plan health services staffing requirements (it's not like the army: a provincial government cannot simply tell the forces of medical personnel where they should go). Governments can tinker with payments systems; but only if the payments are adjusted upwards (because the political costs of cutting medical salaries are generally quite onerous). Alternative payments systems, for example, were introduced in Ontario in 2001 (family health networks, based on capitation) and in 2003 (the family health groups system, which is based on an enhanced fee-for-service system allowing physicians to collect extra payments for off-hours or preventive work). But a study published in 2009 showed that those patients utilizing the alternative systems were generally better off in terms of both health indicators and socioeconomic status (Glazier et al. 2009). This somewhat diminished the point of the practice, which was to expand access to physicians for those unable to find general practitioners. Statistically, it is not the healthier or wealthier patients who tend to have such problems with access.

The second problem lies in having the right information at hand to make useful predictions. This can, in turn, be divided into issues underlying *modelling* and *data* information. Finding an appropriate model is crucial in forecasting the number of health care professionals necessary to provide consistent, efficient, and good quality service. But which model works best? Supply-based models start with the status quo (such as current physician-population ratios) and project forward based on this information. In terms of utility it is not the most accurate basis for allocating future distributions (a wealthy urban area with a relatively large number of physicians doesn't necessarily have the most optimal number if less populated or poorer areas are desperately wanting), but it is useful politically insofar as it is the political baseline from which an area's representatives can most effectively begin (*decreasing* the physician-population ratio in an area with a well-heeled, educated, cohesive, well-organized, and likely well-connected population, e.g., will be seen as a political non-starter). Needs-based planning, in contrast, starts by looking at the health indicators of a population and attempts to set personnel levels accordingly. It gives a better indication of how health human resources should be allocated, but there are some issues regarding which indicators ought to be used (higher age and lower income, e.g., can be correlated to higher health needs, although the link can vary dramatically).

Needs-based planning, however, may not take into account the supply side of the equation: medical staff may not wish to go into these areas, nor may political officials see these areas as a good investment of political capital. Other models (such as benchmarking) have been developed to determine the best means to allocate health human resources. But all models depend on the existence of data to make accurate predictions. This is especially the case when human resource strategies increasingly focus on integrated and collaborative systems. The idea of 'collaborative health care' has been gaining momentum for decades (see Chapter 3), and is prevalent in most countries to some degree. It is based on the premise that access to a wide spectrum of health professionals (dieticians, psychologists, post-natal nurses, dental hygienists, etc.) can take the pressure off the demand for physicians. This makes good sense when looking at an individual 'integrated health care centre.' But when thinking about what is needed for an *entire system* of integrated health centres across each province, the problem becomes much more challenging. This is because we have 'limited information on those professions that are self-regulatory such as pharmacists, midwives, chiropractors etc. and none on those professions that are not regulated. As policy-makers consider integrated delivery models, overlapping scopes of practice and increased use of other health professions, these information gaps are critical' (Kazanjian et al. 2000; Fooks et al. 2002: 12).

A third set of obstacles to effective health human resource planning include the complexity of the policy area and the fragmentation of those who must be involved in the process. The recruitment of health professionals is tied in to the design of the health care system as a whole: any attempt to construct a comprehensive primary care, long-term care, or home care program, for example, would have to involve an evaluation of the numbers and types of health professionals available, as well as a long-term training plan to recruit individuals in the necessary areas. Reform of the public health system in Canada, for example, has been difficult because of the lack of comprehensive accreditation for public health professionals (and the dearth of schools of public health in which to train potential public health workers). As Fooks et al. (2002) argue, implementation of health human resource strategies has been made more difficult to the extent that it has been treated as a separate policy area rather than one that is inextricably linked to other reform initiatives. The very complexity of long-term health planning, they add, often defeats the comprehensive approach that is required for an effective, well-coordinated system.

Structurally, the system of federalism on which Canadian health care services are provided is also responsible for the fragmentation of health human resource planning. Each province is responsible for training its own personnel, and each province does so in conjunction with an autonomous professional regulatory agency (e.g., provincial colleges of physicians and surgeons and colleges of nursing) which may have different requirements and standards in each jurisdiction. The problem of coordination is exacerbated by both the scarcity of many types of health professionals and the free movement of these professionals between jurisdictions. Wealthier provinces will be able to offer higher salaries and poorer provinces will have more trouble retaining the staff that they are able to recruit. Occasionally wealthier provinces are accused of actively 'poaching' health care workers: in 2007, for example, the Calgary Health Region advertised across Canada for their nursing recruitment drive, leading to acrimonious responses from health regions throughout the country.

In addition to the competition between jurisdictions, the expansion of types of health professions as well as the expansion of duties for existing health professionals has meant greater competition between professional organizations. Should pharmacists be able to write prescriptions? Should dental hygienists be able to practise without supervision by dentists? Should midwives be allowed to deliver babies independently? Should nurses have a greater role in providing primary health care? These are all policy questions that involve not only the well-being of patients being treated but also the well-being of the profession as a whole. Professional organizations guard their regulatory power carefully, and they are not quick to cede this authority to others. Many health care analysts argue that the reform of health service delivery has been constrained by physicians' associations, notwithstanding 'the fact that we know outcomes for people have been positively associated with nurses working in advanced practice roles' (Tomblin Murphy and O'Brien-Pallas 2002: 7). Regulatory authority is the primary means that professional organizations have to control the way in which their disciplines are practised (and to protect patients from questionable treatments), but it is also the source of these organizations' political influence.

Few changes to the health services system in any province, for example, are made without due consultation with the college of physicians and surgeons of that province; and where the professional associations are fragmented, their bargaining power is usually diminished.

Unsurprisingly, doctors are the most politically powerful group of health care providers. They are well-organized politically (more so within than between provinces), and their professional associations generally have key decision-making roles in each province (including the establishment of fee schedules, drug formularies, clinical guidelines, and so on). Threats to withhold their services are generally effective in getting their demands met. A less visible source of political influence, however, is the ability to enlist public opinion against a government, especially in forcing a provincial government to endorse (or to back away from) a particular policy move (a public statement by a college of physicians and surgeons that it no longer believes that the current government is able to protect the health of its citizens, e.g., could prove fatal to a sitting government). Physicians can also be enlisted by pharmaceutical companies to pressure governments to add particular drugs to provincial formularies or to place more resources in areas where their drugs are well represented.

There are occasions in which the doctors' political voice has less impact: the move towards regionalization, for example, has in many provinces been implemented despite protests by physicians' groups. Moreover, notwithstanding the strength and organization of professional medicine in Canada, the professional associations are not monolithic. There are, for example, some cleavages in the profession on the basis of gender or age. But the more evident tensions within the profession itself are largely based on specialization, with some specialities (usually geriatrics, psychiatry, and emergency medicine) generally finding themselves more marginalized within the discipline than others. This is often reflected in the fee schedules negotiated for each specialization by the physicians' negotiating committees. When clear differences in interests exist between one group of physicians and others, the ability of certain specializations (especially smaller ones) to promote and defend their interests becomes much more restricted. Thus the difficulty of retaining rural physicians is, to a certain extent, related to their lack of dominance within the larger medical profession itself.

The past decade has seen a flurry of activity in the attempt to coordinate health human resource planning. Provincial and territorial leaders in 2000 released a communiqué committing themselves to a 'more collaborative' approach regarding the 'education, training, working conditions and recruitment and retention initiatives' for health professionals (Fooks et al. 2002: 14). Both the Atlantic Provinces and the Western provinces (in conjunction with the northern territories) have developed their own health human resource planning bodies. Nationally, the primary body for coordinating health human resource planning, the Federal/Provincial/Territorial Advisory Committee on Health Delivery and Human Resources (ACHDHR) was created in 2002. The 2003 Accord on Health Care Renewal included the rearticulation of support for collaborative planning, and in 2005 the ACHDHR released its *Framework for Collaborative Pan-Canadian Health Human Resources Planning* (revised in 2007). This 'action plan' established four overarching goals, including strategies to achieve specific outcomes. These goals are the following:

1. To improve all jurisdictions' capacity to plan for the optimal numbers, mix, and distribution of health care providers based on system design, service delivery models, and population health needs
2. To enhance all jurisdictions' capacity to work closely with employers and the education system to develop a health workforce that has the skills and competencies to provide safe high-quality care, work in innovative environments, and respond to changing health care system and population health needs
3. To enhance all jurisdictions' capacity to achieve the appropriate mix of health providers and deploy them in service delivery models that make full use of their skills
4. To enhance all jurisdictions' capacity to build and maintain a sustainable workforce in health safe work environments. (ACHDHR 2005: 11)

All of these objectives are laudable, and each objective reflects current thinking on what must be done for health human resource planning (integrated system design, needs-based planning, team-based service delivery, and cross-jurisdictional collaboration). Nonetheless, the political obstacles remain difficult to overcome. As the Health Council of Canada concludes, in health human resource policy design 'the reality is that planning remains fragmented': 'Except for some valuable efforts in regional collaboration, each province and territory does its own planning, without the benefit of pan-Canadian information needed for reliable decision-making. The result is burnout in the workforce and continued competition between jurisdictions for health care providers – and continued public frustration with wait times, uncoordinated care, and finding appropriate providers' (Health Council of Canada 2008: 28).

A fourth difficulty is the 'clash of cultures' between health service reform and health human resource objectives. Public service administrative reforms of the 1990s were strongly influenced by business models focusing on efficiency and user-based accountability (see Chapter 3). While private sector models were less influential in the health care sector than in other areas of the public service, there was a clear emphasis on moving away from health services designed on the needs of health care providers towards one based on the needs of the client population itself. There is little dispute that a health care system should be designed in the best interests of those for whom it is established. But neither should improvements occur at the expense of those working within that system. Thus there is discernible tension between reformers attempting to improve the overall capacity and efficiency of health services and professional associations which argue that such reforms are self-defeating because they undermine the ability of health care professionals to work effectively within these systems.

One of the most important aspects of health human resources is job retention. Health professionals are generally highly mobile, and the attrition rate of some groups of health professionals is quite high. Job retention itself in the health professions is frequently determined by job satisfaction. A major determination of job satisfaction, in turn, is professional autonomy. But professional autonomy has multiple dimensions, and each health profession manifests autonomy in a slightly different way. Professional autonomy most clearly exists in a clinical sense in the health professions, and it is based on clinical expertise and experience and, in many cases, on professional self-regulation. A second form of autonomy is that of economic influence over services and incomes. But a third manifestation of autonomy, which is becoming much more relevant in discussions of job satisfaction and retention, is control over 'the broader context in which professional practice takes place' (Randall and Williams 2009: 55; see also Schulz and Harrison 1986).

Issues of professional autonomy play out differently across the health professions. While physicians' autonomy has been based on historical factors (especially the professional independence and self-regulation negotiated during the introduction of public insurance in Canada in the middle of the twentieth century) as well as on clinical expertise, nurses' autonomy has been a more hard-fought achievement. Traditionally, nurses' roles were based on social expectations of female service, deference, and the duty to care. This changed radically with unionization and professional self-regulation, although for historical reasons, the nursing profession remains more fragmented than medicine in terms of professional representation. Further, while physicians' associations generally tend to work closely with governments at the policy-making stage, nurses' organizations are not as closely consulted and therefore their political role tends to be more oppositional. The type of work done by nurses is also qualitatively different than that of physicians; they do not simply do less of the same thing. For example, there is more emphasis, in nursing, on the interpersonal aspects of 'care,' rather than simply biomedical treatments (although, interestingly, female physicians also tend to report that they place more emphasis on such interpersonal dimensions of care).

These characteristics become significant when looking at the kinds of reforms implemented within health care systems in the past two decades. Health service reform has been based on the business-oriented theories of 'new public management.' The problem, as Armstrong and Armstrong (2002: 5) succinctly note, is that business practices 'fail to recognize the specific characteristics of care work.' The care-based model emphasizes 'skill acquisition, continuous learning through practice, clinical autonomy, accountability through judgements based on evidence, as well as peer or (less often) citizen review, and collaboration through teams with complementary skills.' The business-based model of nursing 'emphasizes a division of labour based on quickly learned tasks, accountability through evidence-determined practices and managerial control, and substitution of lower-skilled for higher-skilled providers, as well as flexibility in assigning providers to tasks' (ibid., 6). While the two models do exhibit some overlap, nurses increasingly report that reforms in health care organization and work design 'have been designed to emulate industrial models of productivity improvement, rather than to address nurses' concerns' (Aiken et al. 2001: 51). Thus nurses find themselves working part-time rather than being able to find secure full-time employment; they have no say in scheduling shifts; they spend more time on administrative matters than on personal care; they are expected to perform functions for which they are overqualified; they are not given enough time adequately to address the needs of each individual patient; they are given little or no opportunity to participate in decision making; they face hostile or indifferent management; and so on.

In an administrative system in which outcomes and results must be quantified and measured, a profession in which quality of interpersonal care is emphasized becomes difficult to defend and promote. However, this point also underscores the fact that the ultimate interests of health care professionals and patients are generally not mutually exclusive. Obviously there is competition for resources – if doctors and nurses are paid more, does this mean there will be fewer beds or fewer MRI machines available? But not all human resource issues are resource-based. Focusing on the 'broader context in which professional practice takes place' may be a more useful strategy in the long run than offering financial incentives (such as raises or bonuses) which some health care systems can ill-afford. Social, organizational, and professional aspects of work design may have more success in recruiting and retaining health care personnel across the professions. In policy terms, focusing on factors like skill mix, autonomy in patient care, flexible work arrangements, and opportunities for collaboration 'all improve job satisfaction and the likelihood of maintaining labour force attachment' (Fooks et al. 2002:11).

Ironically, there is evidence that provincial governments' policy choices have had precisely the opposite effect. In a study examining how Ontario's managed competition reforms in the home-care sector affected the professional autonomy of rehabilitation workers, Randall and Williams (2009) conclude that the imposition of business-based models lowered the sense of control that workers had over their ability to provide good-quality care. In conditions where an emphasis on 'service volume and the drive to reduce unit costs had trumped quality,' fewer individuals were drawn to the home-care sector, which meant that the market drove up wages to address these shortages. Deteriorating working conditions led to 'some countervailing gains in terms of job mobility and wages' (66). Thus, the authors point out, the perverse result of a business-oriented strategy to decrease costs was actually 'fewer services at higher cost' (66) with, one would assume, a dissatisfied and unstable workforce.

In conclusion, human health resource issues reach far beyond merely hiring more doctors. The biggest variable, and the factor with the biggest potential for change, is the reorganization of the system in which physicians and other health professionals work. It involves the restructuring of disciplinary boundaries, the integration of facilities, the way in which health care workers are treated, the way in which information technology can be utilized, and so on. There are also issues of ethical recruitment, data collection concerning each profession, and the statistical modelling used to make long-term plans. It also involves thinking about the way in which overarching health system delivery (including primary care and long-term care) should be structured. Of course, we can also hire more doctors. But then there must be a discussion of the trade-offs that will result. Do we pay more for a higher doctor-population ratio, even though there is no clear evidence that this will result in better health outcomes, or that new doctors will work in underserviced areas? Or will doctors simply agree to work for less? Countries such as France, Greece, Finland, or the Czech Republic, all of which have far more doctors than Canada, also pay them much less (there's a question for the next president of the Canadian Medical Association). Much debate over the way in which health services are staffed depends on the collection of statistical information that is still in its infancy – is the use of non-physician health professionals clinically effective and cost-effective? But much of the intransigence over change also comes from political competition between professional groups (e.g., over regulatory power) and between political jurisdictions – why should *we* train more nurses or physicians if *you* just poach them from us when they graduate? Not least, it also comes from the destructive simplicity required by modern electoral campaigns – no emergency physician at your local hospital? Just elect us – we'll hire more doctors!

7 Drugs and Drug Policy

Lucentis is a drug that was approved by Health Canada in 2007 to treat wet macular degeneration (WMD). Usually WMD occurs in older individuals, who are generally insured for pharmaceuticals under provincial health plans. The drug is considered to be quite effective. It is also extremely expensive, costing approximately $2,000 per individual per month. Before Lucentis (ranibizumab) was approved, however, doctors used a drug called Avastin (bevacizumab) to treat the same condition. Avastin is approved only to treat colorectal cancer, but has been widely used off-label for the treatment of WMD by doctors who have reported successful results. It costs approximately $150 per patient per month. The first question that arises here is whether provincial departments of health should cover the higher cost of Lucentis (thereby limiting the amount of funds available for other health care services) or offer only Avastin, a drug that has not been studied as rigorously as Lucentis for WMD. According to the *British Journal of Ophthalmology*, because Lucentis is substantially more expensive than Avastin, it would also have to be considerably more effective to justify the additional expense. Researchers have calculated that this level of effectiveness is not evident (Raftery et al. 2007).

The second question is what political dynamics underlie the administrative issues determining which drug should be covered under provincial health insurance. The Canadian National Institute for the Blind (CNIB) has been lobbying for governments to cover Lucentis. The CNIB has also received a substantial grant from Novartis, the company that markets Lucentis. Interestingly, the company that makes Lucentis – Genentech – also produces Avastin. But Avastin is generally manufactured in larger doses for the treatment of colorectal cancer; for use in

WMD it must be sent to compounding pharmacies to repackage the drug to be injected directly into the eye. In 2007 Genentech halted delivery of Avastin to these compound pharmacies, obliging eye doctors to use Lucentis when supplies of low-dosage Avastin became less available (the company later relented under pressure from ophthalmologists). Genentech also refused to fund clinical trials for Avastin, noting that the higher cost of Lucentis was related to the design and testing of Lucentis to make it as safe and as effective as possible for WMD (the high doses of Avastin used in the treatment of cancer can increase the risk of heart attack and stroke, but it is unknown whether the smaller doses used for WMD pose the same risks). The wealthier provinces have been quicker to cover Lucentis; the smaller provinces have been more cautious in doing so and have therefore faced a tremendous amount of political pressure in their consideration of coverage. The media have been quick to print stories of individuals denied coverage of Lucentis. But there is much less explanation by the media that the drug that *is* covered may be more cost-effective.

This particular debate may well be settled soon: in 2008, the National Eye Institute in the United States announced a new study undertaking a comparison of the two drugs in the treatment of WMD. It hopes to report its findings in 2011. But the story of Lucentis and Avantis highlights the crucial role that new pharmaceuticals play in the provision of health care, and in the political dynamics underlying the development, marketing, prescribing, and utilization of these drugs. Next to hospital costs, spending on drugs is the largest category of health care expenditure in Canada. Total spending for pharmaceutical products in Canada reached approximately $30 billion by 2009 (CIHI 2010: 6), with costs escalating every year. Much of health care itself is increasingly defined by the use of therapeutic drugs: where many medical conditions were once treated through invasive surgical procedures or long hospital stays, modern drugs have dramatically restructured the delivery of contemporary health services by facilitating treatment on an outpatient basis. This has been a very positive trend, as a brief consultation with a physician who prescribes a course of drugs is significantly less expensive than a protracted hospital visit. Nonetheless, the rise of pharmaceutical-based medicine has had two considerable implications for Canadian health care.

The first has been the shift in treatment costs from the public to the private sector. The Canada Health Act (CHA) was designed at the very cusp of the pharmaceutical revolution, and it reflects the way that health care was provided in the first half of the twentieth century. In that period many conditions (such as a removal of cancerous tumours) required extensive surgery, which in turn, meant long convalescent periods under medical observation. Other conditions (like tuberculosis or psychosis) had no effective intervention, and treatment consisted of institutionalized segregation and monitoring. The focus in either instance was on hospitals as the front line for medical treatment, and this emphasis is reflected in the articulation of the Canada Health Act, which ensures that hospital visits are publicly insured. Pharmaceuticals are not insured under the CHA. Medically necessary drugs are provided free at point of delivery to patients only within hospitals: once individuals are treated on an outpatient basis, they are generally required to fund their own course of drug treatment. Sixty-two per cent of therapeutic drugs in Canada are bought within the private sector, either out-of-pocket or through private insurance policies (CIHI 2010: 10). Thus, as drugs are increasingly prescribed, as drug costs increase, and as outpatient treatment is emphasized, there is a substantial 'creeping privatization' of health care in Canada. There have been many attempts to include publicly insured drug costs within the CHA (e.g., Romanow 2002), but the political barriers to expanding an already beleaguered public health care plan are substantial.

The second implication of the pharmaceutical revolution for Canadian health care is the balance of political power held by pharmaceutical companies. By 2015 the global market for prescription drugs is expected to reach U.S.$897 billion (*Pharmaceutical Online*, 2 July 2009), and the global pharmaceutical industry is heavily concentrated within ten to twenty multinational corporations. Both the size and the international mobility of these companies mean that the regulation of this industry is extraordinarily difficult. It is made even more problematic by the nature of the product, as modern pharmaceuticals are (unlike shoes or toasters) highly complex entities, requiring a high level of expertise to evaluate their efficacy, safety, and cost-effectiveness. They are often discussed in an emotionally heightened context, given their potential to save (or destroy) human lives. Few would deny the utility of modern pharmaceuticals. But on what terms do we accept them? In what ways are the pharmaceutical corporations able to exploit their economic and political influence, and what mechanisms can be employed to achieve a suitable balance between technological innovation and political oversight?

The Debate over Pharmacare

One of the most often cited reasons for the superiority of European models of health care over Canada's public health care system is the fact that most people in most European countries have at least some drug coverage. Many Canadians do not; and media stories of anguished individuals being forced to choose between buying medically essential drugs or providing for their families are not uncommon. This problem is especially pronounced in Atlantic Canada, where 27 per cent of residents only have partial coverage against catastrophic drug costs (Metge and Sketris 2007: 136). The discussion over whether to provide publicly insured, universally accessible drugs is as old as the current health care system: the 1964 Royal Commission on Health Services (which served as the blueprint for Canada's health system) also recommended moving towards a national pharmacare framework, in which approved pharmaceutical products would be placed in a public formulary and would be covered for all Canadian citizens. But the government chose to wait for drug prices to stabilize before designing such a system. It waits still. In the early 1970s, the spending on drugs hit a high of 2 per cent of total health care spending, causing much concern. By 2009 the share of total health spending dedicated to drugs reached 16.4 per cent (CIHI 2010: 3).

The call to establish a national pharmacare program was sounded again in 1997 by the National Forum on Health and in 2002 by the Romanow Commission Report. While the provincial governments attempted repeatedly to persuade Ottawa to commit to pharmacare, the federal government refused this on the grounds of cost. The provinces themselves were divided in their support for pharmacare: while Saskatchewan and British Columbia remained enthusiastic, Ontario and Newfoundland had much less interest in pursuing the policy. Pharmacare reappeared on the agenda as part of the 2004 *10-Year Plan to Strengthen Health Care*. A Federal/Provincial/Territorial Ministerial task force was charged with developing a National Pharmaceuticals Strategy to establish a collaborative policy on therapeutic pharmaceuticals. Since 2006 there has been no official communication of progress on this task (MacPherson and Kenny 2009).

This is not to say that Canadians are uninsured for drug coverage. Approximately a third of Canadians are covered publicly for pharmaceuticals, and roughly one-half of working-age Canadians have employment-based private drug insurance (Morgan 2008: 206). Politically, this is part of the problem. Those who have drug coverage do not see phar-macare as an urgent policy area; while those with no coverage often have a weak political voice. The political barriers are also reinforced by regional disparities, as the provinces with better provincial plans would not want to participate in a national program that was less robust than their own, nor would they be happy to subsidize the program for the poorer provinces.

Drug coverage for individuals outside of hospitals is currently deter-mined by each province, and the programs and coverage between provinces differ substantially. Some provinces (such as British Columbia, Manitoba, and Saskatchewan) have public needs-based pro-grams, where individuals who cannot afford their prescription drug costs have coverage. Other provinces (such as Nova Scotia and the Yukon) have public pharmacare programs for seniors, regardless of their health status or income. Quebec has a 'mandated' system, which means that everyone is required to purchase premium-based drug insurance, either public (for low-income residents and seniors) or pri-vate (generally through their place of work). While the Saskatchewan government promised to improve universal coverage in 2007 (by lim-iting co-payments), they were defeated in the provincial election and the proposal has evaporated. Catastrophic drug coverage, a policy espoused by both the Romanow and Kirby commissions, has been implemented differently in each province, with no coordinating frame-works or benchmarks between them. But if substantial drug coverage already exists in Canada, what's the problem? There are three reasons that pharmacare has remained on the political agenda for so long, and will continue to do so.

The main barrier to the implementation of a national pharmacare strategy has always been *the issue of cost*. Current estimates for a Canadian pharmacare program range from between $7 to $12 billion per year (CBC 2004) and $8 to $19 billion per year (Marchildon 2006: 104). A national pharmacare system, however, also has the ability sharply to lower drug costs. Just as a system of private insurance for health services keeps prices high because of the administrative costs, marketing and advertising expenses, the need to produce profits, and the diminution of buying power due to fragmentation, dependence on private drug insurance also allows costs to remain higher. Where a sin-gle buyer purchases product from a manufacturer, it is able to demand better prices than numerous small purchasers. New Zealand, for exam-ple, has been able to use its purchasing power to cut its drug budget by almost half, while Australia's Pharmaceutical Benefits Scheme is able to keep drugs prices well below those in Canada (Lexchin 2007a: 265). Not only is a single purchaser able to negotiate lower prices on drugs, but it is more rigorous in the drugs it selects, demanding proven performance and cost-effectiveness to get a place on the national formulary. (It is noteworthy that Medicare, the largest single purchaser of drugs in the United States, is forbidden by law to use its purchasing power to negotiate lower prices with drug companies.) Canada's buying power is fragmented between thirteen provinces and territories, which purchase half of the drugs Canadians use; the federal government, which is responsible for discrete populations such as Aboriginal groups and those in the military; numerous private insurance companies, which purchase over a third of these pharmaceuticals; and countless individuals, who pay directly out of pocket. 'Even allowing for increased use of prescription drugs by groups now not covered at all or under-covered,' argues Lexchin, a national pharmacare system would mean that 'total spending on medications would actually *drop* by between 9 and 10 per cent because of lower administrative costs and the lower prices that could be achieve through national bargaining power' (2008: 266; original emphasis).

The argument for a national pharmacare strategy also mirrors the justification for a national 'medicare' program in terms of *equity* as well as cost containment. To the extent that drugs are now a substantial and integral aspect of medical treatment (as was access to physicians and hospitals in the last century), tolerating inequality across region and income level flies in the face of having a public health care system at all. Individuals in some provinces, such as those in the Atlantic region, simply do not have access to the same level of pharmaceutical care as those in other provinces, unless they can afford private health insurance for drugs, or can pay out of pocket. A recent study published in the *Canadian Medical Association Journal* developed various hypothetical 'avatars' with specific conditions, then calculated how much their drug costs would be in each province. The same senior citizen with a heart condition would pay over $600 in British Columbia for the required prescription drugs, compared with $400 in Alberta, over $1,300 in Saskatchewan and Manitoba, less than $200 in Ontario, almost $900 in Quebec, under $100 in New Brunswick, close to $400 in Nova Scotia, under $100 in Prince Edward Island, and $1,300 in Newfoundland. A 40-year-old with high blood pressure, who lives on social assistance, would pay nothing in British Columbia, Alberta, Manitoba, Prince

Edward Island, or Newfoundland and Labrador, but would have to pay $8 in Saskatchewan, $8 in Ontario, $200 in Quebec, $16 in New Brunswick, and $20 in Nova Scotia (Demers et al. 2008). Moral suasion regarding the unfairness of this situation becomes diluted, of course, when it involves real costs to fix. But, as Marchildon (2006) points out, pharmacare could also address a third axis of inequity (beyond that between individuals and between provinces). This axis of inequity is the vertical fiscal imbalance. To the extent that all provincial leaders are solidly unified in their position that Ottawa has the funds to pay for health care while the provinces have the responsibility, pharmacare would be an effective means of redistributing health care funds vertically while being 'of particular benefit to "have not" provinces that can least afford such a rapidly growing program' (ibid., 102).

A third reason presented by proponents of pharmacare is that a national pharmaceuticals strategy has the capacity to facilitate *coordination* of various aspects of pharmaceutical policy that are currently addressed through a number of agencies and committees at federal, provincial, and territorial levels. The federal government, explains Marchildon, 'has virtually all the regulatory tools, while the provinces are responsible for designing, administering, and funding their respective prescription drug subsidy plans. Alone, neither order of government is capable of addressing the financial sustainability problem or initiating thoroughgoing change in drug utilization patterns' (2006: 97). One aspect of the disjuncture between regulatory and purchasing functions focuses on the utilization of particular drugs. Some drugs, for example, are released on the market early and require 'post-marketing' surveillance; some expensive drugs that are heavily marketed have no real improvements over cheaper existing drugs; and so on. A national pharmacare system with a single formulary would be much more efficient at communicating prescribing guidelines to physicians (Lexchin 2008: 263).

Since 2002 Canada has had a Common Drug Review, exercised under the authority of the Canadian Agency for Drugs and Technologies in Health (CADTH). The purpose of the process is to evaluate the clinical- and cost-effectiveness of new drugs (in comparison with existing drugs) and to provide advice to the eighteen publicly funded drug plans in Canada. It has no regulatory authority. In January 2009 Ottawa announced the creation of a Drug Safety and Effectiveness Network, the purpose of which is to monitor the safety of prescription drugs *after* they have received marketing approval. This is especially important given that the approval process for new drugs can be 'fast tracked' under recent regulatory changes. Notwithstanding these developments, there is little progress in the development of a pan-Canadian pharmaceuticals strategy (Health Council of Canada 2008). This means that there is still little coordination between the active players in this area. There is, for example, no articulation of how the Drug Safety and Effectiveness Network will interact with Health Canada's proposed progressive licensing framework for newly approved drugs; nor is there any coordination between the active provincial pharmaceutical strategies (such as Ontario's Transparent Drug System for Patients Act) and the Common Drug Review, which means that these systems could potentially end up acting at cross-purposes (MacKinnon and Ip 2009).

The question invariably arises: if a national pharmacare program is such a good idea, why don't we have one? The most evident reason would seem to be cost. However, as noted above, there are good reasons to suggest that pharmacare would be an effective means of *controlling* costs. A more specific explanation of the cost barrier is that it does not fit the political timetable particularly well. A solid majority government confident of at least two terms in office might consider the implementation of a pharmacare program to be a reasonable political investment, as the up-front costs could be justified over time with reference to a slowdown in the rate of growth over a period of years. A minority government of any stripe fighting for survival, especially during inauspicious economic times, would see no conceivable political payback for such a scheme. Furthermore, cost is not the only consideration for provinces. Shifting provincial plans to a federal level also means giving up sovereignty in a relatively substantial area, regardless of the cost savings. Many provinces, despite the expense involved, prefer being in control of important policy areas. In some cases (such as Quebec) this is done on principle; in other cases provinces are wary, given the lessons of history, about the untrammelled capacity of the federal government to require provinces to shoulder more of the costs by unexpectedly backing away from established programs. Ottawa, for its part, is leery (again given historical experiences) of committing itself to a program that seems to augur continual and unrelenting cost increases, and that has the potential to cause even more disputational headaches from querulous provinces. The majority of individual Canadians who have drug coverage do not see the point of major policy implementation to keep what, from their perspective, is the status quo;

and others are opposed on the grounds that a more rigorous public plan would limit the variety of drugs available to them by excluding either brand-name drugs in favour of generics, or expensive new generation drugs (that may not, in fact, perform substantially better than older, less expensive ones). Finally, governments at both the federal and provincial levels are often wary of offending pharmaceutical companies themselves. A national pharmacare program could be effective both because of its relative strength as a purchaser and because of its access to a large body of clinical and academic expertise which can evaluate drugs independently of corporate claims. But when pharmaceutical firms are seen as 'good corporate citizens' by governments (providing jobs, taxes, and publicity) there is much less willingness to step on their toes by implementing a program that would disadvantage such strategic corporate allies.

Regulating the Pharmaceutical Industry

Canadians spent a total of $25.4 billion on prescription drugs in 2009: an average of almost *$70 million per day*. This amounted to $755.62 per person annually, although the regional variation reflected a high of $908.20 per person (in Newfoundland) and a low of $571.11 per person (in the Northwest Territories). The total figure represented an increase of $1.4 billion over the previous year, despite the fact that an increasing percentage of prescription drugs were generic rather than brand-name products (CIHI 2010). That drug utilization is becoming a dramatically larger component of health care costs is one reason to keep a sharp eye on the production and marketing of pharmaceuticals. It is useful to keep in mind how important it is for pharmaceutical companies to have high-performing drugs in their inventory: the most profitable drug firm in Canada, Pfizer, had three of the most popular drugs in 2009; the next most profitable company, Apotex (a generic drug manufacturer) produced six of the most commonly prescribed drugs; the third most profitable, AstraZeneca, had only two on the list, but one of these is a popular cholesterol-lowering drug. Novopharm, the fourth most profitable, also had only two drugs on the list, but one is a generic form of the popular anti-depressant Effexor (see Tables 7.1 and 7.2).

Another reason to scrutinize the pharmaceutical industry carefully is the spate of high-profile court cases that have begun to document some of the more dubious practices of the pharmaceutical corporations themselves. Perhaps the most visible of these legal battles has been

Table 7.1 The Top 20 Dispensed Drugs in Canada, 2009

Rank 2009	Name of Drug	Use	Total Prescriptions 2009 (000s)	% Change over 2008
1	Lipitor	Cholesterol lowering	15,440	2.9
2	Synthroid	Hypothyroidism	12,133	5.8
3	Crestor	Cholesterol lowering	7,711	26.7
4	Norvasc	Antihypertensive	5,958	−22.9
5	Ratio-Salbutamol H	Asthma	4,552	−1.6
6	Novo-Venlafaxine Xr	Antidepressant	4,399	−6.0
7	Apo-Ramipril	Antihypertensive	4,328	−11.2
8	Apo-Furosemide	Diuretic	4,041	−1.5
9	Nexium	Excess stomach acid	3,534	14.1
10	Actonel	Bone metabolism regulator	3,216	10.2
11	Plavix	Antiplatelet	3,068	6.9
12	Novamoxin	Penicillin/antibiotic	2,701	19.4
13	Apo-Hydro	Diuretic	2,678	−10.0
14	Ativan	Tranquillizer	2,677	1.0
15	Adalat Xl	Antihypertensive	2,619	−12.9
16	Apo-Lorazepam	Tranquillizer	2,603	3.9
17	Celebrex	Antiarthritic	2,534	1.3
18	Apo-Amitriptyline	Antidepressant	2,485	−3.1
19	Tylenol #3	Analgesic	2,478	−9.9
20	Coversyl	Antihypertensive	2,359	25.1

Source: IMS Health, 2010b.

Table 7. 2 Top 10 Pharmaceutical Corporations in Canada, 2009

Rank 2009	Company	Purchases by Pharmacies and Hospitals ($ million)	% Change over 2008
1	Pfizer	2,541	−1.2
2	Apotex	1,607	5.7
3	AstraZeneca	1,399	4.7
4	Novopharm	893	7
5	GlaxoSmithKline	841	−0.4
6	Novartis	799	14.2
7	Schering-Plough	743	92
8	Roche	673	7.9
9	Jannsen-Ortho	610	0.3
10	Merck Frosst	551	10.6

Source: IMS Health, 2010b.

over Vioxx (rofecoxib), an anti-inflammatory painkiller produced by Merck that was claimed to have fewer gastrointestinal side effects than existing analgesics. An academic study performed in 1996–7 showed some evidence that the drug might involve some cardiovascular risk, but Merck persuaded the scientists to 'soften' their clinical interpretation of the results. The company then submitted its initial set of studies to the U.S. Food and Drug Administration (FDA) in 1998 without any attempt to evaluate cardiovascular risk. A clinical trial of Vioxx set up in 1999, involving over 8,000 patients, was implemented with no standard operating procedure for gathering data on possible cardiovascular side effects, and without the participation of a cardiologist on the monitoring board. The subsequent data was, according to the lawsuit, manipulated by Merck to minimize cardiovascular side effects. Sceptical academic scientists faced pressure from the company, and the journal articles appearing in support of the drug were later found to have been written by authors other than those whose names were appended to them. Evidence presented in court also showed that Merck set up a journal, the *Australasian Journal of Bone & Joint Medicine*, solely for the purpose of publishing studies supporting the claims of its drug. Facing a class action lawsuit from 30,000 individuals, Merck settled the case in 2007 for U.S.$4.85 billion, later facing an additional lawsuit from shareholders (Krumholz et al. 2007; Moynihan 2009). A study published in the *Annals of Internal Medicine* in 2009 argues that heart risks for those using Vioxx became apparent in internal drug studies as early as 2000, but that Merck waited until 2004 to withdraw the drug. Had this information been publicly accessible, comment the study's authors, cardiovascular risk associated with the drug could have been identified much earlier (Ross et al. 2009).

A second case involves Paxil (paroxetine), an antidepressant marketed by GlaxoSmithKline (GSK) for use in adolescents, even though its own research indicated the drug had no specific benefits for this group and even resulted in an increase in self-harming behaviour. An inquiry by a BBC investigative journalism program presented evidence that the company manipulated the research and marketing of the drug and paid large amounts of money to promote the product, and even 'lied to the media when pressed about the product's side effects' (Collier 2007: 209). In 2004 the state attorney of New York filed a civil suit against GSK, charging the company with 'repeated and persistent fraud' for concealing clinical study results. GSK agreed to a U.S.$64 million settlement in April 2007. In 2008 a major academic spokesman for GSK, Charles

Nemeroff, lost his position as chair of the Department of Psychiatry at Emory University for failing to disclose more than U.S.$800,000 he had received from GSK between 2000 and 2007 (Dyer 2004; Tanne 2009a).

A third case concerns the pharmaceutical corporation Eli Lilly, whose drug Zyprexa (olanzapine), its best-selling drug, boasts total sales of over U.S.$30 million. In 2007 the attorneys general of Florida and California filed civil investigation demands to determine whether Eli Lilly had concealed data indicating a serious risk of side effects. The company was also required to disclose internal documents to ascertain whether the company was deliberately marketing the drug for a medical condition (dementia) for which it was not approved. One of the company's internal memos stated that 'dementia should be the first message' to general practitioners, even though the FDA now warns that the drug can increase the risk of death in individuals with dementia. In 2005 Eli Lilly agreed to a U.S.$700 million settlement with 8,000 claimants, and in 2007 the company announced a settlement with another 18,000 claimants for a sum 'not expected to exceed $500 million' (Dyer 2007). In 2009 Eli Lilly was found guilty for illegally marking Zyprexa for off-label use, and was fined U.S.$1.42 billion.

Two issues must be considered here in tandem: why do pharmaceutical industries have the influence they do, and how do they use their influence to maintain their position? All business organizations seek profits; that is, by definition, what they do. But drugs and drug companies are different. Large multinational companies have the resources to engage in behaviour that small ones do not (by, for example, exercising their 'mobility threat' to take their business – and potentially lucrative tax payments – elsewhere; or by engaging large teams of expensive legal counsel; or by engaging in extraterritorial activity, which involves the head office controlling the activity of its international branches). It is fitting that large multinational corporations must endure greater scrutiny because of this (Levitt 1970; Gilpin 1975). Canada's largest drug company, Pfizer, for example, has a global worth greater than the domestic listed equity market of many countries (Henry and Lexchin 2002: 1591). Pharmaceutical corporations are also different because of the nature of what they produce: as drugs have a much greater potential impact on consumers than, say, basketballs or barbeques, regulatory standards must be able to protect those who buy and use these products. Thus, while pharmaceutical companies should not be expected to operate like public service organizations, they must expect to be treated with a high level of scrutiny and to meet a high level of accountability.

Like other corporations, the pharmaceutical industry experienced a rapid period of growth from the 1980s, due in part to a period of economic restructuring that included the lowering of relative corporate tax rates, deregulation, and the growth of international trade. At the same time, the industry was successful in medicalizing conditions, from shyness to premenstrual irritability to sexual languor, which previous generations had viewed more as aspects of character than as illnesses to be treated. Relatively stable from 1960 to 1980, pharmaceutical sales tripled between 1980 and 2000, becoming by far the most profitable industry in the United States (Angell 2005: 3). But regulation of the pharmaceutical sector has not been easy. For over two decades the ideological paradigm (ushered in by the 'new right') assumed that self-regulation is both effective (what company would engage in practices that would alienate its own customer base?) and integral to economic growth. Scrutiny of the drug industry is also difficult given the high level of technical knowledge required to evaluate the product and the limited number of people with the expertise to judge the merits of particular drugs.

In the past, physicians were seen as the front line of defence against problematic drugs, but given the huge increase in the number of drugs and the number of people prescribed drugs (as well as physicians' increasing patient loads), it has become unrealistic to expect doctors to maintain an encyclopedic knowledge of all current drugs, including potential side effects or the thoroughness of clinical trials. As Sketris et al. (2007) observe, Canadian physicians in 2005 had 322 million patient visits in their offices (of which 94% resulted in handwritten paper records), and they wrote 400 million prescriptions dispensed by pharmacies. They could prescribe from 22,000 products on the market, and saw the introduction of twenty-four new active products on the market that year, with sixteen more substances reported. They could stay up to date on 300,000 clinical trials by reading 1.8 million papers published in 2004 (ibid., 8). Depending on doctors alone to keep vigil over the safety and effectiveness of the drugs they prescribe is both unreasonable and ineffective.

Pharmaceutical policy in Canada is further weakened by the fragmentation of political jurisdictions, both regional and regulatory. While provinces are responsible for paying for many drugs (through their hospitals and drug plans), Ottawa has full competence to set laws and standards governing the pharmaceutical industry. Thus, in 2008, when the federal government announced its intention to further expand the patent protection of brand-name drugs, provinces charged that the move would put severe economic strain on their health care budgets by preventing them from accessing cheaper generic copies of these drugs. The provinces were not consulted on this measure prior to the announcement, and were given half the usual time to respond to the policy announcement. In reply, Ottawa declared that the move was important to meet 'the pharmaceutical industry's need to have confidence in Canada as a place to invest in research and development' (Galloway 2008: A8).

Pharmaceutical policy in Canada is also determined by two factors that have shaped Canadian policy for over two hundred years: proximity to the United States and regional politics. American foreign policy was the key influence on Canada's drug policy during the Free Trade Agreement of the mid-1980s. The United States became concerned that Canada's 'weak' protection of intellectual property rights threatened the American pharmaceutical sector, and appointed the president of Pfizer to lead the American trade advisory panel. Patent protection for pharmaceuticals consequently played a large role in the bilateral talks over free trade, and in 1987 the Conservative government passed a bill strengthening patent protection in exchange for American support of the Free Trade Agreement. Despite dissatisfaction from many provinces, support from Quebec on patent protection was strong, as several pharmaceutical companies were located in Montreal, and the federal government was quite cognizant that failure to protect this sector could jeopardize its (then-sizeable) majority of seats in Quebec (Harrison 2004).

How the Pharmaceutical Sector Maintains Its Influence

The political influence of multinational pharmaceutical corporations is considerable, but it is not absolute. Nor is it the source of all problems related to the inappropriate use of drugs. Not all suboptimal prescribing practices, for example, should be seen as the result of nefarious corporate plotting (while the widespread use of Demerol in certain jurisdictions goes against effective prescribing practices, e.g., the drug industry has little to gain from its continued use). There are many variables that determine prescribing practices (see, e.g., Sketris et al. 2007). Moreover, the (largely domestic) field of generic drugs is becoming an increasingly important player given the increasing volume of generic drug sales (the cost of generic drugs is higher in Canada than in any developed country in the world except for the United States: see PMPRB 2007; Competition Bureau Canada 2008). Other private sector players, such as corporate pharmacy chains, also have an impact on government policy. Notwithstanding this, pharmaceutical companies can be powerful political players who have numerous ways of leveraging their influence.

There are four broad strategies that pharmaceutical companies employ in exercising their influence: financial, political, commercial, and scientific. In the first, drug firms use their economic resources to obtain their objectives; in the second, they become political actors and attempt to change the playing field (e.g., through favourable regulatory reforms). Commercial strategies focus on marketing and advertising tactics. The last stratagem is based on the scientific nature of drug testing and reporting: here, the issues focus on research design and the communication of results.

FINANCIAL INFLUENCE

The *financial influence* of corporations simply depends on the way in which these firms use their economic clout. This ranges enormously. On the one hand, it can be almost trivial, such as the way the publishing company Elsevier offered $25 Amazon gift cards to academics if they posted five-star reviews of its medical text on the book company's web site (Mooney 2009). On the other hand, it can be patently illegal, as in the way that Bristol-Myers Squibb paid physicians (in the form of 'consulting fees' and expenses) to induce them to purchase drugs produced by the company (Tanne 2007). But in between these two extremes there are a number of greyer instances of drug firms exerting influence through the dispensation of funds. The question has been the extent to which these industry handouts affect the behaviour of those receiving the funding, and whether this behaviour conflicts with the objectives of safe and effective health care provision.

There are at least six different funding relationships that pharmaceutical companies target. The first involves academic centres (including scientists); the second focuses on students within these institutions; the third looks at physicians and other health care professionals directly; the fourth revolves around industry-run educational seminars for health care providers; the fifth concentrates on academic or professional journals; and the sixth targets patients' advocacy groups.

To appreciate the impact of pharmaceutical firms on academic medical centres, one must understand the way in which academic institutions have been funded historically. Most regulatory mechanisms were developed at a time when universities – especially in Canada – were funded largely through public sources. But by the late 1980s, at the same time that free trade was negotiated and patent protection was increased, government monies decreased as a proportion of medical research funding, and pharmaceutical firms, flush with rising profits, rapidly increased their share of funding, giving rise to 'university-industry partnerships' (Schafer 2004). The problem was that universities increasingly began acting like private firms, with the transparency and accountability provisions popular in the new public management literature being conspicuously absent from university governance. As universities became able to profit directly from research conducted in their faculties, the rhetoric of 'intellectual property rights' and corporate security dominated discussions of transparency, due process, objectivity, individual safety, and public good; for a more detailed discussion of this trend see Downie and Herder (2007).

The turning point for universities in Canada occurred in 1996, when a medical researcher at the University of Toronto began having doubts about the safety of a drug she was evaluating in a clinical trial. But when Dr Nancy Olivieri articulated the need to inform patients receiving this drug as part of the clinical trial (as required by the university hospital's ethics board), the pharmaceutical company funding the study (Apotex) disagreed, noting that she had signed a confidentiality clause in her funding agreement with them. They refused to allow her to release this information. She did so regardless. Apotex threatened her with legal action and revoked her funding. The University of Toronto, rather than supporting her academic freedoms and protecting the well-being of her patients, relieved her of her position as head of the Hemoglobinopathy Research Program. Five years later, the College of Physicians and Surgeons of Ontario cleared her of all misconduct, concluding that 'Dr Olivieri ceased to administer [the drug] in a timely and expedient way, and in a manner which was in the best interest of her patients' (Viens and Savulescu 2004). In the course of this acrimonious dispute, it came to light that the University of Toronto was negotiating a twenty million dollar donation from Apotex. This was in addition to the company's ongoing funding of research performed at the university. It was also disclosed that the president of the University of Toronto had lobbied the prime minister of Canada in 1999 on behalf of Apotex (Schafer 2004). Just as the Olivieri case was being resolved, the University of Toronto became the focus of another case involving yet another large pharmaceutical company with ties to the university. A noted psychiatrist who had been hired to head the university's Centre for Addiction and Mental Health was dismissed a week after giving a talk at the university in which he expressed scepticism regarding the efficacy in using Prozac to treat adolescents and underlined the need for further investigation in this area. Just prior to his dismissal, Eli Lilly, the company manufacturing Prozac, donated $1.5 million dollars to the university's Centre for Addiction and Mental Health (ibid.).

The adverse publicity did lead the University of Toronto and other academic institutions to scrutinize contracts between researchers and industry partners more closely for potential conflicts of interest and to permit disclosure of risk when necessary. But it does not address the more opaque and intransigent problem of self-regulating behaviour on the part of institutions who depend so heavily on funding from the pharmaceutical industry. The issue is the extent to which any academic institution will stand up to a commercial interest on whom it is financially dependent. The problem exists for both academic administrations (those who govern the university as a whole) and individual researchers. Even the most morally fastidious scientist must be aware that, in a highly competitive research funding environment, research outcomes that undermine the commercial viability of a firm's product may also affect both his own prospects for receiving further funding from the company and career advancement within the university. Clear evidence that a drug has adverse side effects may be easy enough to declare with good conscience. But a more insidious problem exists when niggling anomalies arise which might, for an independent researcher, bear further investigation. For a scientist dependent on commercial funding, the intellectual curiosity in examining such outliers and anomalies might understandably be counterbalanced by an appreciation that such investigations might not be well received by those sponsoring the research. It is simple to leave well enough alone when the costs of curiosity are so pronounced. But, to the extent that scientific discovery is driven by the investigation of such anomalies, the commercialization of academic research shapes the direction of scientific discovery itself.

A further dynamic shaping the behaviour of medical research is the way in which academics are rewarded professionally as well as financially. An academic's curriculum vita is judged according to the number of publications he or she produces (which, as explained below, presents a motivation to append one's name to ghost-written articles) and the number of research dollars one can attract. Because scholars are so frequently compared and evaluated for a number of different reasons (promotion, tenure, and the awarding of research grants or prestigious chairs) it is useful to be able to reference quantitative indicators in making such decisions. What is lost, however, is the qualitative influence of a scholar's work: an academic who writes a book that shifts the way in which a discipline views itself, for example, may simply not be able to compete with an academic who receives vast sums from a pharmaceutical firm for developing a lucrative 'me-too' drug that has few advantages over older versions of the same drug. A scientific researcher with more grant dollars next to his name is often judged to be a better scholar, regardless of the merits of the research itself.

A second manifestation of the financial influence of pharmaceutical companies is the targeting of medical (or dental, pharmaceutical, or nurse practitioner) students with various forms of largesse. This can be either indirect (buildings and classrooms are named after corporate donors, plaques on walls recount the generosity of firms towards capital costs, classroom materials bear corporate logos) or direct (companies give students everything from pizza to textbooks to electronics to full scholarships). Does this affect the way that future doctors (or dentists, or pharmacists, or nurse practitioners) will view these corporations? A recent study published in the *Archives of Internal Medicine* found that 'subtle exposure to branded pharmaceutical promotional items influences implicit attitudes of medical students toward pharmaceutical brands' (Grande et al. 2009: 890). Senior medical students at the University of Pennsylvania (which has a policy of restricting gifts from drug firms to students) and the University of Miami (which does not) were asked to make clinical decisions regarding two similar drugs (Lipitor and Zocor). Students at the University of Miami were casually exposed to promotional items with the Lipitor logo (such as clipboards and notepaper) immediately prior to determining their results, while students at the University of Pennsylvania were not. Results showed that medical students exposed to the promotional material for Lipitor were much more likely to come to more favourable clinical conclusions about the drug. The Association of American Medical Colleges established a Task Force on Industry Funding of Medical Education, which called for a 'zero-tolerance approach to industry handouts' on the grounds that they compromised the 'autonomy, objectivity, and altruism' of medical professionals (Kondro 2008: 1651). In 2007 the American Medical Student Association (AMSA) developed an annual 'PharmFree scorecard' which gives letter grades to U.S. medical schools based on their policies regarding the influence of pharmaceutical corporations. Of 146 medical schools polled, only six received grades of 'A,' and twenty-three refused to respond (in 2009, the AMSA posted this scorecard online: see http://www.amsascorecard.org/). A WHO study looking at the way in which pharmacy and medical students were educated about drug promotion across several countries found that 'the lack of importance of drug promotion in medical and pharmacy education stands in stark contrast to the large volume of drug promotion targeting health professionals, and the body of empirical evidence indicating that promotion affects behaviours, health care quality and costs' (Mintzes 2005: 29).

A third strategy by pharmaceutical firms is to target practising physicians directly. While most physicians likely consider themselves to be objective and impervious to suggestion, numerous studies have found an unconscious bias of doctors towards companies that give them gifts. These handouts can take the form of meals, travel, golf club memberships, and so on. They can also take the form of free samples, a practice many general practitioners appreciate because it allows them to provide pharmaceutical treatments to patients who otherwise might not be able to afford them. Groves et al. (2003) compiled the results of forty papers published between 1986 and 2002 discussing the effects of drug samples on prescribing behaviour. 'Within the pharmaceutical industry,' state the authors, 'sampling is a critical driver in the production and adoption of new products' (ibid., 26; see also Spurling et al. 2010). It remains the most influential form of marketing by pharmaceutical companies. Researchers who have studied industry gifts to physicians explain that 'receiving gifts is associated with positive physician attitudes toward pharmaceutical representatives. Physicians who request additions to hospital drug formularies are more likely to have accepted free meals or travel funds from drug manufacturers. The rate of drug prescriptions by physicians increases substantially after they see sales representatives, attend company-sponsored symposia, or accept samples. The systematic review of the medical literature on gifting by Wazana found that an overwhelming majority of interactions had negative results on clinical care' (Brennan et al. 2006: 431). Pharmaceutical corporations have sophisticated modelling techniques which allow them in many cases to track the prescribing habits of individual physicians, and they employ cutting-edge marketing research to persuade physicians to prescribe their drugs. Nonetheless, corporate influence is simply one of several factors that affect the prescribing behaviour of physicians. Other variables include the nature and location of a physician's practice as well as the gender, age, and training of the physicians themselves; for a thorough discussion of physicians' prescribing behaviour, see Groves, MacKinnon, and Sketris (2009). Nevertheless, the pharmaceutical industry still views physicians as lucrative consumers and lobbies heavily to maintain its ties to physicians. In 2007, for example, U.S. senators Chuck Grassley and Herb Kohl introduced their Physician Payment Sunshine Act, which would make public all corporate handouts over U.S.$25, with fines from U.S.$10,000 to U.S.$100,000 for failing to disclose gifts received. Within a year, lobbying by the drug industry weakened the proposed bill to increase the disclosure threshold and to lower the penalties for non-reporting.

A related strategy is the practice of funding educational seminars for physicians. Physicians are expected to engage in a certain number of hours per year of 'continuing medical education' (CME), which gives them the opportunity to keep up with current treatments, practices, and products. But this process is potentially quite expensive, and pharmaceutical companies have become involved in the 'education' of doctors. While some of these educational programs can be run by non-profit groups or academic institutions, most are organized by private, for-profit 'continuing medical education companies' or 'speakers' bureaus,' which are, in turn, largely funded by pharmaceutical corporations (in the United Kingdom, e.g., about half of all continuing medical education has been funded by the pharmaceutical industry). These firms can, in turn, select the speakers that are used for the seminars or presentations given to physicians by the continuing medical education company. For example, a brochure given to drug firms by one CME company (HealthEd) assured drug firms that for less than $10,000 they could 'work with us to determine a topic that is on message for your product area' (Moynihan 2008a: 416). Rarely are the physicians attending such talks told of the direct involvement by the pharmaceutical industry in these CME programs. In 2000 alone, the drug industry sponsored 314,000 events in the United States specifically directed at physicians (Brennan et al. 2006).

A similar practice is the use of 'key industry leaders' or key opinion leaders by pharmaceutical companies to provide 'information and expertise' to fellow physicians. These key industry leaders generally specialize in the treatment of a particular condition, and they are courted by drug firms who often pay them between U.S.$2,500 and $3,000 or more to lecture on current treatment practices in their area of specialization.

Slides are often prepared for them by the sponsoring drug company. Defenders argue that the use of experts is vital in providing 'analysis, critique, and guidance to other doctors regarding the appropriate placement of a drug in clinical practice' (Buckwell 2008: 1404). They maintain the independence and integrity of the key opinion leaders, and point out that it is not in the interests of the pharmaceutical industry to have their products used improperly.

But claims of a free lunch are generally met with scepticism. Drug firms use sophisticated software to track the effect that key industry leaders have on the sales of their product in order, as one marketing study explained, to avoid 'wasting money on the wrong people' (Moynihan 2008b: 1403). Why has it taken so long to address this phenomenon? There is an assumption, based on the historical 'agency' model of physicians' roles, that doctors have not only the expertise but also the integrity to act in the best interests of patients at all times; however, this model was constructed well before pharmaceuticals played such an integral role in medical treatment, and well before the therapeutic drug industry became such a powerful player. Most individual physicians likely do have a strong sense of their own autonomy and clinical judgment. But pharmaceutical firms have access to an incomparable level of financial sweeteners, both in cash and in kind – clinicians can earn U.S.$25,000 per year in 'advisory fees' in promoting a company's product (Moynihan 2008b). Key industry leaders also receive visibility, influence, and prestige within their profession, as well as the additional income. How common is this practice? After facing pressure to disclose payments made to key opinion leaders, Merck listed payments of U.S.$3.7 million made to 1,078 American medical experts between July and September 2009 alone (Tanne 2009b).

The 'quid pro quo' is rarely stated explicitly, but it is understood. One assistant clinical professor of psychiatry recounted how he found himself promoting his sponsor's drug overenthusiastically, and when he began to be more moderate in his views a drug company representative visited him to inquire about his 'less enthusiastic' presentation. The experience made him aware how even those who engage in such activities with no intent at deception 'can nevertheless be slowly seduced into questionable behaviours, such as making pumped-up claims of drugs' effectiveness while failing to give full weight to side effects' (Lenzer and Brownlee 2008: 20). Also complicit in this practice, argues Angell, are the physicians attending such presentations who become used to the largesse at their disposal; these individuals recognize that, without the vast sums spent by the pharmaceutical industry in continuing medical education, they would likely have to bear these costs themselves (2005: 147).

The glare of publicity in the past few years has had an effect. Calls for transparency have increased substantially, as have demands that voluntary codes of practice be made mandatory. Critics are pushing for a greater clarification between 'consultants' and 'marketers' (there are clear laws preventing drug firms from marketing their products 'off-licence,' or for purposes for which official approval has not been given, although industry-paid 'consultants' can recommend the off-licence use of drugs without sanction). In July 2008 Pfizer announced that it would no longer be funding private for-profit continuing medical education companies; and in March 2009 the Royal College of Physicians in the United Kingdom published a report calling for continuing medical education to become independent of pharmaceutical sponsorship. This was followed by a report by the committee on conflict of interest of the U.S. National Institutes of Health, Institute of Medicine, that a mandatory national reporting program should be established to catalogue all industry payments to physicians, researchers, universities, and health institutions, and that a new system should be implemented for funding accredited continuing medical education free of industry influence (Lo and Field 2009).

But there are still other areas in which the pharmaceutical industry attempts to use its financial influence. These include, respectively, the financing of academic journals and the sponsorship of patient advocacy groups. Journals rely on the pharmaceutical industry in a number of ways: for advertising revenue, for the sponsorship of 'supplementary issues,' and even for content itself: between two-thirds and three-quarters of clinical drug trial results published in the largest American medical journals (*Journal of the American Medical Association, Annals of Internal Medicine,* and *the New England Journal of Medicine*) were funded by pharmaceutical firms (Smith 2005). Nevertheless, it should be noted that medical journals were among the first to organize against the influence of the pharmaceutical industry and to resist their decline into what the editor of the *Lancet* has called 'information laundering operations for the pharmaceutical industry' (Horton 2004). In 2005 the International Committee of Medical Journal Editors began to establish steps to ensure the integrity of published articles, including publishing details concerning potential conflicts of interest by the authors (especially whether they are funded by the firms whose drugs they investigate), requiring authors to be fully accountable for all information published, and requiring all drug trials submitted for publication to have been registered (more on this below).

Pharmaceutical companies also fund non-profit patient advocacy groups. The assumption is that 'there is nothing inherently wrong with patient groups taking money from the drug industry provided that it does not put them under pressure to adopt a position that they would otherwise not choose to take up' (Kent 2007: 934). Still, the issue of transparency remains problematic. Pharmaceutical firms have used patient support groups to add a veneer of impartiality to their marketing campaigns, or as allies in political campaigns. The question, again, becomes the extent to which such groups will become sufficiently dependent on such funding that they may 'look the other way' when troubling questions regarding the performance of their sponsor's drug arise (Mintzes 2007). Pharmaceutical sponsorship of patient groups may also bias groups' support for treatment options available to patients: an organization funded by a company manufacturing high blood pressure medication may not be inclined to tout the advantages of diet and exercise; while a group supported by a firm marketing antidepressants may decide not to promote the virtues of talk therapy as a treatment for mild depression. 'Is it coincidence,' asks one researcher, 'that pharma-funded groups focus their criticism of government on issues like "drug lag," formulary access to new drugs and the ban on direct-to-consumer advertising, while groups independent of the industry critique government partnerships with industry that have weakened the government's monitoring of drug safety and misleading claims?' (Batt 2005: 12).

POLITICAL INFLUENCE

The ability of pharmaceutical companies to exert a tremendous degree of economic leverage is the most obvious manifestation of their influence. But they also exercise considerable political power in their ability to affect a change on the social and political environment within which they operate. In 2003 confidential documents from the American pharmaceutical industry's trade association, the Pharmaceutical Research and Manufacturers of America (PhRMA), were published by the *New York Times*. These documents detailed how PhRMA intended to use its influence. U.S.$73 million was earmarked for lobbying at the federal level, and U.S.$49 million was targeted for the state level. But an additional one million dollars was to be used 'to change the Canadian health care system' (Angell 2005: 215). PhRMA also hired Gordon Gibson, the former American ambassador to Canada, to lobby the Canadian government to resist easing rules concerning the importation of cheaper Canadian drugs to the United States (Beckel 2009a).

The most straightforward way that pharmaceutical companies attempt to influence political decisions is through campaign financing. In the United States, pharmaceutical corporations make huge contributions to political parties. But in Canada, corporations are not allowed to make contributions to registered federal parties, although individuals owning or working for corporations can – in 2006 a federal Liberal candidate drew unwanted attention when it was reported that his campaign had received thousands of dollars in the names of children under the age of 18, including three whose parents were pharmaceutical industry executives (CBC 2006).

A more opaque method of political influence is the 'revolving door' phenomenon, in which executives from the pharmaceutical industry gain positions of influence in areas such as regulatory boards, academic institutions, and lobby firms. In Canada, for example, Merck Frosst hired the public relations firm Knowlton Hill to convince the federal government to buy its HPV vaccine Gardasil. Knowlton Hill utilized a number of its registered lobbyists for the task, including Ken Boessenkool, Prime Minister Stephen Harper's former senior policy adviser; Bob Lopinski, who once worked at the Ontario premier's office; and Jason Grier, former chief of staff to Ontario Health Minister George Smitherman. Ottawa agreed to spend $300 million to provide Gardasil to the provinces, even though some clinicians have argued that the money would have been more effectively spent if it had been used to improve cervical cancer screening (which could have the same epidemiological result as the vaccination program). Knowlton Hill, which represents such clients as Canada's Research-Based Pharmaceutical Companies (Rx&D), Merck Frosst Canada Ltd., and Pfizer Canada Inc., also hired Ian Brodie, who was until recently the prime minister's chief of staff. Capturing influential positions is a crucial means of setting the policy and institutional framework within which the pharmaceutical industry must work. One of Canada's few independent drug advisory bodies, the Therapeutics Initiative at the University of British Columbia, faced closure when a report recommended its 'replacement.' The task force that wrote the report consisted of some members connected to the pharmaceutical industry, one of whom who was a chief lobbyist for the industry in Canada (Moynihan 2008b).

The main goal of this strategy is 'regulatory capture,' in which the pharmaceutical industry uses its influence to ensure a favourable regulatory regime (see Abraham 2002a, 2002b). In Canada regulatory capture has been institutionalized in a form of 'clientele pluralism,' in which the country's drug regulatory agency becomes dependent on the industry for funds and for expertise. In some cases, the government works directly with the industry to develop policies, laws, or regulations (such as setting standards for manufacturing or codes for marketing practices); in other cases the industry directly funds the body that is supposed to regulate it (Lexchin 2001). In many instances (such as the government's announcement of regulations to speed the approval process to get drugs on to the market) the precise form of industry influence is much more opaque. In the United States corporate donations to politicians and political parties are big business (see Chapter 11).

The pharmaceutical industry is also involved in setting clinical guidelines. In the United States the development of guidelines determining how drugs should be used is not centralized but depends on the involvement of professional organizations or societies representing medical specialties, many of whom are funded directly by the pharmaceutical industry. Well over half of 192 authors of clinical guidelines surveyed reported ties to the companies whose drugs were being considered within these clinical guidelines (Baird 2003). The ability to expand prescribing guidelines means that more drugs can be prescribed for more conditions more often. While Viagra, for example, was initially developed for men with erectile dysfunction due to other underlying conditions (such as diabetes or prostate surgery), the drug is now commonly prescribed for 'any degree of erectile dysfunction, including rare or transitory failures to achieve or maintain erections' (Lexchin 2006: 430). This also illustrates the practice of 'evidence capture,' in which an interested party can define what constitutes proof that a particular condition exists, or that only a specific course of treatment is indicated. This is especially problematic with conditions such as heart disease, diabetes, or obesity, where pharmaceutical companies have little incentive to measure expensive new drugs against programs based on nutrition and exercise.

An even more troubling aspect of corporate behaviour is the attempt undertaken by firms to neutralize and discredit those who are critical of pharmaceutical companies' claims or tactics. Evidence disclosed in an Australian court in the trial of Merck (over their marketing of Vioxx) included company e-mails referring to 'a list of "problem" physicians that we must, at minimum, neutralize.' 'Neutralizing' referred, in some cases, to providing large sums of money to physicians for their research or as payment for lectures to entice them not to speak out. But in other cases it referred to attempts at discrediting the reputation of physicians and research scientists who were critical of pharmaceutical companies and their products. Another e-mail written by a Merck executive spoke of the need to 'seek out' critical voices 'and destroy them where they live.' The practice of academic stalking is varied; it can consist of threats to withdraw funding to institutions if critics are not brought into line, or it can employ other individuals in the same field to undermine and discredit the academic reputation of outspoken critics. Another document released at the Australian trial of Merck was a letter by a prominent professor of medicine at Stanford University who complained to the chief executive of Merck about 'a consistent pattern of intimidation' (Moynihan 2009: 849).

COMMERCIAL INFLUENCE
The marketing strategies employed by the pharmaceutical industry can also reinforce its influence. For example, because of a loophole in U.S. law, drug manufacturers can pay generic drug manufacturers not to produce cheaper generic clones of expensive drugs once the patent expires. Another tactic is direct-to-consumer advertising, which entices consumers to persuade their physicians to prescribe drugs that may not be necessary or may even be harmful. In the United States, pharmaceutical firms spent over U.S.$5 billion on direct-to-consumer advertising; and regulatory oversight of drug advertising is not particularly stringent. In New Zealand, the only other developed country that permits direct-to-consumer advertising, commercials are 'not independently assessed for balance or the scientific validity of the claims unless someone complains' (Toop and Mangin 2007: 694). But the target audience is generally not well enough informed to be able to launch effective complaints, and the process is time-consuming enough to dissuade many complainants. In Canada there are certain restrictions against pharmaceutical advertising to the general public (a commercial can discuss the condition and make a suggestion to 'talk to your doctor,' or it can reference a particular drug, but it cannot do both in the same commercial). In 2005 a Charter challenge was launched by CanWest Mediaworks, who argued that the statutory prohibition on direct-to-consumer advertising amounted to an infringement of their right to freedom of expression, but the case was indefinitely suspended in 2009 because of the company's financial

difficulties. Yet another tactic is 'stealth advertising,' in which viewers are not aware that a company has paid to promote its product. These can include the 'help seeking ads' noted above, which may appear as public service announcements; interviews with celebrities in which a product name arises in conversation; product placement; or even, some argue, uncritical journal articles.

Another marketing strategy is off-label marketing, in which pharmaceutical companies deliberately sell products for purposes for which they have not been approved. This is an illegal practice, but it is not uncommon because the fines imposed on drug companies are not always commensurate with the profits they stand to gain from the sale of drugs used off-label. (While physicians can prescribe drugs for purposes other than those approved by regulatory agencies, drug firms cannot actively promote these drugs for such purposes.) In 2009, for example, Pfizer was fined U.S.$2.3 billion for the off-label marketing of four drugs. The *New York Times* has commented that $2.3 billion represents less than three weeks of Pfizer sales (3 September 2009). This should also be viewed against the backdrop of sales worth U.S.$44.2 billion in 2008 alone. In 2004 Pfizer paid a U.S.$430 million settlement for the off-label marketing of Neurontin; but some have argued that off-label profits for the same drug amounted to U.S.$10 *billion* (Murphy 2009). Others suggest that pharmaceutical firms simply build potential fines into the cost of marketing drugs.

Because drugs are so much more lucrative when they are under patent (as they face no competition), it is in the interests of drug companies to extend the patent as long as possible. This process, often called 'evergreening,' attempts to renew or lengthen the patent period through a number of different strategies. Canada has, over time, experienced a lengthening of the legal patent period for pharmaceutical products. Bill C-22, passed in 1987, guaranteed seven years of patent protection; while Bill C-91, passed in 1993, extended this period to 20 years. Drug companies can also extend patent protection for individual drugs by developing 'me-too' products, which are very similar although not exactly the same as older variations: they may, for example, consist of a different concentration, delivery system, designated usage, or even colour and shape. If a brand-name company charges that a generic drug producer is violating the patent, an automatic 24-month extension of the patent is granted.

Often marketing strategies conflict with larger public health objectives. Drugs are generally developed – and even manufactured – according to profitability, not need. Antibiotics, for example, are a low-profit area because they are taken only for a brief period (usually 3 to 10 days) while 'lifestyle drugs' which address personality traits or a low-level sense of malaise can be taken indefinitely. Eli Lilly, for example, coloured Prozac pink and purple and marketed it to women for 'premenstrual dysphoric disorder,' charging consumers much higher prices than the generic form of Prozac now available. Bayer marketed Yaz, a contraceptive, for premenstrual dysphoric disorder as well as for acne, even though the drug contained drospirenone, which can lead to an increased risk of serious heart problems and other health issues in some individuals. In 2009 the U.S. Food and Drug Agency (along with the attorneys general of 27 states) required Bayer to change its advertising campaign; but the drug, which made U.S.$616 million for Bayer in 2008, is still widely advertised as a lifestyle drug for young women in the treatment of irritability, anger, 'markedly depressed moods,' and acne (Singer 2009a). The phenomenon of lifestyle drugs received much attention in 2007, when Australian artist Justine Cooper developed an advertising campaign for Havidol ('have it all'), which promised to alleviate symptoms of 'dysphoric social attention consumption deficit anxiety disorder' (DSACDAD). The mock YouTube campaign included glowing testimonials, a slogan ('when more is not enough'), and a list of side effects (including 'inter-species communication, dermal gloss, excessive salivation, and terminal smile': http://www.youtube.com/watch?v=sQw_cdhXGco).

SCIENTIFIC INFLUENCE

The debate over research bias and publication bias is at the heart of the current criticism of pharmaceutical companies, as it addresses the fundamental core of what constitutes scientific truth. Until the catalogue of dubious practices became documented by clinicians, medical journals, academics, and others there was an implicit trust in the veracity of the 'scientific method' clearly to determine what worked and what did not. One of the key standards of scientific proof is the condition of replication: an experiment, to be persuasive, needs to be able to show similar results when performed by other investigators using similar methods. In clinical trials, often involving thousands of individuals, replication is usually foregone in favour of a review of results. But this assumes full access to data, a thorough understanding of experimental design, and the objectivity of reviewers themselves. These conditions frequently do not exist, and there have been many problems in the collection, interpretation, and communication of the research results used to sell and prescribe quite powerful and expensive pharmaceutical products.

Intellectual issues can be divided into two categories: *research bias* and *publication bias*. Research bias involves manipulating the research design or data in order to come to a particular result. Clinical trials (which come after long periods of laboratory and animal studies) are generally divided into three phases: 'phase one' looks at the effects of the drug in healthy volunteers; 'phase two' uses patients who have the condition the drug is designed to treat; and 'phase three' generally expands the patient base onto a much larger scale. Occasionally 'phase four' studies, which involve post-marketing surveillance, are required for drugs that have been fast-tracked to market. Research bias can occur at any stage of the investigation.

One example of research bias can be found in *the composition of the group* under investigation: are drugs approved for use on women or children actually tested on women and children? And when drugs are targeted for seniors or those with severe health problems, are they tested on patients with multiple health problems (the condition many actual patients would have), or patients who only manifest the condition under investigation? The research design of clinical trials was developed in an academic environment, and it was constructed to determine the relations of causality as clearly as possible. Thus seniors with multiple health issues are commonly not included in clinical trials because their poor health clouds the direct determination of causality – which effect did *this* drug have on *this* condition? Critics point out, however, that drugs are often used in conditions that are anything but clear, and they argue that clinical trials focusing on explanatory models should at least be supplemented by trials focusing on pragmatic treatment situations (Zwarenstein and Treweek 2009).

Another question about the composition of the group asks whether the subjects actually *have* the condition under investigation – e.g., if the drug is used to treat 'severe acne,' do the participants actually have 'severe' as opposed to 'moderate' acne? Yet another basic question concerns *the trial size:* a positive result in a group of only twelve individuals is hardly as robust as a positive result in a group of twelve hundred. Also important is knowing how many participants left the group while the study was in progress (many individuals leaving a trial could indicate that they could not tolerate certain side effects, which would be important in understanding the full nature of the drug under investigation).

Another example of research bias is the use of *inappropriate compara-tors*. If a drug is only compared with a placebo, or dummy pill, rather than with drugs currently in use to treat a condition, we have little sense of the practical efficacy of the drug. If a simple dose of acetylsalicylic acid (Aspirin) is much better at treating a condition than a placebo, then the fact that a $100 pill is also 'much better' than a placebo does not say much for the drug under investigation (except that it is an expensive means of treating that condition). On the other hand, if the drug is only compared with the current treatment option but not with a placebo, then we do not have a sense of how effective *either* of these drugs is at treating the condition. If one drug under investigation ('Credulenza') is found to have slightly fewer side effects than the current treat-ment drug ('Dollarmycin') in treating condition X, there would seem to be good reason to approve the drug. But if both Credulenza and Dollarmycin show very little improvement over a placebo, the grounds for rushing the new model to market are substantially diminished. The case of Diane-35, a drug marketed both as a form of birth control and as an acne treatment, shows how the comparator drug used in two trials was not even approved for use in Canada; while a third trial compared the drug with one used specifically for birth control, but not for acne (Mintzes 2004).

What reviewers must also determine is the concentration and dosage of comparator drugs. Is drug A more successful only because it was tested against a weaker concentration or smaller amount of drug B? They must also note what constitutes a measure of 'success': is it clear superiority over placebo or existing drugs, or is it 'non-inferiority' (i.e., equivalence) to current treatment? To what extent are 'data' quantita-tively measurable, and to what extent are they dependent on the sub-jective reporting of research subjects (or the subjective observation of researchers themselves)? Are 'surrogate markers' (which indicate effec-tiveness in one area by exhibiting effectiveness in a separate but caus-ally related area) used in place of first-hand evidence?

A third category of research bias involves the *research design*. The gold standard in clinical research is generally a double-blind, randomized model, in which neither the subject nor the clinician knows which drug a subject is receiving, and in which a subject has an equal chance of being selected to receive the drug or its comparator(s). Yet the prac-tice of drug companies submitting 'surveillance' studies or 'open-label' studies (where subjects and clinicians know exactly what drug is being used) in support of its products is not uncommon, especially in phase four studies. Another problem with research design is length of time. If a drug is only studied for a period of six months in a clinical trial, it may not give an accurate indication of what the side effects may be after a period of one or several years.

Many clinical trials are no longer performed in academic environments, but in 'contract research organizations,' private businesses that run clinical trials for corporate clients. Often the drug companies control the collection and the collation of the research data themselves, fragmenting the research teams so that even the investigators themselves only have access to data subsets and cannot get a sense of the larger picture (Baird 2003). Clinicians, whether employed by contract research organizations or not, are often not given rigorous instruction as part of their medical training in the development of clinical trial design in any case. However, there is a movement to increase the capacity of clinical scientists, including CIHR's Clinical Research Initiative.

These forms of research bias are compounded by *publication bias*, which is the tendency for articles submitted for publication to favour the interests of those funding the research. In the past half-dozen years, innumerable studies have documented the tendency for published research sponsored by pharmaceutical firms 'to produce results favouring the product made by the company sponsoring the research' (Lexchin et al. 2003; see also Baird 2003; Garattini and Bertele 2007; Yank et al. 2007; Wang et al. 2010). An analysis published in the *Journal of the American Medical Association* in 2008 examined seventy-four FDA-registered studies of antidepressants. The lead author, a former FDA officer, used the Freedom of Information Act to gather the data submitted to the FDA by drug companies. The authors found that only three of the thirty-eight negative studies were published, while thirty-seven of the thirty-eight positive studies were published. Thus the results of nearly all of the trials of antidepressants were reported in the publications as positive. Of these published studies, however, FDA analysis *of the same studies* only determined half of the outcomes to be positive (Turner et al. 2008). This bolsters a 2002 study of FDA reviews (also secured through a Freedom of Information request) that showed that placebos were 80 per cent as effective as the six most widely prescribed antidepressants (Kirsch and Moore 2002, cited in Angell 2005: 290). Another study published in 2008 compared data given to the FDA on a wide range of drugs, and also found that only the positive results tended to be published in academic journals (Lee, Bachetti, and Sim 2008). Interestingly, access to drug firms' clinical trial data in several cases has become available because the firms are in litigation for other reasons (thereby making internal documents publicly accessible). For example, Pfizer and Parke-Davis were brought to court for illegally marketing the drug gabapentin for off-label use. This allowed researchers to examine the firms' internal drug trial results more closely. They concluded that the clinical trials conducted by the company did not represent information published in the public domain (Vedula et al. 2009; Steinman et al. 2006).

This practice, of reporting only positive results, is known as 'selective reporting.' It means that those who read the journals have a very skewed perception of what works, how well it works, and what the best options are. If the only three published articles on 'Placebozene' are glowing, the attitude of clinicians will likely be much different than if they had also read the ten reviews critical of Placebozene that were not published. It is also possible selectively to report the data that are published. The most notorious instance of this was Celecoxib, the makers of which pooled data between subgroups over varying periods of time in order to come up with positive findings (Lexchin 2004). A related publication bias is multiple reporting, where the positive result of a drug study may be written up (either individually, or pooled with other studies) so that the results are published more than once. This way, when all the positive studies are compiled, the total tabulation of positive results is misrepresented.

Another common practice has been that of ghost writing. In this instance, medical writers (who are hired by contract research organization or pharmaceutical companies themselves) write up the clinical trials, but are given little or no formal recognition for the task. Clinicians with established names are paid to append their names to the document, which is generally given to them in a completely written format. In return, they receive payment and an addition to their list of 'publications.' Between 1998 and 2005, for example, the pharmaceutical company Wyeth paid a medical communications company to draft twenty-six papers emphasizing the benefits and limited the risks of taking hormone replacement therapy. Wyeth's hormone drugs, Premarin and Prempro, brought in sales of close to U.S.$2 billion in 2001 (Singer 2009b). Wyeth did not disclose its direct payment to the firm employing the authors. The prosecution of Merck (over its marketing of Vioxx) in the New Jersey Superior Court in 2005 allowed researchers access to a database of over 20,000 Merck documents, including internal and external correspondence, reports, and presentations. An analysis of how 'Merck used a systematic strategy to facilitate the publication of guest authored and ghost written medical literature' subsequently appeared in the *Journal of the American Medical Association* in 2008. The researchers concluded that articles appearing in medical journals had been 'frequently authored by Merck employees' but that they had 'attributed first authorship to external, academically affiliated investigators who did not always disclose financial support from Merck, although financial support of the study was nearly always provided' (Ross et al. 2008: 1806).

Regulatory Reform in Canada

Understanding the politics of drug regulation in Canada first requires understanding who the players are. There are three sets of actors: governmental, industry, and independent or quasi-independent not-for-profit 'watchdog' bodies. The players are represented schematically in Figure 7.1.

The major actor for Health Canada is the Health Products and Food Branch, which plays a similar role to the FDA in the United States. This government department, under the direct control of Health Canada, is divided into four units. The most important of these is the Therapeutic Products Directorate (formerly the Drugs Directorate), which is the regulatory body for drugs derived from chemical manufacture. The other units are the Biologics and Genetic Therapies Directorate, which regulates biological and radiopharmaceutical products, including vaccines; the Marketed Health Products Directorate, which addresses post-marketing drug surveillance; and the Health Products and Food Branch Inspectorate, which deals with compliance and enforcement. These four units of the Health Products and Food Branch together determine the 'efficacy, safety, and quality of manufacture' of pharmaceuticals, including clinical trial authorization and drug licensing.

The issue surrounding the Health Products and Food Branch, and especially the Therapeutic Products Directorate (TPD), is the extent to which it has been 'captured' by the pharmaceutical industry. During the fiscal crisis of the mid-1990s Health Canada decided to recoup costs by placing the funding burden on the pharmaceutical companies, whose profit margins were considerably higher than Ottawa's. Drug companies now pay the TPD for their services, and especially for the evaluation of their products for regulatory approval (current fees range from $143,800 to $212,000 depending on the product). It is clear that the new procedure has led to faster approvals and a higher proportion

Figure 7.1. Key actors in the regulation and monitoring of pharmaceutical products in Canada

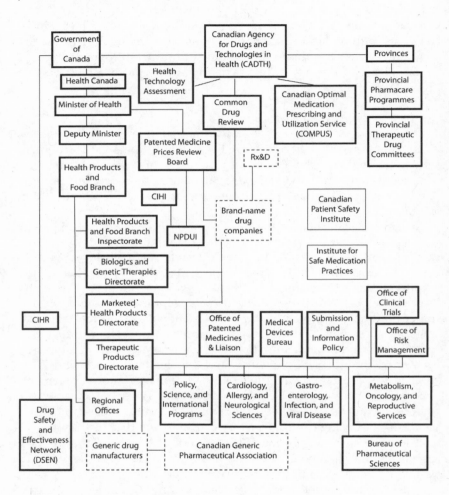

of drugs approved, both of which are in the interests of the pharmaceutical industry (Lexchin 2006). What is not so clear is the extent to which these regulatory bodies weigh the interests of the pharmaceutical companies over those of the public because of the dependence of the regulatory bodies on the user fees collected from the drug industry (which provide over a third of the funding for the TPD). This is not uncommon: 70 per cent of the budget for Europe's drug regulatory body, the European Medicines Agency (EMA), also comes from large pharmaceutical companies (Garattini and Bertele 2007: 3). Critics question whether the faster approvals are thorough enough to catch possible side effects; whether effective monitoring is taking place (especially post-marketing); and whether the evidence provided by industry is analysed sufficiently rigorously. While few would assert that the governmental regulatory agencies are in the 'back pocket' of the industry, it does raise questions about the extent to which such changes encourage a more permissive regulatory approach, in which the balance of doubt (are these potential side effects worrisome enough to reject the drug application?) has shifted in favour of the pharmaceutical industry.

Compounding the problem is the lack of transparency in the approval process. While Health Canada has the legal right to demand whatever information it requires from drug firms regarding their products, government officials still depend on the data presented by the industry. The Therapeutic Products Directorate does not conduct independent, systematic reviews for each product. Moreover, the public has no access to the information provided to regulators for approval of their drugs, and so the basis of approval (or the existence of dissenting or critical voices in the regulatory process) is unknown. Even unapproved applications are not disclosed. This information is kept from the public for two reasons: first, because industry demands 'commercial confidentiality' in order to protect its intellectual property rights; and second, to meet the trade-related intellectual property right measures imposed by international trade agreements. But critics respond that the FDA publishes a much greater range of information on drugs submitted than does the TPD, and that there is no reason Canada could not at least disclose as much information as its neighbour. Moreover, they argue, commercial confidentiality cannot (and does not in law) preclude the public interest and that even trade-related intellectual property rights can be superseded when necessary to protect the public. Whenever drugs are taken off the market because of serious side effects or complications, the question is raised whether such a drug would have made it to market had the regulatory unit been more independent and the approval process more transparent.

A second government body involved in the regulatory process is the Patented Medicine Prices Review Board (PMPRB), which is an independent quasi-judicial tribunal. This means that it technically has more autonomy than the Health Products and Food Branch, but it is still in the end answerable to the minister of health. The PMPRB was established in 1987, after Bill C-22 ended the practice of compulsory licensing (giving drug companies more freedom from competition). Given the strengthened monopoly status of the pharmaceutical firms, the PMPRB was established to protect consumers and keep drug prices down. The PMPRB regulates the prices of patented drugs (prescription and non-prescription) sold in Canada by setting the maximum non-excessive price firms can charge; and it reports on, but does not regulate, the price of generic drugs. It limits the price of new drugs introduced to market, and it also ensures that the prices of existing drugs do not surpass the rate of inflation. Because of these limits, brand-name drugs in Canada are approximately 40 per cent cheaper than in the United States. While the role of the PMPRB is to keep prices down, it does not determine 'whether the product provides reasonable value for money' (Tierney et al. 2008: 432). This is the function of the Canadian Agency for Drugs and Technologies in Health (CADTH).

The CADTH (until 2006 the Canadian Coordinating Office for Health Technology Assessment) stands at even greater arm's length from the government than the PMPRB. Funded by federal, provincial, and territorial governments jointly, it is an independent, not-for-profit body charged with providing 'credible, impartial advice and evidence-based information about the effectiveness of drugs and other health technologies to Canadian decision-makers' (http://www.cadth.ca/index.php/en/home). Most importantly, the CADTH oversees the Common Drug Review, launched in 2003, which analyses the cost-effectiveness and clinical efficiency of drugs submitted by manufacturers and determines whether they should be listed on federal and provincial formularies. Unlike the PMPRB, the Common Drug Review compares the cost and efficacy of new drugs with those already on the market. The Common Drug Review streamlines the drug evaluation process for both governments and manufactures, which otherwise would have to conduct the reviews individually. In 2008 another oversight body, the Drug Safety and Effectiveness Network (DSEN) was established under the auspices of the Canadian Institutes of Health Research (CIHR) to monitor drugs already on the market, including those under independent clinical trials. The National Prescription Drug Utilization Information System (NPDUIS) is an initiative which involves the development of a database collecting prescription claims (run under the auspices of CIHI) and the production of analytical reports based on these data (for which the PMPRB is responsible). Drug monitoring is also conducted more peripherally by non-governmental, independent not-for-profit organizations such as the Institute for Safe Medication Practices, an internationally based group focusing on safe medication use, and the Canadian Patient Safety Institute.

The other key players are the pharmaceutical firms themselves. They are usually grouped into two separate categories: the multinational corporations that manufacture brand-name drugs and the (often domestic) firms which produce generic drugs. The former is represented by the umbrella organization Rx&D (Canada's Research-Based Pharmaceutical Companies), and represents almost all of the large pharmaceutical producers. The Canadian Generic Pharmaceutical Association (CGPA) represents approximately 15 per cent of the pharmaceutical industry, and it was developed following the suggestions of a civil servant that it would be a useful counterfoil to the established brand-name lobby (Ritchie 1973: 101). It does not, however, include Apotex, the largest generic drug manufacturer. Other relevant groups (not listed in Figure 7.1) include the Canadian Association of Chain Drugstores, the Canadian Pharmacists Association, and the Canadian College of Clinical Pharmacy. Certain units of Health Canada (and especially the Therapeutic Products Directorate) also communicate directly and frequently with international drug regulatory bodies (such as the FDA).

Since 2000 the pharmaceutical sector has begun to face an unprecedented demand from the public for greater accountability. This was led in the first place by clinical insiders who were aware of the massive level of conflicts of interest occurring between those selling drugs, those testing drugs, and those prescribing drugs. By September 2001, a dozen of the most respected medical journals internationally (including the *Canadian Medical Association Journal*) began to refuse publication of articles unless authors signed a legal document attesting that they had seen all the relevant data, that they were responsible for the clinical trial about which they reported, and that the decision to publish rested with them. This was followed in 2004 by another declaration by key medical journals that trial results would not be published unless the trial had been registered. In this way, results from the trial could be tracked in order to monitor selective reporting, as all trial results – including negative ones – would be on record. In 2003 there were two major drug registries: the International Standard Randomized Controlled Trial Number Register (ISRCTN) and ClinicalTrials.gov, maintained by the U.S. National Institutes of Health. By 2007 so many trial registries existed that concerns were raised regarding standardization and monitoring of these sites. Thus in March 2008 the CIHR held a key meeting in Ottawa for all international stakeholders (clinicians, researchers, reviewers, medical editors, consumers, manufacturers, and funders, as well as regulators) to discuss the Public Reporting of Clinical Trials Outcomes and Results (PROCTOR). While Canada has played a key role in the development of clinical trials registries (such as the development of the 'Ottawa Statements'), there is currently no requirement by Health Canada that drugs under development in this country must be registered. Canada's largest public funder, the Tri-Council Agency (which funds the natural sciences, medicine, and the social sciences) does require clinical trial registration, but this is only for publicly funded research. In the United States, however, the Food and Drug Administration Amendments Act of 2007, or FDAAA, now requires that pharmaceutical companies register *all* drugs that are subject to FDA regulation. Notwithstanding this, however, a 2009 study revealed that less than half of 323 clinical trials were properly registered, and that one-quarter of the total clinical trials were not registered with the National Institutes of Health at all (Mathieu et al. 2009).

For several years, Health Canada has been attempting to overhaul its framework for the licensing and regulation of therapeutic products. Regulation often lags behind technological innovation, and Canada's regulatory framework (predominantly the Food and Drugs Act of 1953, but also the Hazardous Products Act of 1969, the Radiation Emitting Devices Act of 1969, and the Quarantine Act of 1970) has lagged behind the regulatory regimes in many other countries. The government of Canada's regulatory authority in the area of emerging technologies is currently quite limited, as is its ability to regulate drugs once they have been given marketing approval (the maximum fine against drug manufacturers for some infractions rests at $5,000; which, for many pharmaceutical firms, has the disciplinary force of a parking ticket). The problem is that regulatory reform is being designed within a context in which large pharmaceutical firms are – both directly and indirectly – key players. Their interest lies in moving new products from clinical trials to market as quickly as possible, while the regulatory body, Health Canada, is expected to ensure that all products available to Canadians are as safe and as effective as possible. But the wider political context is important as well: the pharmaceutical sector has for several decades been a major driver for economic growth. This includes not only brand-name drugs, but also generics, biologics (therapeutics based on the metabolic activity of living organisms, such as vaccines, blood and blood products, hormones, interferon, gene therapies, and even snake venom), and bio-similar products (generic forms of biologics). Thus the pharmaceutical industry has its own supporters within key government departments (including, but not limited to, Industry Canada); and the regulatory dance (to what extent should physical risk be balanced against economic growth?) has been choreographed according to the relative influence of these primary interests. In 1998, for example, the 'conditional notice of compliance' (NOC/c) was introduced as a means of balancing a faster approval time with the ability of Health Canada to regulate a drug after receiving marketing approval. Approval time has sped up; but there is, according to critics, less indication that the conditions stipulated by Health Canada are being rigorously monitored (Lexchin 2007b; Bouchard and Sawicka 2009). In 2004 Health Canada began to issue a 'Summary Basis of Decision' for each approved drug, which explains the reasons, based on the drug's relative risks and benefits, for which the regulatory agency accepted the compound for public use. Again, however, there is criticism that this information is too limited to provide adequate protection to the wider public (Lexchin 2004). In 2007 Ottawa announced the establishment of the Drug Safety and Effectiveness Network (DSEN), which provides data and research studies for drugs already in use. The most sweeping regulatory reform regarding drugs, Bill C-51, was introduced in April 2008, and attempted to develop the concept of 'progressive licensing.' This is the idea that all drugs have a 'life cycle' (like tadpoles or marmots), from molecular development through to clinical trials, approval, and marketing, but also including the increased knowledge about the drug following its widespread use, and possibly the removal of the product from the market, or the development of superior drugs used to treat similar conditions. Progressive licensing is designed so that regulatory oversight can be applied at any point in the drug's life cycle, and not only prior to approval. Bill C-51 died when a federal election was called in September 2008, and regulatory reform remains in limbo. (In contrast, the FDA in the United States released in May 2010 a draft proposal for greater transparency in drug regulation, including the disclosure of which drugs are being considered for approval; whether, when, and why a drug has been withdrawn from the approval process; whether any major safety concerns have arisen regarding the compound; and any reasons the regulatory body would have for denying approval for a product.) International regulatory oversight is, currently, more promising than domestic developments in pharmaceutical regulation. This includes the development of inter-jurisdictional regulation of the pharmaceutical industry. One of the strengths of brand-name drug firms has historically been their multinational nature, allowing them to play states (and their regulatory regimes) against each other. Since September 2009 the FDA and its European counterpart have begun working together to monitor clinical trials and drug marketing across both jurisdictions, but Canada is not formally part of this network.

Another growing development has been the restriction of largesse by pharmaceutical companies to medical students and physicians. This has, however, been both very fragmented (each medical school has its own policy) and discretionary (many guidelines are voluntary). While the more recent trend is for academic health institutions to insist that their members disclose industry ties to *them*, this information is rarely made available to the wider public (Tanne 2010). Nevertheless, conflicts of interest are much more carefully scrutinized than they ever have been; and some pharmaceutical firms have been proactive in developing their own 'codes of practice' (PhRMA introduced its 'Code on Interactions with Healthcare Professionals' in 2008), including disclosing speaking fees to academics and clinicians. Both the U.S. Task Force on Industry Funding of Medical Education and the U.K. Royal College of Physicians have strongly articulated an end to industry handouts: the chair of the former, a former Merck president, baldly stated that such practices 'have helped to create an insidious "sense of entitlement," if not an outright reliance on graft within the medical profession' (Kondro 2008: 1651).

But it may be that the influence of pharmaceutical firms has begun to wane for other, larger reasons. One is the financial meltdown that began in 2008 and which signalled an acute public scepticism of the principle of self-regulation that had informed corporate governance since the early 1980s. This was subsequently exacerbated by the lax oversight of deepwater petroleum extraction which resulted in the environmental disaster in the Gulf of Mexico in 2010. No longer does the argument 'trust us – would we ever do anything that would hurt our own industry?' inspire confidence in the general public. Here the egregious behaviour of Vioxx manufacturer Merck was likely a tipping point, especially after public access to court documents revealed that corrupt practices were much more substantial and systematic than most people had expected. The other factor is the performance of the industry itself. From 1980 to 1987 the average pre-tax rate of return on equity for pharmaceutical companies in Canada was an astounding 36.8 per cent, compared with an average of 14 per cent for Canada's manufacturing industry; from 1988 to 1995 the comparison was 29.6 per cent to 10.7 per cent (Lexchin 1997). But now profits are down because so many 'breakthrough' drugs are at the end of their patents, and there are few products in the pipeline to take their place. Nearly sixty new molecular entities were produced by pharmaceutical firms in 1996 at a cost of U.S.$15 billion; ten years later the industry spent over U.S.$40 billion for twenty new molecular entities. Less than a handful of firms make over 10 per cent of current revenues from drugs less than five years old (Smith 2007). In Canada in 2009 there were twenty-two new drugs introduced. Of these, only one was a 'category 2' drug, which is a drug 'that provides a breakthrough or substantial improvement.' All others were 'category 3' drugs, which 'provide moderate, little, or no therapeutic advantage over comparable medicines' (PMPRB 2009: 9).

Drug firms are quick to acknowledge their poor performance, and they use it to justify the argument that they are becoming over-regulated. If restrictions do not loosen, they argue, they will have little to spend on research and development, and their capacity to produce innovative, life-saving products will be undermined. Certainly, there *have* been major advances in improving patients' quality of life through new pharmaceuticals. But critics have little patience for this defence. In the first place, they point out, the pharmaceutical industry is simply not innovative: most innovation in the United States, argues Angell (2005: 57), 'is sponsored by the National Institutes of Health (NIH) and carried out at universities, small biotechnology companies, or the NIH itself.' Once the drugs are licensed, the large firms buy the licences 'just before they are ready to enter large-scale clinical trials'; the NIH itself found in one survey that sixteen of the seventeen key scientific papers leading to the discovery and development of five top-selling drugs came from outside the industry (ibid., 65). This means that taxpayers pay twice for their drugs: once through the research supported by their tax dollars, and again in purchasing the drug itself. Moreover, the amount of industry money targeted at research and development (R&D) is much lower than what the industry spends on marketing and administration. The top ten American drug companies, for example, spent just over 14 per cent on research and development in 2002, kept 17 per cent as profits, and spent 31 per cent on marketing and administration (Angell 2005: 48). Gagnon and Lexchin (2008: 32) reinforce this estimate, calculating that 'pharmaceutical companies spend almost twice as much on promotion as they do on R&D.'

The same trend exists in Canada, although the dynamics are somewhat different. Bills C-22 (1987) and C-91 (1992) extended the period of patent protection for brand-name pharmaceuticals, thereby eliminating much potential competition from generic drug manufacturers. Drug firms had lobbied hard for such protection, arguing that the profits were necessary in order to maintain a significant level of research and development in Canada. In exchange for patent protection, Canada demanded that the brand-name pharmaceutical industry commit 10 per cent of sales specifically to R&D. But manufacturing output by drug firms was actually cut back after this legislation took effect, and the industry increased its spending in the area of marketing and sales, citing the need to compete in a globalized economy (Kondro 2006b). The umbrella organization for brand-name drug firms (after pointedly changing its name from the Pharmaceutical Manufacturers' Association of Canada to Canada's Research-Based Pharmaceutical Companies in 1999) aggressively campaigned to change the definition of 'research and development' to include clinical trials. According to the Patented Medicine Prices Review Board, clinical trials represent over 76.8 per cent of applied research and development, while other 'non-basic' research (generally the cost of drug regulation submissions) comprised another 20 per cent of the 'research and development' produced in Canada. Innovative research and development, then, comprises a minute percentage of pharmaceutical firms' sales. Even *including* clinical trials and drug submission costs, the industry has failed to meet the 10 per cent floor for research and development for several years: as the 2009 PMPRB Annual Report notes, the ratio of R&D expenditure to sales revenue among all patentees was 7.5 per cent in 2009, down from 8.1 per cent in 2008. 'This is the lowest ratio since 1990, and also represents the seventh consecutive year it has been below 10%' (PMPRB 2009: 37).

Regulatory reform has been quite substantial in the pharmaceutical sector over the past decade. To what extent is the industry *still* under-regulated (or over-regulated)? The industry retains considerable influence in its ability to fund physicians, researchers, students, and institutions. While the Olivieri incident made academic institutions scrutinize their protocols more rigorously, it has not led to the restriction of access by pharmaceutical companies to students, researchers, or clinicians. Rather, institutions instead attempt to 'educate and sensitize' students (however briefly) to issues surrounding commercial conflicts of interest (Ferris et al. 2004). Academic detailing (where academic teams with expertise on drug utilization, clinical efficacy, and cost-effectiveness offer an outreach service to professional physicians to present impartial information) is currently practised in five provinces (British Columbia, Alberta, Saskatchewan, Manitoba, and Nova Scotia). The practice of clinical trial registration has become more regularized and standardized. Various limits are placed on industry funding of continuing medical education (including full disclosure), although this varies across institutions, jurisdictions, and subfields. Often 'codes of practice' remain discretionary, with no clear understanding of what the consequences of violation may be. Expecting transparency and account-ability in research and education is substantial progress, but it does not address deeper and more endemic conflicts. To what extent does dependence by regulators on fees paid by industry affect the objectivity and impartiality of regulation? Will regulatory agencies benefit from the number of applications they process, and the speed in which they can perform this task, or will the quality of investigation be compro-mised (e.g., will subtle anomalies in research data or procedure be over-looked)? To the extent that industry is by far the largest funder of phar-maceutical research, will the research agenda of individual researchers or even academic institutions be (subtly or otherwise) influenced by the corporate goals of the multinational companies that fund them? Will researchers focus on the burgeoning market in 'lifestyle drugs' in place of unprofitable products that save lives? Will they actively pursue a potential problem in drug development if it may jeopardize their com-mercial funding sources? To what extent do researchers practise self-censure because of their recognition that commercial funding may end if positive results do not ensue?

In Canada, the discussion is complicated because of the role played by generic drug manufactures. Generic drugs normally cost far less than brand-name drugs, and they account for an increasing amount of spending on pharmaceuticals in Canada. The prices for generic drugs in Canada are not regulated, however, as are brand-name drugs, and they are generally higher compared with international generic drug prices. There are a number of reasons for this. The first is purely politi-cal: two generic drug companies, Apotex and Novopharm, dominate the industry in this country. Apotex is the second-largest drug manufac-turer in Canada, behind Pfizer, while Novopharm is the fourth-largest (IMS Health 2010b). As biomedical industries become key economic players, national governments are keen to encourage domestic firms in this industry who can compete as global players. Another reason is the structure of generic pricing in Canada. Generic drug companies com-pete not for doctors' attention but for that of pharmacists. This has led to a practice of 'rebates' (or 'trade allowances') whereby generic drug manufacturers offer rebates of 40 to 50 per cent of the nominal price to pharmacists to stock their products. But pharmacies charge their cus-tomers (and customers' insurance plans) the *full* price, not the price after rebates. Given that pharmacies have an incentive to buy the highest-price generic drugs offering the largest rebates, normal market competition is ineffective. Regulation of the price generics offer is complicated, however. The actual cost of manufacturing generic drugs is unknown, as it is proprietary information held by private companies. Moreover, just as brand-name drug companies argue that they need high profits to facilitate research and development, generic drug companies maintain that they require a certain profit margin to litigate against brand-name firms. Large brand-name pharmaceutical companies are loath to relinquish profitable patents, and often engage in 'evergreening' practices solely to extend the length of their patents. A manufacturer or generic drugs must spend significant amounts in litigation in order to wrest the expired patent away from the brand-name company; but once it is successful in doing so all generic companies are free to manufacture the newly off-patent drug. There is no guarantee that the dollars spent in litigation can be recouped by manufacturing the subject of the litigation. Any attempt at over-regulating generic drug prices could undermine the very existence of generic drug firms; for more detailed discussions of the dynamics of generic drug pricing in Canada, see Hollis (2009) and Competition Bureau Canada (2008). But, as with brand-name drug companies, the issue of *how much profit is necessary* to keep a company producing their products is a largely subjective one, and the evidence needed to make a conclusive judgment remains proprietary information that few companies willingly disclose.

Larger ideological issues also cloud regulatory debates. Governments are increasingly obliged by international trade obligations, as well as by the strategic attempt to attract profitable industries, to protect the commercial confidentiality and 'intellectual property rights' of the pharmaceutical industry. The extent to which refusal to allow public access to this information (e.g., the outcomes of drug trials) compromises public safety is not clear. Moreover, to the extent that health is seen as a business rather than as a public good, governments often believe that their own political viability coincides with the corporate health of successful firms. As the life sciences industry (especially biotechnology) increasingly challenges the manufacturing industry as a key economic driver for developed countries, governments will be even more inclined to favour the interests of this sector. This is occurring at a time when the overall fiscal health of developed states is less than robust. The clear alternative to industry dominance – publicly funded research and surveillance – keeps receding in the distance. Codes and regulations concerning transparency and lines of accountability are cheaper to maintain than large-scale publicly funded research institutions; but funding still exerts a powerful influence that is difficult to control effectively. The multinational structure of large pharmaceutical corporations also allows them to engage in extraterritorial behaviour (such as the actions by GlaxoSmithKline, Pfizer, and AstraZeneca against Canadian pharmacies exporting drugs to the United States). Ongoing scrutiny is better than no vigilance at all, but the sheer size and sophisticated marketing ability of large multinational industries should never be underestimated.

8 Mental Health

Mental health care is not simply a subset of health care; it is qualitatively different from it. Rarely in any country does mental health
receive the same emphasis that general health services do. But in
Canada many major developments in health care policy have actually been *detrimental* to mental health care. The structure of the health
care system in Canada often works at cross-purposes to mental health
care; however, attempts at health care reform are themselves subject
to so many political minefields that policy makers seldom consider
the effects of reforms on mental health care when developing new
policies. Like general health care services, mental health policy is also
highly political. But the politics of mental health care are still more
complex than those underlying general health care services, involving
the complicated and intractable issues of citizenship (inclusion in and
exclusion from social communities), selfhood (the capacity to make
autonomous choices), and political autonomy (the legal status of self-
governing behaviour).

While academics have begun to dig more enthusiastically into the
political terrain of health care itself, the politics of mental health policy
remain largely neglected. Very few books on the subject are written
by political scientists, using the tools of their discipline; and most of
these are out of date (including Connery's 1968 study of the politics of
mental health in six urban areas of the United States). None addresses
the complex political nature of mental health policy in Canada, except
for some province-specific accounts (e.g., Simmons 1982). While the
debate over what mental health *is* shifts as frequently as the debate
over how to treat it, the fact that it plays an increasingly prominent
role in health care expenditure alone means that policy makers will be

forced to grapple with the way in which it is provided. The larger social issues surrounding the meaning of citizenship and inclusion will also manifest themselves into political pressures to which officials will have to respond. This chapter will examine why mental health care has taken the form it has, with particular focus on the political tensions that exist within this policy area in Canada.

Paradigms and Politics in Mental Health Care in Canada

Many of the factors that have structured the evolution of mental health policy in Canada are common to most developed nations. These include the emergence of new psychotropic drugs and the subsequent move towards deinstitutionalization; the influence of new public management theory and its effect on health policy, including regionalization, accountability, and an emphasis on quantifiable results (see Chapter 3); the fiscal pressures on states which have led to many common patterns of growth and retrenchment; and the trends in thinking about both mental health (including moral therapy, psychotherapy, the anti-psychiatry movement, and biomedical schools of thought), and the place of disadvantaged individuals within society (influenced by Christian beliefs, liberal values, feminism, postmodernism, and even postcolonial schools of thought). But the two variables that have distinguished Canadian mental health policy, and that determine the parameters for any potential reform, are federal political structures (see Chapter 2) and the Canada Health Act (see Chapters 1 and 4).

Pastoral Asylum and 'Moral Therapy' (Mid-1800s to Mid-1960s)

The models presented here are abstract representations. They are not mutually exclusive – it is possible to find examples of several models within the same jurisdiction – but they do represent the chronology of thinking about mental health care through recent history. It is important, from a policy perspective, to remember that existing models can shape the political landscape in ways that limit (or expand) the kinds of reform options that may be viable in the future (this idea is often presented in theories of 'crystallization' or 'path dependency'). The establishment of discrete asylums for the treatment of the mentally ill, for example, constrained mental health reform for a long time in Canada despite the emergence of evidence indicating the obsolescence of the asylum model.

Approaching the treatment of the mentally ill from a systematic, scientific perspective was a nineteenth-century phenomenon. In Canada, the first 'lunatic asylums' were established in Quebec, Ontario, and the Atlantic provinces between 1845 and 1857. Prior to this, the mentally ill were frequently kept in poorhouses or penitentiaries. Individuals with psychiatric conditions were generally not segregated from other inmates; and when they were (as in one Newfoundland facility used in the early 1800s) the conditions were 'comparable to a dungeon, with patients chained and food provided at the end of a pole' (Sussman 1998: Table 1). Occasionally the mentally ill, if harmless, were allowed to 'wander at will'; but given the harsh conditions of frontier life (including severe winters and insecure food supplies) this was likely a solitary, brutish, and short existence for those allowed to evade incarceration. Those kept within the domestic sphere often fared little better. Individuals with severe psychiatric conditions were often chained or confined for years without respite; and they were beaten, baited, humiliated, or simply neglected (Shorter 1997).

The idea underlying mental asylums was to develop a humane alternative; a protected environment based on the principles of comfort and concern. 'The calm that the psychiatric patients enjoy,' wrote an early nineteenth-century physician, 'far from the tumult and the noise, and the mental rest [*repos moral*] conferred by removal from the businesses and domestic problems, is very favorable to their recovery. Subject to an orderly life, to discipline, to a well calibrated regimen, they are obliged to reflect on the change in their life. The necessity of adjusting [*se contenir*], of behaving well with strangers, of living together with their companions in suffering, are powerful allies in achieving restoration of their lost reason' (quoted in Shorter 1997: 19).

The establishment of asylums in Canada was a serious undertaking, and spending on mental hospitals between 1845 and 1902 exceeded expenditure on medical hospitals and prisons combined (Wright, Moran, and Gouglas 2003). But, as with similar institutions in Europe and the United States, the romantic ideal of asylum treatment was short-lived. The populations of mental hospitals increased exponentially with little change in resources directed to them. This was due to a number of factors, both biological (including the rapid increase in syphilis, which resulted in severe psychiatric conditions, and possibly the sudden increase of schizophrenia as well) and social (including the disruption caused by increasing patterns of urbanization and immigration). The early efforts of pioneering psychiatric reformers had, by the beginning of the twentieth century, become a system of warehousing the mentally ill in largely decrepit facilities run by overburdened staff. In the early 1920s, Ontario physicians C.K. Clarke and Clarence Hincks, under the auspices of the newly created National Committee for Mental Hygiene (later to become the Canadian Mental Health Association), undertook a survey of the conditions of Canada's major mental asylums. The results were shocking, even by the standards of the day:

> In a survey of the first asylum in New Brunswick, Hincks found one group of insane people who were put to bed in boxes filled with hay. Wooden slats were then nailed on top. All boxes except two were secured at night; these belonged to patients designated as trustees. Their job was to deal with any noisy inmates by urinating through the slats.
>
> In a Halifax asylum, a man was kept in an unheated room year-round. The staff were somehow convinced he could not feel the cold. In the Edmonton Institute, imbecile children were rolled in long strips of cotton with their arms and legs bound. They were then piled on shelves. (Lajeunesse 2002: 68)

The grim conditions of such institutions became even more pronounced as the Depression and the Second World War diverted both attention and resources away from mental hospitals. Physicians already in short supply in psychiatric hospitals were drafted into active duty; even after the war, developments in social policy designed to accommodate demobilization often overshadowed interest in mental health reform (Grob 1991).

The shift in a new treatment paradigm is often supposed to have happened in the early 1950s, when the development of effective new drugs presented alternatives to the standard treatments of sedation and restraint. It was the Second World War, however, that served as the impetus for a new paradigm change in the treatment of mental illness. Screening for active service in the United States had revealed a startling statistic: 1.75 million men were deemed unfit for service due to 'neuropsychiatric reasons,' while 1.1 million psychiatric admissions for those in active service during the war focused attention on the role of environmental stressors in the manifestation of mental illness. This was the first major instance of the 'normalization' of mental illness. In opposition to the common view encompassing the two solitudes of 'healthy' and 'mentally unfit,' wartime experiences drove home the fact that anyone subject to egregious conditions could succumb to mental illness (and could, with proper treatment, possibly recover). Thus the wartime experiences of young psychiatrists 'in successfully treating neurotic symptoms in noninstitutional settings (and presumably preventing the onset of more serious psychotic symptoms) created an alluring model that would contribute to the postwar transformation of the speciality' (Grob 1991: 17).

But the institutionalization of the 'asylum' model for over a century also established a policy legacy that determined the way in which Canadian mental health care would be delivered for decades after most provincial psychiatric hospitals were demolished. The treatment of mentally ill patients in an environment segregated from other medical hospitals did result in the professionalization of psychiatry, but it also served as an enclave for mental health elites, often with their own agenda. This did not always fit with the models of reform that began to develop by the middle of the twentieth century. While medical hospitals were organized and run locally, for example, mental hospitals were governed by a provincial board. This meant that psychiatrists often had direct influence on policy making at the provincial level. It also meant that the profession could more easily protect their interests by continuing the asylum model, where their influence was concentrated, rather than supporting a community-care model, where their influence would be far more dispersed. At the same time, the institutional bifurcation of the medical profession between psychiatric and non-psychiatric physicians further emphasized the fragmentation of the mental health system, a development which was to have a lasting legacy on the mental health system (Mulvale et al. 2007).

The Second World War may have produced a coterie of professionals who were willing to challenge the paradigm of therapeutic asylum, but it was the advent of effective biochemical treatments which caught the attention of policy makers. Prior to the development of chlorprozamine (an anti-psychotic drug) and lithium (an anti-manic drug) treatments for psychiatric patients were labour-intensive and expensive, while results were uneven and unpredictable. The mental asylums of the first half of the twentieth century were visibly different institutions from the sterile urban treatment centres of the twenty-first. Large, sprawling complexes of graceful Victorian buildings rose out of rural woodland or dusty prairie, surrounded by acres of carefully tended lawns, exquisite flower beds, and perfectly groomed shrubbery. These immaculate landscapes were tended by crews of patients, endlessly digging, weeding, and pruning through the short summer months. This was not employment, but therapy; and was often much preferred to more invasive alternatives.

A common treatment at this time was hydrotherapy. Patients in tubs, their heads protruding from secured tarps, were exposed to alternating baths of warm and cool water. Stronger patients could brace against a powerful jet of water from a standing position. Other treatments (especially for severe forms of syphilis) focused on the use of the patient's own body temperature to fight the disease. Heat boxes – long black cabinets similar in appearance to iron lung machines – were used to raise patients' body temperatures; but such equipment depended on having qualified staff trained to use it, and thus often went unutilized. Malarial fever treatments, where patients were injected with the malaria parasite, were considered effective treatments: a consistent temperature of 103 degrees or above for ten to twelve hours was generally deemed sufficient to arrest progress of the disease. However, malaria treatment was very labour intensive as it required medical and nursing staff to monitor patients' temperatures (and other symptoms) very carefully. Another common treatment during this period was to induce a coma through the injection of insulin, as patients were often found to be much improved when emerging from such a state; but this also required a great deal of close observation. Those with more severe conditions could receive surgical treatments (including bilateral trans-orbital or prefrontal lobotomies) or electroconvulsive therapy. These, along with sedation and restraint, were the standard treatments available for psychiatric patients until the 1950s.

Psychotropic drugs were used throughout the twentieth century, but were generally limited to sedatives such as paraldehyde, often given to patients in chocolate syrup. Chlorprozamine, discovered in 1952, was in use in Canadian mental hospitals by 1957. Chlorprozamine was a chemical so harsh that by 1960 nurses handling it were told to wear masks and rubber gloves. Nevertheless, the results were dramatic: patients who had been incapable of even basic discourse for over three or four decades could be found, after treatment, having tea and chatting with the nurses. Aggressive patients were calmer, which meant less damage to the facilities and less physical harm to the staff. There was much concern about the high cost of the drug, which amounted to $2.50 per patient per day. But the buzz about the drug was compelling; and one Alberta hospital cut the patients' clothing allowance in order to fund an experiment with the drug (Lajeunesse 2002). Chlorprozamine was not the first instance of psychopharmacological treatment during this period; LSD was also used in Canadian psychiatric hospitals in the 1950s (notably, but not exclusively, in Saskatchewan: see Dyck 2007), as were amphetamines and lithium; for more detailed discussions see Healy (2002) and Shorter (2009).

Deinstitutionalization (Mid-1960s to Mid-1980s)

Much debate exists regarding the precise reasons for the trend towards deinstitutionalization (Davis 2006). By the early 1960s the population of psychiatric hospitals across Canada had risen to their highest levels, and the facilities themselves, most of which had been built at the turn of the twentieth century, had disintegrated to the point that massive capital costs would be required to restore them. The concept of community-based care that grew out of the Second World War had developed into an articulate school of thought with numerous proponents who argued that therapeutic community-centred care would be both more effective and more humane. The attention on civil rights (especially in the United States) had a profound effect on the relationship between human rights and mental health law in Canada, especially concerning involuntary incarceration and, in Alberta (where at least one institution lined patients up for routine sterilizations), the legal basis for physical integrity. Given the presence of these factors, the development of drugs that alleviated the need for much labour-intensive therapeutic treatment merely facilitated the political decision to release patients into the community. The pivotal year for mental health restructuring was 1963, when both the United States and Canada released major documents outlining the need to shift mental health care away from asylums into the community. On signing the Community Mental Health Centers Construction Act, President John F. Kennedy declared that 'reliance on the cold mercy of custodial isolation will be supplanted by the open warmth of community concern and capability' (quoted in Davis 2006: 105). In Canada, the report *More for the Mind* (Tyhurst et al. 1963), released the same year, called for the transfer of patients to both community care facilities and general hospitals, and for the rationalization of services scattered across departments to be restructured in order to provide a greater continuity of care.

This restructuring had already been occurring on a small scale in Canada for some time. In 1948 the system of Dominium Health Grants allocated five million dollars as part of a shared-cost funding system for the establishment of psychiatric units within general hospital facilities

(Mulvale et al. 2007). This was the prototype for the development of the Hospital Insurance and Diagnostic Services Act of 1957 which, along with the 1966 Medical Care Act, served as a template for the Canada Health Act of 1984. Ironically, these two pieces of legislation (along with the subsequent Canada Health Act) were to have much more effect on the nature of mental health care policy than any mental health strategy would have.

In the first place, the two pieces of legislation clearly distinguished what would and would not be subject to federal-provincial cost-shared funding. Physician visits, of course, would be funded whether they took place in the community (private practice) or in hospitals. But other mental health workers, including psychologists, social workers, psychiatric workers, occupational therapists, or addiction counsellors would not be subject to shared-cost payment plans. In other words, treatments occurring in psychiatric wings of general hospitals would cost provinces half the amount that the same treatments would cost in the community, as the remaining half would be funded by the federal government. It is hardly surprising, given this funding structure, that provinces would attempt to provide as much mental health care in hospitals as possible rather than in 'non-institutionalized' settings, which had been the very point of deinstitutionalization.

The federal-provincial funding system had a number of important secondary effects on the development of mental health care. As explained in Chapter 7, neither the Hospital Insurance and Diagnostic Services Act nor the Medical Care Act covered prescription drugs procured outside of hospitals. Thus the more that psychiatric treatment focused on pharmacological therapy, the more treatment costs were shifted onto patients themselves. And, to the extent that individuals with severe psychiatric conditions were often unable to secure the employment that would allow them to buy the drugs they needed, access to effective treatment in many cases actually diminished considerably.

The funding system also had negative effects on the provision of human resources in mental health care. The care of psychiatric patients is qualitatively different from the nursing of non-psychiatric patients, and the nursing staff in general hospitals were not usually trained to care for severely mentally ill patients. However, as patients moved from provincial mental hospitals to psychiatric wings of general hospitals, psychiatric nurses in some provinces often did not want to make the transfer from psychiatric to general hospitals or community clinics. This was because many had only a two-year 'psych nurse' training accreditation rather than qualification as a registered nurse (RN) with post – basic training in psychiatry. When they sought employment outside of psychiatric hospitals they did not have the same status as RNs and, in many cases, were demoted from being nurses to acting as ward aids. Psychiatrists, too, often preferred working in mental hospitals, as their influence on mental health policy was more direct than it would be were they 'just another doctor' within the general hospital system. Because clinical psychologists were not remunerated by public insurance as private practitioners, and because the places for clinical psychologists in hospitals were strictly limited, psychotherapy was usually limited to those who could afford it. This, in turn, led to an increasingly class-based system of mental health care, where poorer individuals remained in custodial care in the remaining provincial psychiatric hospitals, while those with more resources could seek private care by psychologists.

The new system of public health insurance also had lasting effects on the capacity of the health care system to move towards a more integrated model of health care. Public health insurance in Canada was achieved only by ceding professional self-regulation to physicians. This meant that physicians retained a more direct role in health policy making at the provincial level, one that other mental health professionals did not enjoy. This has tended to reinforce the model of 'medical dominance' within the mental health system. Describing the process of health policy making in Ontario, Mulvale et al. write that 'physicians learned to protect the OHIP [Ontario Health Insurance Plan] funds from encroachment by other provider groups and to lobby against any reforms that might reduce existing privileges' (2007: 376).

From 1965 to 1981, the population of mental asylums in Canada fell by 70 per cent (Nelson 2006). Rather than community reintegration, however, the result was often the segregation of the mentally ill within smaller institutions, in poor-quality housing, or on the streets. A large part of the problem was that there was no financial incentive or political motivation to provide community care. But another problem was that there had been no clear conceptualization of what was *meant* by 'community care.' For the first half of the twentieth century what community support existed in Canada was provided by organizations such as the Canadian Mental Health Association (CMHA). This body, in turn, largely depended on the volunteer activity of upper- and middle-class housewives (Fingard and Rutherford 2008). However, precisely at the time that the policy of deinstitutionalization placed thousands of individuals in the community, these same women were turning away from a lifestyle of domestic and volunteer work to one of paid employment. The implicit assumption of political officials (with some exceptions) underlying the policy of deinstitutionalization was that it would be much cheaper to maintain. They were correct: by 1990, only 3 per cent of provincial mental health budgets were allocated to community support (Mulvale et al. 2007: 378). But this also reflected the paucity of mental health services provided in the community, and it certainly was not the result that had been envisaged by the original proponents of a community care model.

Coordinated Community Services (Mid-1980s to Mid-1990s)

By the middle of the 1980s, a body of literature had developed which attempted to address the gaps in the system of community care province by province. Several ironies had become apparent throughout the 1970s and 1980s: while the impetus of reforms developed in the 1960s had been to achieve the rationalization and continuity of care for the mentally ill, the only real systematic continuity of care (including treatment, housing, nutrition, occupational therapy, and lifestyle training) existed in the old mental hospitals. The segregation of mentally ill from the larger population not only remained, but it was moved to even more dangerous environments.

By the 1980s funding had begun to follow patients into the community. 'During the late 1980s,' observes Nelson, 'all of the provinces except Saskatchewan spent 68% or more of their mental health budgets on institutional services ... However, from the late 1980s to 1998, provincial spending on community mental health increased thirteen-fold from $8 million to $113 million, with several provinces making significant progress in reallocating resources from hospitals to community-based services' (2006: 250). This statistic, however, omits the tremendous political tensions underlying individual policy changes. On the one hand, for example, there was the development of 'not in my back yard' lobbies at the local level to prevent halfway houses, counselling facilities, and other community services from locating in many residential or business communities. On the other hand, however, there was the equally strong lobby by communities serving the large mental hospitals not to dismantle them. These large institutions were often the source of stable employment for local residents, from skilled occupations such as nursing or occupational therapy to unskilled employment in the kitchens, housekeeping facilities, and on the wards themselves. One early example of this phenomenon was in Saskatchewan, where Premier Tommy Douglas, whose Master's thesis in 1933 had addressed the social problems associated with mental disorders (Dyck 2007), had throughout the 1950s developed a relatively enlightened mental health policy for the province. Douglas's own constituency of Weyburn, however, also housed a large mental asylum, and Douglas had no intention of alienating his political support by closing it. Even as late as 1996, mental health funds were directed towards such remote rural psychiatric facilities as the Alberta Hospital Ponoka, despite the plethora of reports and studies agreeing on the need for funds to be directed into community services; but the hospital stood squarely in the riding of the provincial government's minister of health, who was equally cognizant of the fact that his political survival rested with the interests of his constituents, and not the province's mental health lobby (Lajeunesse 2002).

By the late 1980s, the nature of community health care began to be analysed and defined much more thoroughly than it had been for the previous two decades. A series of 'best practices' in mental health reform began to be articulated. Two predominant aspects of this were the development of 'case management' and 'assertive community treatment,' both of which were designed as an attempt to provide seamless mental health care. *Case management* looks at mentally ill individuals within the context of their community, including housing, employment, education, legal matters, and other services in addition to the issue of proper medical treatment. Case managers act as system navigators for mental health care users, coordinating care on an ongoing bases as necessary for each particular case. Often this service is provided by social workers. *Assertive community treatment* (ACT) is designed for 'intensive users' of the health care system: generally those with serious and persistent illnesses or functional impairment (Davis 2006). Rather than expecting these individuals to seek out and visit case management workers, ACT teams visit mental health users on their own home base in order to provide necessary supports or to assist in the acquisition of skills. ACT programs have been evaluated as 'superior for improving clinical status and reducing hospitalization' (PHAC 2002); and such models, in conjunction with crisis response services and ongoing housing supports, are seen as cost-effective methods of providing mental health care services (Federal/Provincial/Territorial Advisory Network on Mental Health 1997).

Recovery and Empowerment (Mid-1990s to the Present)

Perhaps the most potent political shift at the beginning of the twenty-first century was the challenge to traditional epistemology. The earliest manifestation of this was the 'third wave' of feminist thought which argued that the ways in which women understood knowledge was qualitatively different from that of men. One example commonly given was in the practice of medicine, where female nurses 'knew' certain aspects of their patients' health (attitude, personality, mannerisms, physical idiosyncrasies) much better than physicians, even though this knowledge was dismissed or devalued in relation to the overarching biomedical knowledge possessed by male doctors. This idea of 'situated' knowledge was expanded by postmodern theorists, who argued that 'truth' always had to moderated and filtered through complex social relations, and would therefore reflect the particular power relations of that context. The observation that truth was defined by power was echoed by the postcolonial theorists, who argued that dominant social values and beliefs were internalized by the disenfranchised, making them reinforce the conditions of their own oppression.

Such themes resonated with those using the mental health system. An earlier tradition of 'critical' or 'anti' psychiatry had developed during the period of social activism in the late 1960s, but with the intellectual armature provided by continental political thought a 'neo-critical' school of thought developed that had a clear impact on mental health policy making. This approach is characterized by a number of interrelated themes. First, it accepts the postmodern assertion that oppression is perpetuated by the articulation of categorical dualities (good/bad, progress/stagnation, and so on). Mental asylums established in remote locations had removed the mentally ill from the human landscape for over a century; this, in turn, reinforced the perception of a sharp bifurcation between 'healthy' and 'mentally ill.' Current thinking attempts to present mental illness as a common and ongoing manifestation of the human condition rather than a terminal state experienced by an unfortunate set of 'others.' Policy reform thus involves the integration of the mentally ill into all facets of social life. Earlier attempts at deinstitutionalization had merely led to a more informal but equally devastating form of segregation: the mentally ill resided in the community, but were not a part of it.

A second key aspect of the 'recovery' movement is the privileging of experiential knowledge. Professionals, according to this account, should have no monopoly in determining 'what is best' for users. Despite their lack of specialized, scientifically oriented knowledge, consumers of mental health care nonetheless have a sense of what is important to them, what is necessary to maintain a sense of dignity and self-respect, and what kind of treatment would fit well with their lives. In policy terms, stakeholders' groups (such as the Canadian Mental Health Association) are increasingly consulted in the design and evaluation of policies and treatment programs. A third characteristic of this movement addresses the power balance between consumers and providers of mental health care services. Case management and assertive community treatment may have proven effective in managing mental health, but the very qualities that made them effective also had the potential to make them more intrusive and coercive. 'Mental health' in a modern liberal social context means the development of autonomy and assertiveness (rather than, say, the qualities of submissiveness and acceptance that would have been seen as the proper state of mind for most medieval Christians). This means that mental health care users must take an active role in the provision of care; they are participants rather than subjects. Related to this is the development of 'peer support' mechanisms, so that mental health resources (and thus relations of power) are not structured in a hierarchical fashion but rather in a more diffused manner.

The theoretical articulation of this position is, of course, much simpler than its practice. The nature of severe mental illness often means that individuals are in a poor position to make complex judgments of what constitutes their best interest. In such cases, much comes down to the perceptiveness, experience, and sensitivity of each individual care provider. Overall, the 'recovery' model does not replace the 'coordinated community service' system, but simply presents a different approach to the provision of these same services.

Political Obstacles to Mental Health Reform

Canadian mental health care seems poised on the cusp of a new era. Like the rejuvenation of other health services triggered by the 2003 Health Care Accord and the push for new approaches and technologies articulated in the 2004 *10-Year Plan to Strengthen Health Care*, mental health services would seem to be entering into a period of sustained restructuring. A collaborative report on mental illness in Canada was presented under the auspices of the Public Health Agency of Canada in 2002, while the Canadian Alliance on Mental Illness and Mental Health published *A Call to Action* a year later. The 2003 federal/provincial/territorial accord reaffirmed funding increases for acute community mental health services and case management programs. On the heels of the Romanow and Kirby reports into health system reorganization came a sister document in 2006 (*Out of the Shadows at Last*) which discussed the need to reinvigorate Canada's mental health care system. Convergent with this was the Canadian Collaborative Mental Health Initiative (Phase One, 2005–06; Phase Two, 2007–08), which attempted to establish the groundwork for interdisciplinary collaboration. In keeping with the Canadian way of doing things, federal/provincial/territorial collaboration on mental health policy was facilitated by the establishment of the Pan-Canadian Planning Committee for Mental Health Promotion and Mental Illness Prevention (under the auspices of PHAC). Following the recommendations of Michael Kirby's Senate report on mental health care, the Mental Health Commission of Canada (MHCC) was established in 2007, and in 2009 it released a draft framework for the development of a comprehensive national strategy on mental illness and mental health.

And yet, for all the activity, little attention has been focused on the structural barriers for change underlying attempts at mental health reform for the past half-century. Nor has there been a systematic analysis of the way that reforms to general health care services affect and impede the provision of mental health care services. Very few mental health reforms are seen as substantial successes; most innovative programs are developed in a very localized setting rather than as part of an overarching policy. Ontario, in particular, has gamely attempted to address mental health reform, but its record of twenty reform documents in twenty years simply exemplifies its 'history of largely failed attempts to achieve widespread mental health reform' (Mulvale et al. 2007: 4, see also Forchuk et al. 2007). Even a comparison of the broad brush strokes of the 1963 document *More for the Mind* and the 2006 report *Out of the Shadows at Last*, with their similar emphasis on the need to address the stigmatization of the mentally ill and to integrate them into the community, seem remarkably similar. Notwithstanding the real progress made in thinking about how one ought to approach mental health care, policy reform in mental health care seems more like a continuous reiteration of policy goals than an attempt to understand why these goals remain so difficult to achieve.

Table 8.1. Top Ten Reasons for Physician Visits in Canada, 2009

Reasons for Physician Visits	Total Visits
Hypertension	20,657,890
Routine general medical exam	10,491,640
Diabetes	9,746,500
Depression	8,580, 910
Anxiety	6,366,280
Acute upper respiratory infection	6,296,420
Normal pregnancy supervision	4,954,970
Hyperlipidemia	4,747,670
Inner ear infection	4,501,330
Urinary tract infection	3,526,790

Source: IMS Health, Canadian Disease and Therapeutic Index, 2010.

Table 8.2. Top Ten Therapeutic Classes in Canada, 2009

Rank	Therapeutic Class	Total Prescriptions (000s)	Change over 2008 (%)	Dollar Value of Prescriptions Dispensed (000s)
1	Cardiovasculars	74,458	4.0	3,273,482
2	Psychotherapeutics	61,233	5.4	2,368,428
3	Gastroitestinal/ Genitourinary	33,542	8.1	1,875,357
4	Cholesterol agents	31,839	6.8	2,594,714
5	Hormones	26,147	2.9	1,022,490
6	Analgesics	25,252	14.2	1,026,467
7	Anti-infectives, systemic	24,738	1.0	887,468
8	Diabetes therapy	21,360	5.9	908,471
9	Neurological disorders	20,008	7.3	1,095,030
10	Diuretics	17,524	2.0	181,222

Source: IMS Health, Canadian Disease and Therapeutic Index, 2010.

Not just difficult to achieve, but arguably, progress towards these goals has been worsening. In 2009 depression and anxiety were among the most common reasons Canadians visited their family doctors. The two conditions often overlap or exist concurrently; and diagnoses of the two often vary according to historical period and culture. If considered together, they are the second most common reason that

Table 8.3. Total Patient Days and Average Length of Stay (Days) Related to Mental Illness, 2004–5

Province	Psychiatric hospitals		General hospitals		All hospitals	
	Total patient days	Average length of stay	Total patient days	Average length of stay	Total patient days	Average length of stay
Newfoundland and Labrador	79,915	61.6	41,626	20.0	121,541	36.0
Prince Edward Island	4,559	18.1	13,296	8.7	17,855	10.0
Nova Scotia	51,057	91.5	71,363	17.9	122,420	26.9
New Brunswick	62,529	275.5	136,372	25.3	198,901	35.4
Quebec[a]	NA	NA	882,410	22.0	NA	NA
Ontario	1,150,418	86.7	676,012	12.1	1,826,430	26.4
Manitoba	98,571	172.0	182,872	24.6	281,443	35.1
Saskatchewan	110,944	511.3	79,953	12.0	190,897	27.7
Alberta	241,355	84.2	302,607	16.7	543,962	26.0
British Columbia	363,060	616.4	386,804	15.0	749,864	28.5
Yukon	–	–	1,483	6.8	1,483	6.8
Northwest Territories	–	–	6,931	13.6	6,931	13.6
Nunavut	–	–	308	2.4	308	2.4
Canada	2,162,408	108.9	2,782,037	16.6	4,062,035[b]	27.5

Source: Hospital Mental Health Database 2004–5, Canadian Institute for Health Information.
[a]Data from Quebec's psychiatric facilities were not included in 2004–5 due to a data quality issue identified by the province.
[b]Total for all hospitals does not include Quebec data.

individuals visit physicians, hypertension being the first (Table 8.1). Psychotherapeutics are the second-most prescribed (and second-most expensive) class of drugs in Canada after cardiovasculars (Table 8.2). There is little indication that severe mental illnesses are declining: notwithstanding the move to treat severe mental illnesses in the community, one in seven hospitalizations in Canada involves patients diagnosed with mental illness (Table 8.3). The problem is not that we don't know what needs to be done. The problem is that we don't know how to achieve these policy goals. What are the barriers to effective reform?

The first structural barrier is the legacy of 1867. Most articles addressing mental health reform note that Canada is the only developed country without a national mental health strategy. The main reason for this is that mental health is under provincial jurisdiction and, legally, the federal government is *not allowed* to regulate policy in this area (see Chapter 2). We now have a Canadian Commission on Mental Health but, importantly, it has no legal jurisdiction to make policy. Rather, it has been set up in order to coordinate the real political players: the provinces. Given that the CCMH cannot simply legislate new policy directions, it must work hard to entice all the individual political jurisdictions into some cooperative framework. The CCMH is doing this by facilitating discussion between governments and stakeholders (the 'mental health strategy'), establishing an anti-stigma campaign, and funding research projects. This is all it can do.

Canada can never have a 'national' mental health policy; the best it can achieve is an integrated mental health policy. The strategy for achieving collaboration across political jurisdictions is, arguably, best suited not for the Mental Health Commission but for the Public Health Agency, which is responsible for coordinating numerous aspects of health policy across provincial boundaries. Until the establishment of the MHCC, PHAC did take responsibility for the attempt to facilitate communication across jurisdictions through its Pan-Canadian Planning Committee for Mental Health Promotion and Mental Illness Prevention. But if history is any judge, the prospects for a highly integrated mental health system are poor. Most of the 'pan-Canadian' frameworks established in the past decade are moribund (such as the Pan-Canadian Healthy Living Strategy and the Pan-Canadian Pharmaceuticals Strategy); those that resolutely survive (the Pan-Canadian Public Health Network) have faced ongoing criticisms over the failure clearly to designate proper authority and to streamline processes effectively (see Chapter 5). The framework of federalism further exacerbates the difficulty of providing an integrated mental health care system because two key policy fields in addressing mental health needs – housing and employment – are themselves fragmented and uncoordinated (Forchuk 2007). Each province has its own housing policy and its own employment strategy; rarely are the two coordinated *within* each province let alone *between* provinces. To add a layer of complexity, the federal government also has a presence in each of these fields, including the Canada Mortgage and Housing Corporation, Employment Insurance, the Canada Pension Plan (disability support), and Health Canada (in helping to fund general hospitals, regulating psychopharmaceuticals, and establishing mental health legislation relating to the Criminal Code, among other areas).

The second structural barrier is the legacy of 1957. The move to set up a shared-cost system of health services that excluded community treatment put in motion a set of political decisions that would, in time, effectively disadvantage mental health services as other health policies developed. Physician, hospital, and diagnostic services were built on fifty-cent dollars (at least until 1974) and provinces, quite sensibly, pushed health care in this direction. But this meant that many psychological services immediately became twice as expensive for the provinces; and it partly explains the low levels of these services in the wider move to deinstitutionalization. Moreover, because community services were often seen as municipal concerns while psychiatric hospitals were run at a provincial level, political officials at all three levels had different interests (and a great deal of motivation to shift financial responsibility whenever possible).

The development of the Canada Health Act in 1984, and its earlier prototypes, also fragmented mental health services by segregating the regulation of mental health providers. Fifty years later, this has imposed severe difficulties in the attempt to provide collaborative care within the area of mental health. The remuneration of physicians as private players but not psychologists, social workers, psychiatric nurses, or occupational therapists means that accessible mental health care has remained physician-driven, institutionally oriented, and expensive. The political agreement to permit the self-regulation of physicians has given them more ability than any other stakeholder group to shape policy. It has reified the professional dominance over other health care providers, with the effect that other cognate groups (such as clinical psychologists with doctoral degrees) have no prescribing privileges, even though they often have a better understanding of the etiology and presentation of psychiatric disorders than do general practitioners. It has also meant that the alternative to biomedical treatment – psychotherapy – has remained unregulated. 'In all Canadian provinces,' note Bourgeault and Mulvale, 'psychotherapy is not a controlled act and there are no restrictions on who can provide it' (2006: 489). While this may be beneficial for those who have enough money to access psychotherapy privately (and enough good sense to choose their psychotherapist wisely), it means little quality control in the provision of talk therapy, and consequently good reason for provinces to refuse to pay for it.

Obstacles to mental health reform are also being thrown up by current shifts in health policy reform. As described in Chapter 3, the paradigm of governance in health policy has strongly been informed by new public management principles. After twenty years of reforms based on these ideas, the general consensus is that the provision of health care services should be informed by three overarching principles: evidence-based care, integration, and accountability. But how well do these principles fit with the reform of mental health care?

One of the most emphatic shifts in public administration in the past two decades has been the move to results-based management, including the collection of data, the use of benchmarks and performance indicators, the articulation of business plans, and the demand for evidence-based care. In many respects this has been a very constructive strategy for general health care. Inefficient or outdated techniques and treatments have been eliminated, administrative accountability has been systematized, and the sheer volume of data has allowed researchers better to understand the manifestation of illnesses. But the emphasis on evidence-based decision making and the quantification of treatment evaluation has had mixed consequences for mental health care. While more rigorous investigation into psychopharmacology has led to a wider selection of drugs that work (and a better sense of which drugs do not work), the focus on quantifiable evidence has, unsurprisingly, privileged those treatments which more easily lend themselves to quantification. Thus, while random controlled trials can (if done properly) provide a valid sense of relative efficacy compared with other drugs (or no drugs at all), it cannot as easily provide rigorous evidence concerning other therapeutic techniques (and it raises the question whether commercial enterprises would be willing to fund them if they *did* challenge biomedical treatments). This is especially relevant for mental health care, where the evaluation of the symptoms as well as the success of treatment unavoidably requires a larger subjective component. There is good evidence to show that psychotherapy does work well in treating mental illnesses (Paris 2008), but beyond this it is difficult to quantify the nature of talk therapy. Do only certain kinds of therapeutic discussions work (such as cognitive behavioural therapy) or is any form of interpersonal activity helpful (talking to a priest, visiting a sweatlodge, phoning a psychic hotline)? Is it the nature of the discussion or the simple chemistry between individuals that is relevant? How is it possible to know that the therapeutic relationship itself, rather than external factors (a patient wins a scholarship or falls in love), have been the effective variables in a successful treatment? In an evidence-based environment, where the treatments must be able systematically to show positive results, regimes based on more ineffable dynamics have difficulty competing with easily comprehendible and measurable treatments. Thus, when 'best practices' evidence is required for a treatment to qualify for public funding (or insurance coverage), certain treatments will be given priority over others. The perception of indefinite cost liability also arises with psychotherapeutic approaches. One can only take so much Paxil at a time; but psychoanalysis can take a lifetime. And while there is current evidence that ten to twenty weeks of cognitive therapy is optimal, seven pills per week still cost less than one hour with a qualified psychotherapist.

The dilemma over whether to utilize orthodox medical treatments or 'fuzzier' psychosocial techniques does not simply involve debates over funding. The move towards biomedical approaches in psychiatry ('depression is just like an ulcer') has been useful in the attempt to destigmatize mental health. One is not a lesser person for developing cancer; neither should one be diminished by a diagnosis of depression. Both are likely the interplay of biochemical processes, social or environmental factors, and heredity. Yet this approach only reinforces the idea of mental illness as a biomedical condition requiring a biomedical treatment. It is difficult to have it both ways.

Finally, the focus on quantifiable outcomes and efficiencies in treatment often begs the question of how one measures efficient treatment. If providers are paid according to how much they accomplish and how well they have accomplished it (as in British reforms), the intractable nature of mental illness again makes results-based management more problematic. If a surgeon can implant so many sets of tubes in children's ears, and if the children no longer succumb to ear infections, then success can be measured relatively simply. Policies in this case can be directed to reward those who provide more surgeries with more positive outcomes. But, again, mental health care does not lend itself so easily to measurable outcomes. A psychiatrist who treats a higher number of individuals who no longer need her services after six months might also be seen as having a higher success rate. But it could also mean that most of these patients could more efficiently be seen by a GP or psychologist, so that the psychiatrist could focus for a longer time on a fewer number of more intractable cases. Rewarding 'successful outcomes' on this account would be highly counterproductive.

A second major focus of the new public management paradigm is integration. From a distance, the move towards regionally integrated service delivery would seem to augur well for mental health care, which more than any other health care sector depends on a high level of coordination across jurisdictions. Yet the political dynamics underlying the process of restructuring themselves can throw up a number of obstacles to integration. The case of Ontario's move towards health care restructuring from the late 1990s to the early 2000s is a cautionary tale. As Wiktorowicz (2005) explains, the Health Services Restructuring Commission (HSRC) established by the Ontario government had executive authority to develop and implement policy autonomously, but had no jurisdiction over community services. The Mental Health Implementation Task Forces (MHITFs) established in 2001 had more capacity to think about the integration of mental health care with community services, but they had only an advisory role. Moreover, the more powerful political interests (such as the Ontario Hospital Association and the Ontario Medical Association) were quite vociferous in their resistance to amalgamation, and especially to the idea of seeing their budgets transferred, out of reach, to community services. The MHITFs were seen to be more pliable than the OHA and OMA, and the transition funds that were seen as essential to providing community services as the psychiatric hospitals discharged their patients were not realized. 'As devolution fundamentally alters who makes decisions and oversees control of funds,' notes Wiktorowitz, 'it entails a bargaining process, and is not simply a juridical act. Without such devolution, regions lack the instruments of authority needed to develop models of coordinated care among the organizations that provide mental health services. Sequential shifts in the locus of planning to the nine task forces, and seven regional ministry offices, made program development a moving target' (2005: 405). The same kind of political dynamic has been witnessed in other provinces, where health service integration in practice has produced no significant transfer of funds to mental health care (e.g., Block et al. 2008). While the move towards regional integration is theoretically promising, without proper legislative oversight regarding *how* integration is to be achieved the current relations of power in the distribution of health care resources will simply be reproduced in the new structures of delivery.

The third aspect of new public management that has had a tremendous effect on the way in which health service provision has been organized is the principle that individuals should have more say in the kind of health care provided and in the way in which it is delivered. This would seem to fit well with the recovery and rehabilitation model. But it is worth remembering that the experiments with the concept of citizen engagement throughout the 1990s came to nothing. Rather, jurisdictions became aware of why they did *not* want to open up health care policy making to the wider community (Chapter 3). To the extent that the idea of individual control over health care provision still has legs, it remains most influential within market-oriented proposals for health care provision. This may, in fact, have most impact on the provision of mental health services, which already have a robust private sector component (especially for psychologists). But a commercial model of mental health care would do little to help the vulnerable populations who need them the most.

In conclusion, the mental health care sector is perhaps the area of health care most affected by political power struggles. Yet it is also the area in which thorough analyses of these dynamics of power have been least studied. The obvious reason for this is that mental health care disproportionately affects the politically dispossessed, and those with fewer economic and political resources have, in turn, more difficulty in becoming politically organized. Political change is also more difficult in this area because of the lack of political solidarity that has been built on the public funding framework for hospital, physician, and diagnostic services. The mental health care system has been more sharply bifurcated between public and private spheres because of the institutionalization of mental health into discrete asylums for much of the twentieth century. Unlike general health care services, which have been for the most part sharply restricted to the public sector, two of the most widely used mental health services – psychotropic drugs and psychological counselling – are readily available in the private sector. This, in turn, means that those who can afford such services (also those who generally have a stronger political voice) have no reason to seek substantial reform, while those who cannot afford these services are often too disenfranchised to have much political impact. Inpatient mental health care is almost exclusively provided under the auspices of the public health system (a common point for all individuals regardless of socioeconomic background). But the more that mental health care is provided in the community, the more it becomes passively privatized: those who can, access good quality private care. But those who cannot must depend on community services which are themselves subject to a political struggle within policy-making circles.

Mental health advocates must not be complacent in thinking that the wider policy trajectory towards health service integration will automatically alleviate the ongoing problem of funding shortages for

community health care services. If anything, it will make the allocation of health care resources even more opaque by placing them within
autonomous regional administrative units (such as local health integration networks or district health authorities) which may or may not
have transparent decision-making structures. Collaborative health care
systems may also fail mental health users by making accountability for
community services more difficult to identify. The political strategy of
mental health care advocates has been to attempt to broaden the grassroots support for constructive mental health policies and reforms. This
is not necessarily a bad tactical plan. But proponents of a more robust
mental health care system must also remain vigilant of the way in
which administrative reforms extend or obstruct the provision of mental health services within new decision-making structures. For political
activists it may be a very prosaic task. But given the way in which larger
health care policy choices have constrained the development of mental
health care in Canada throughout the twentieth century, it may be a
sensible strategy.

9   Beveridge Systems: Britain, Sweden, and the Internal Market

'Beveridge' and 'Bismarck' systems are the two dominant health care models in Europe, while a third model, mandated private insurance, typifies the Netherlands, and is the basis of the U.S. health care reforms. Beveridge systems, named after the British economist whose 1942 report established the foundation for Britain's modern welfare state, are funded through general taxation. In this way, all individuals contribute to a public health insurance system, and all individuals are covered. As health care funding comes from general tax revenues, individuals' contributions are determined by income, rather than health risk. In some systems, a portion of citizens' income tax is earmarked for health care; in others, income tax contributions are simply directed to a general revenue fund, which is then used to finance health care spending. Bismarck systems, named after the first German chancellor, who in 1883 created the first formal social insurance system, are based on social insurance contributions. Employees, through payroll deductions, and employers jointly contribute to sickness funds, which are private not-for-profit bodies formally independent of, but highly regulated by government. As in a Beveridge system, contributions are made according to income, not health status. In reality, pure types of these models are rare. Many countries employ some mix of these systems: general tax-based systems can also impose payroll taxes; social insurance systems can direct general tax revenue into health care funding.

A Note on Comparing Health Care Systems

The comparison of health care systems can itself be a very political act. Given how complex these systems are, it is extraordinarily easy to find aspects of any system that illustrate its superiority. It is also simple for detractors to find poor indicators for each country. This is why most cross-national surveys have become very careful about rankings: they are still done, but now they generally target very specific indicators (e.g., mortality, spending per capita, waiting times, numbers of doctors, acute beds, or CT scanners per capita). The World Health Organization's World Health Report for 2000, *Health Systems: Improving Performance* is a notorious example of the complexity involved in attempting to rank health care systems. Most Canadians were quite surprised to find that their health care system was ranked thirtieth out of 191 states, behind star performers such as San Marino, Malta, and Andorra. Critics of the Canadian health care system had a field day.

The WHO survey is constructive in understanding the issues and distortions that can arise in cross-national comparisons. For example, a major component of the survey was the assessment of systems' 'responsiveness to the expectations of the populations they serve' (Anderson and Hussey 2001: 227). Unsurprisingly, France and the United States fared well in this measurement, as both systems (among other things) allow individuals to access specialists without a referral from a family doctor. This makes health consumers happy. But, from an epidemiological perspective, it is also a very inefficient and expensive means of providing health care. Thus certain countries whose systems were costly and inefficient were actually *rewarded* by employing this indicator. Another issue was that the 'fairness of financing' indicator looked at whether different income groups used the same percentage of their income on health care. But, as Deber (2004) has pointed out, because progressive and regressive situations were treated symmetrically, highly redistributive systems that shifted the burden of illness to the affluent were scored as *less fair* than those that imposed more uniform costs. Further, the survey attempted to keep some major non-health variables as similar as possible in order to make the comparisons of health care systems more equivalent. For example, it attempted to ensure that health care effectiveness was due to the health services themselves, rather than because some countries' populations were better educated. But controlling for education meant that countries with better education levels were penalized: 'The suspicion that better rankings on health-system performance reflected lower education rather than better healthcare appears supported; it is noteworthy that all four countries receiving the highest ranks for overall performance showed relatively low educational levels, which boosted their rank (by between 5 and 26 places) from what they would have obtained looking only at their performance on goal attainment. Conversely, those with higher educational levels have had their rankings substantially depressed (by between 14 and 23 places), seemingly for that reason alone' (Deber 2004: 6).

The Canadian Institute for Health Information (CIHI) has published a very useful study for interpreting health rankings. They suggest four kinds of evaluation to which any health care ranking should be subject. The first is an examination of *which aspects of health and health care* are being considered. Is it just the health status of the population – for example, mortality and morbidity? Or is it also the social determinants of health – including, for example, education, environment, working conditions, and early childhood education? The second set of evaluations address the *specific set of indicators* chosen to make quantitative comparisons between jurisdictions. For example, CIHI uses results on influenza immunization, mammogram screening, and Pap smears to determine the *accessibility* of health care systems, and the rate of Caesarian section combined with the rates of vaginal birth after a Caesarian section to judge the *appropriateness* of health care. Obviously some jurisdictions, especially those with particular health care needs or priorities, might counter that these are misleading or prejudicial sets of indicators. Each set of indicators has its own limitations. Using lung cancer as an indicator of a health care system's performance, for example, is problematic because the rate of lung cancer is largely determined by historical smoking prevalence rates rather than current behaviour or policies. Likewise, using the rate of breast cancer as an indicator can be problematic because it might simply reflect disparities in screening practices: a better screening system would lead to the reporting of higher rates, while systematic neglect might result in fewer reported cases (CIHI 2008b: 7).

A third focus for evaluation concerns not the kind of indicator, but the *quality of the data* used for the indicator. Are the data outdated, or unrepresentative of the larger population, or too subjective? Or are there simply different ways of calculating the same indicator? CIHI notes, for example, that infant mortality rates are calculated differently across countries: some, like Canada and the United States, record deaths of very premature babies as 'infant mortality,' while others register these cases as 'fetal deaths.' This will skew infant mortality comparisons between countries to some degree. Ideally, states CIHI, 'data should be free from bias, current, complete and represent the population of interest' (2008b: 9).

Finally, one must evaluate the *methodological principles* that are used to interpret the data. For instance, how significant are the gaps between ranking positions: are they trivial or substantial? If the first five entries have very similar rankings, but the gap between the fifth and sixth is quite large, this is important information. 'In horse races,' comments Deber (2004: 6), 'rankings are all that matter – it does not matter whether the victor won by a nose or by several lengths.' But in considerations of the performance of health care systems, the specific *rating* of a jurisdiction is often more useful than its *ranking*. Another variable that might influence results is the composition of a population: an urban catchment area with a high number of long-term care facilities (such as retirement communities) may always score low on health indicators such as mortality and morbidity, but this is not necessarily a good reflection of the quality of the health care services in that area. Or the indicator could be based on small sample sizes, resulting in less confidence in the accuracy of the measure. Or it could be based solely on extrapolation, which was the case in several instances of measurement within the 2000 WHO survey.

Notwithstanding the pitfalls, however, comparisons between countries can be a useful exercise if they are undertaken cautiously. They can, for example, give us a sense of what seems to work, even if it is not always clear *why* some forms of organization tend to work better than others. A notable example of a cross-country survey that eschews simplistic rankings in favour of more nuanced comparisons is a 2007 Commonwealth Fund survey that examined patients' experiences in seven countries (Australia, Canada, Germany, Netherlands, New Zealand, the United Kingdom, and the United States). The survey addressed individuals' 'overall health system views, confidence, access, cost burdens, and perceptions of waste and complexity' (Schoen et al. 2007: 720), and while it utilized self-reported data, it did present interesting comparisons between countries. Germans and Americans, with the most fragmented systems, had the most negative views of their health care systems, while Britons and Canadians had the most positive views of theirs. At the same time, however, Germans and Americans reported that they had the most rapid access, while British and Canadian respondents stated they had the longest waits. The Americans and the Dutch, with the most options for insurance and treatment payment schemes, also spent the most time on paperwork and disputes over payments (ibid., 720, 722).

So cross-country comparisons, while tricky, can occasionally point us in policy directions that might improve the overall performance of our health care system. The 2007 Commonwealth Fund survey, for example, found that individuals in jurisdictions with easy access to a primary care 'home' were more likely to receive preventive care and less likely to encounter coordination problems, while experiencing fewer disparities in care (Schoen et al. 2007: 718). Cross-national comparisons can also give us a strong sense of which practices, on balance, are best *not* duplicated. What is more difficult to determine is whether (and how) the advantages of other countries can be adopted at home. In some cases, the historical institutional structure of a country allows it to develop a particular framework for health care systems. In Germany and the Netherlands, for example, the social insurance system developed from structures and social groupings that had their roots in the medieval guild system. In other cases, such as Sweden, the health care system is a reflection of particular social and cultural values that are unique to that region. In still other cases, the health care framework is a reflection of the particular political and economic constraints that dominated the country's landscape when the health care system was established: Greece and Portugal, for instance, developed modern health care systems when 'entrenched right-wing forces were much more powerful' (Evans 2005b: 282). The current institutional context, too, is vital in considering why, and how well, a given health care system performs: German policy making, for example, is developed in a context of coalition governments and negotiation between federal and Länder governments, so radical change is difficult to impose; policy making in the United Kingdom is much more centralized with fewer veto points and can be shifted with less political effort.

But the question is not simply *whether* we can adopt particular aspects of other states' health care systems. It is also *what the costs would be* to import such changes. What would Canadians have to give up, for instance, to shorten waiting times? We could adopt an American approach and simply encourage as much private health care provision as the market could bear: but then we would compromise the principles of equity, comprehensiveness, and cost containment. Or we could adopt the French or German solution and opt for a more complex system of social insurance: we could retain the principle of comprehensiveness and adopt a slightly different form of equity, but we would still sacrifice cost containment.

Thus the practice of cross-country comparison, while useful in broadening our understanding of what is possible, is no simple or quick fix. Interjurisdictional comparisons, both regional and international, are a mainstay of modern policy making: the utilization of certain information technology systems, the restructuring of management techniques, or the establishment of policy mechanisms are all ways of making existing systems work better. There is, in the utilization of such processes and devices, a hope that positive-sum improvements can be made that will not jeopardize gains in other areas. This does happen. But the more fundamental the change (shortening waiting lists by changing the funding structure of health care, say, rather than employing a computer program to determine a system's excess capacity), the more destabilizing it will be. (This is one reason there are so few attempts at systemwide changes in health care, and it is also one reason for complaints that 'governments just aren't doing anything to solve the problem.') Leaving aside the political capital required for major policy changes, governments (often quite sensibly) recognize that the devil they know is usually a safer political antagonist than the devil they don't know. This brings us back to Aristotle's 'golden mean': the truly difficult task is to determine which precise balance of qualities – equity, efficiency, cost containment, responsiveness, universality, and comprehensiveness – is best for each entity (and which is most politically sustainable). The utilization of cross-jurisdictional comparisons, then, should never be viewed as a simple solution to the deficiencies of our health care system, but rather as a backdrop to understanding the costs and benefits of moving in one particular direction rather than in another.

Britain's Health Care System

Britain's National Health Service (NHS) was the product of two historical events: the Second World War and the election of a majority Labour government. The idea of a comprehensive health care system free at the point of delivery had been part of the Labour Party's position since 1934, but the program was not implemented until the Atlee government was elected in 1945. Historians suggest that the Second World War had an integral role in the establishment of the NHS, as the war had forced officials to coordinate local and voluntary hospitals in order efficiently to deal with air raid victims and other casualties of war. (The Luftwaffe, quipped one historian, had succeeded in months where British politicians had failed for two decades: Webster 2002) The framework for a comprehensive national health service was in place by the end of the war; the main task was then to formalize this structure.

On 5 July 1948 the NHS began operation. It was based on the principles of comprehensiveness, accessibility, universality, equity, quality of care, and central funding. After sixty years, the NHS has been remarkably successful at achieving and maintaining most of these principles. It is highly comprehensive (especially compared with Canada). While co-payments for dentistry, optometry, and prescription drugs were introduced in the early 1950s, they currently comprise a mere 1.3 per cent of total NHS spending. Like Canada, accessibility is diminished by waiting times, rather than economic barriers; although there has been notable recent success in reducing waiting times. The system remains universal for all residents, and quality of care remains reasonably high excepting complaints over waiting times (Delamothe 2008a, 2008b, 2008c). But the primary success of the NHS from a comparative perspective has been its ability to control costs. This is primarily a function of central funding from a general tax base (technically, 8.4% of NHS funds come from 'National Insurance,' but because individuals are not denied treatment if they have not paid this levy, it is generally considered to be an earmarked tax rather than a true form of health insurance). But Britain's success in cost containment has rarely been applauded, as it is also often seen as a symptom of 'underfunding.' Long waiting times are the most politically visible manifestation of underfunding. When governments attempt to respond to accusations of underfunding by pouring resources into health care services, of course, cost containment suffers. One can't have it both ways. Or can one?

What the Thatcher administration brought to NHS reform was the belief that one could 'square the circle' and accommodate both well-funded services and cost containment. What was missing, according to this account, was the principle of *efficiency*. If health care services were provided more efficiently, one could offer better services for less money. This was what led to major administrative reform within the NHS. The first step of this reform was the 1983 Griffiths Report. At this time, the United Kingdom was at the epicentre of the new public management revolution (see Chapter 3). NPM addressed the cost containment/underfunding dilemma by suggesting ways in which 'wasteful spending' could be eliminated within the NHS. By replacing old-style consensus management with devolved decision making and clear lines of accountability, noted the Griffiths Report, spending could be controlled. But by 1987, in the midst of a serious recession and in the face of a ministerial gaffe, Prime Minister Thatcher announced (to the surprise of the medical profession, and even her own ministers) that the NHS would soon be the subject of much more radical reform.

Development of the Internal Market, 1989–1997

These reforms were announced in the 1989 White Paper *Working for Patients*. Designed according to ideas articulated by American NPM theorists (including, most notably, Alain Enthoven), the document proposed the creation of an internal market within the NHS to take advantage of the way in which markets naturally tended to seek out efficiencies. Its points of reference, as with all NPM models, were consumer-oriented service provision and managerial accountability. The system articulated by the 1989 White Paper (also referred to as a quasi, mimic, managed, or regulated market model) established a split between the purchasers and the providers of health care services. It was implemented in 1991 under the auspices of the 1990 NHS and Community Care Act. The 'purchasers' in this system were not the patients but rather general practitioners and district health authorities (DHAs), working in patients' interests. GPs in the NHS were always considered to be independent practitioners, but nonetheless they worked within the NHS and were largely paid on the basis of capitation (the number of people who were registered with the practice) rather than by fee-for-service. Given this existing structure, GP practices with patient lists over a given size were given the option to form 'fund-holding' groups, where they would be given budgets with which they could buy services for their patients. These budgets came from the GPs' district health authority, which also had the ability directly to purchase services from the 'providers' (generally hospitals, but also some community services). Providers were expected to compete with each other to provide services (mostly elective surgery) to the GP fund holders and DHAs. Referencing the theory of comparative advantage, the expectation was that providers would concentrate on their areas of expertise, providing them more cheaply as a result of the economies of scale effect that is inherent in mass production. Purchasers could then shop around to get the best deals on all the services they needed, thereby trimming costs while selecting for quality. The circle could be squared after all. Further, GPs were given an incentive to participate in this system by allowing them to keep a certain proportion of saved costs.

How well did this system work? Two decades later, there is still little agreement on the evaluation of the reforms. Why? 'The first point to make about the evidence concerning the working of the quasi-market,' writes LeGrand (1999: 30) 'is that there is not very much of it, and what there is, with one or two exceptions, is not very helpful.' Remarkably, notwithstanding the NPM emphasis on constant and thorough evaluation at all levels, the Thatcher government resisted commissioning such studies for political and strategic reasons. There were several tentative indications of success: by 1996, about half of England and Wales were covered by GP fund holders, which 'achieved a wide range of benefits for their patients, contracted on a cost-per-case basis, switched contracts between providers, and involved GPs in managing budgets' (Bevan and Robinson 2005: 64). The worry over potential cream-skimming or cherry-picking, in which GP fund holders would refuse to cover high-cost patients, was assuaged when this behaviour failed to materialize (probably because DHAs, and not GP fund holders, were assigned to cover high-cost patients). Nevertheless, administrative costs increased, patients did not end up with more choice (as GPs, quite rationally, began to negotiate block contracts with providers), there were insufficient data effectively to develop pricing information on individual services, and hospitals were limited in their ability to eliminate inefficient services to the extent that their emergency departments required at least some capacity in most medical fields. 'Perhaps the most striking conclusion to arise from the evidence,' surmises LeGrand, 'is how little overall measurable change there seems to have been' (1999: 31).

The reason for this is that the internal market was, in the end, not much of a market. Because both providers and purchasers were run under the auspices of the National Health Service, the NHS itself remained run by the government and the government remained accountable for it. 'Everything that happens in the NHS,' explains Klein, 'is therefore likely to be politicized. Decisions cannot be left to the market, since ministers will be left with the consequences' (1998: 117). Moreover, the incentives put in place to pursue market-based activity were too weak, and the constraints faced by those who wished to do so wholeheartedly were too strong (LeGrand 1999: 33). Neither health authorities nor trust hospitals were allowed to keep any 'savings' they had accumulated through efficiencies. Neither health authorities nor trust hospitals saw failures to meet budgets as hard constraints, as they knew the political pressure to bail them out would be forthcoming were they to encounter dire circumstances. Rather than a health care system based on choice and competition, the NHS had become increasingly dependent on regulation and centralization. By 1997, when the Conservatives handed political power over to the new Labour administration, evaluations of the NHS were incomplete and inconclusive: no one could determine with any certainty whether the NHS had become more or less efficient (LeGrand and Robinson 1994; LeGrand, Mays, and Mulligan 1997; Klein 1998; Bevan and Robinson 2005). 'The British quasi-market in health care,' concludes LeGrand, 'neither succeeded nor failed, simply because it was never tried' (1999: 37).

Retreat and Retrenchment, 1997–2010

If the National Health Service reforms had shown little conclusive evidence of success, neither was there any unequivocal proof of failure. What shifted dramatically under the new Labour government was the rhetoric: 'choice' and 'competition' were replaced by 'partnership' and 'collaboration.' A focus on efficiency became attention to quality. More emphasis was placed on primary health care, evidence-based medicine, and integrated treatment, but these were themes that all countries were beginning to address regardless of their systems of delivery. The essential structure of the NHS, however, remained the same: the trappings of competition resting on an undercarriage of regulation.

Under the Labour government, the purchaser-provider split remained. All general practitioners were organized into primary care groups (PCGs) which included both fund-holding and non–fund-holding GPs. These PCGs were given budgets by district health authorities to meet the needs of their respective patient populations. The logic of this was not only to retain GPs' function as purchasers (for those who chose to do so) but also to impose a dynamic of peer pressure on fellow GPs to make sure that the PCG budget was not exceeded. This was a radical departure from the historical understanding of GPs as independent contractors; but at the same time it gave GPs, collectively, more power over the provision of health services than they had ever enjoyed before (Klein 1998). PCGs and now hospital trusts were allowed to retain savings that they were able to attain through competitive purchasing or providing. At the same time, DHAs lost their purchasing role, but became directly responsible for PCG activity.

In addition to structural changes, the new Labour administration adopted a more stringent regulatory framework based on the NPM principles of performance management. The National Institute for Clinical Effectiveness (NICE) was established in order to set out clear guidelines for safe and cost-effective treatments and procedures, while the Commission for Health Improvement (CHI), and later Monitor, watched the performance of health care providers. Numerous performance indicators were established (first as a series of green-yellow-red 'lights,' then as a star system). This led to much concern that the Labour government was reinforcing the centralization of power over health care services through its new regulatory regime. It was. But if this tactic worried those on the right, those on the left were equally anxious about the government's new policy of encouraging private sector involvement in the provision of health care. This took two forms: the building and financing of medical infrastructure and the running of non-clinical services (public-private partnership or P3 hospitals), and the development of private treatment centres to compete with hospital trusts (trusts were 'not-for-profit,' but they allowed to retain 'savings' to roll back into hospital use). Private medical care (usually for medical insurance and hospital services) has always been allowed in the United Kingdom, but it has been limited. The move to increase capacity by not only encouraging private medical companies (increasingly from outside of the United Kingdom) but also giving them preferential treatment has been considerably controversial.

Notwithstanding all these measures, criticism of the National Health Service remained high and public support was increasingly equivocal. Long waiting times were symbolic of the difficulties that beset the NHS. This led Labour, in 2003, to raise taxes and pour new funding into the health care system. If the NHS were to survive, they believed, 'the funding quantum would have to increase dramatically. Otherwise, the gap between system performance and public expectation would widen, the middle classes would progressively buy their way out, and the NHS would spiral down to become a residualist safety net' (Stevens 2004: 37). Thus the middle of the decade saw another wave of major NHS reform. Medical schools boosted their enrolment by over half; more nurses were hired; hospitals were built; and electronic information technology (IT) systems were put into place. More structural changes were introduced: primary care groups and district health authorities were rolled into a smaller number of larger primary care trusts (PCTs), which were given responsibilities for meeting primary health care targets and budgets of purchasing other health services (Figure 9.1 provides a simplified diagram of how health care services are funded in England).

Performance indicators and diagnostic-related groupings were fine-tuned so that providers could more effectively be given 'payment by results.' High-performing hospitals were allowed to become 'foundation trusts' which gave them even more self-governing autonomy. Further, local accountability was emphasized by making local hospitals accountable to a locally elected hospital board. The principle of devolution, which had been embraced since 1997, meant that England, Scotland, Wales, and Northern Ireland had the ability to design their individual NHSs to their own specifications. By 2003 Scotland had effectively abandoned the idea of a purchaser-provider split, and Wales followed in 2008. This process of decentralization within the health services was driven as much by political considerations as it was by ideological approaches. Centralizing control also meant centralizing responsibility; by decentralizing responsibility for the provision and regulation of services (through regionalization and independent regulatory agencies as well as the internal market), blame for politically embarrassing circumstances could also be avoided.

How Well Has It Worked?

The remarkable thing about the internal market in the United Kingdom is that, after twenty years, there is still no agreement about how successful it has been. On the one hand, many health care indicators have been positive, including substantial drops in waiting times for diagnosis and treatment at both the primary and secondary levels. Patients are treated more quickly in emergency departments, more screenings for major diseases are taking place, and fewer individuals are dying from cancer and heart disease (Klein 2007). That Britons themselves are reasonably satisfied with the NHS may be reflected in the fact that the number of individuals purchasing private health insurance has fallen since 2002 (Delamothe 2008d). Telling, too, is the fact that a Labour government would, over its entire mandate, refuse to eliminate a mechanism that symbolizes Thatcherite principles of governance. However, these do not amount to substantive evidence that the internal market works *well*. It would be surprising, given the sheer amount of funding pumped into the NHS since 2003, if indicators had not improved substantially. The real question is whether such improvements had anything to do with the internal market, or were simply a reflection of either the larger amount of resources available or the use of performance management systems.

Figure 9.1. How health care services are funded in England

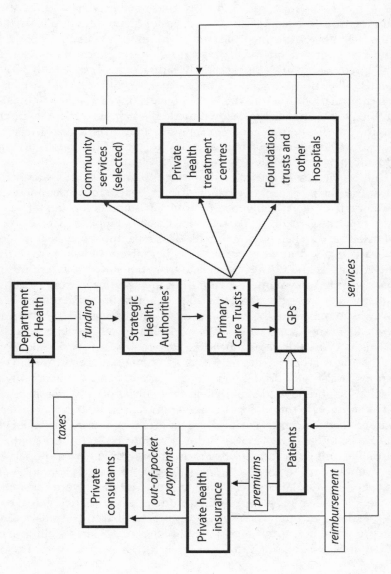

*Primary care trusts and strategic health authorities are to be replaced by GP commissioning consortia in 2013.

The superiority of the British system has, for decades, been its ability to contain costs. But a system that can do so effectively also has the ability to underfund health services (by comparative standards). It is clear that the health care system in the United Kingdom has in recent years been able to maintain equity, quality, and responsiveness, but only at the expense of cost containment. Because of the private-public partnerships (P3s) the government has entered into, it will be liable for costs from these agreements for decades. It will also be locked into contractual agreements with a substantially larger number of health professionals, who are now among the best paid in Europe. The stream of spending that poured into the NHS from 2003 was due to end in 2008; but the global financial meltdown made the halt even more emphatic. Has the internal market generated enough gains in efficiency that it can survive without generous increases in public funding? It is simply too difficult to determine this conclusively before the fact.

One problem with the internal market was that distortions tended to arise. The initial concept of a patient-driven system in which money followed patients never really materialized. GP fund holders (and then primary care trusts) realized (like seasoned Costco shoppers) that they could get better deals when buying in bulk. This meant that a system of block contracts evolved in which providers guaranteed a lower price if they were given a set number of patients to treat. But since providers' income now depended on volume, providers had an incentive 'not only to attract as many patients as possible but also to diagnose and treat them in such a way as to maximize their income. In short,' observes Klein, 'there are, for the first time in the history of the NHS, incentives to over-treat' (2007: 9). This, of course, drives up spending even more. Thus, while GP-driven purchasing was believed to be a means to containing costs through efficiencies, it also produced a countertendency to *increase* costs by giving hospitals an incentive to treat as many patients as often as possible.

The solution to this was to strengthen primary care trusts in order to counterbalance hospital trusts' drive for greater volume. The belief was that PCTs, in order to keep costs down, would try to limit (expensive) hospital admissions and seek as much ongoing treatment as possible in the primary care sector (including strategies of health promotion and illness prevention), where costs are cheaper. Yet there were substantial barriers to this approach. A limited number of 'efficiency gains' have been realized through the exercise of 'practice-based commissioning,' but progress, notes one report, 'has been slow, and is stalling completely in some areas' (Curry et al. 2008: x). There are several reasons for this. The theoretical idea behind practice-based commissioning is that GPs would be making more decisions about treatment options. But there is a tension between PCTs, which must manage budgets, and the GPs *within* the PCTs, who may or may not be given the freedom by the PCTs to make such decisions. It also assumes that GPs have the managerial, as well as medical, expertise to make such market-based decisions on an ongoing basis. This requires them to have reasonable data analysis skills, comprehension of the commissioning system itself, good business acumen, and extra time to devote to business planning in addition to their clinical workloads (Curry et al. 2008). These skills are not,however, taught and are rarely systematically supported, and it is therefore hardly surprising that so few general practitioners take advantage of the opportunities to engage in practice-based commissioning. An additional barrier is the availability of useful data. Good market decisions depend on how well-informed actors are; if this information is missing or misleading, players are much less willing to take risks with their decisions. Further, the more that this information is provided by complex data systems, the more individuals need training in how to decipher and use them. The question at present is whether the roles of GP purchasers can be strengthened to counterbalance the influence of large hospital trusts, or whether the attempt to fine-tune the internal market so that efficiency gains are secured is destined to fail.

The problem with the internal market is precisely the problem with the real market: for it to work effectively, one has to incur risks. If the risks involved in an internal market are too intolerable for political officials, then governments will modify the market mechanisms so that they have no bite. But then they will also be less effective in modifying behaviour. However, if one chooses to impose strict market discipline on the players, both purchasers and providers, then health care services will be subject to the same volatility that the real market faces. Would any government have the fortitude to defend this strategy? Two additional challenges now confront the National Health Service: first, the financial contraction experienced since 2008 means that the NHS is facing 'an era of austerity unlike anything experienced in recent memory' (Ham 2009a: 1024). If the NHS has survived only on additional government funding, then the internal market is dead. If the internal market can produce efficiency gains, then it had better make them apparent soon. Second, Labour may have let the fox into the henhouse with its attempt to use the private sector as a means of increasing capacity in the health care system. By not only allowing but encouraging a proliferation of private treatment centres, patient care and funding may drain away from the NHS as public funding dissolves and NHS services contract.

In May 2010 a Conservative/Liberal Democrat coalition formed a new government in the United Kingdom, and in June 2010 the new government announced plans to strengthen the existing system of GP commissioning. Under the Lansley plan, the 35,000 GPs in the United Kingdom would, by 2013, be divided into approximately five hundred 'commissioning consortia' to purchase all services directly from providers. These GP consortia would control 80 per cent of the NHS's £100 billion budget. Many issues remain, including whether GPs will want to take on greater managerial control, whether most of them will be equipped to do so, how they will remain accountable, and whether (like the regional health authorities in Canada in the mid-1990s) their role as primary decision makers in a period of severe economic cutbacks will be used to deflect criticism away from governments' attempts to decrease spending; for an evaluation of how well the NHS has functioned from 1997 to 2010 see the King's Fund (2010), and for a critical evaluation of the new coalition government's NHS reforms see the Nuffield Trust (2010).

Sweden's Health Care System

Sweden shares many common characteristics with the United Kingdom. Both are largely tax-funded systems, with a small national insurance component. Both are comprehensive systems offering universal access, and both have struggled with accessibility issues based on long waiting lists. Finally, while both are fairly effective at cost containment, such restrictions have in each case led to accusations of underfunding. To encourage more efficient use of resources while maintaining the ability to control costs, Sweden, like Britain, implemented an internal market system in the early 1990s. Intriguingly, these internal markets were introduced by Conservative governments in both countries and have been largely maintained by the social democratic administrations which succeeded them.

There are also substantial differences between the two systems. The most substantial – especially from a Canadian perspective – is that Sweden's health care system is highly decentralized on a regional basis. Swedes will point out that the state has been active in establishing health care since the middle of the eighteenth century (when its first eight-bed hospital was set up to serve, not just the entire country, but Finland as well). The system has shifted, however, from a historically decentralized one to a modern centralized system after the Second World War, and back towards greater decentralization beginning in the 1970s. This highly decentralized structure means that, like Canada, there are difficulties both in making generalizations about the country as a whole and in finding measures that have been standardized between regions. It also means that reforms are frequently begun at a regional level, and (like Canada) adopted nationally when their utility is proven within a discrete area.

As in most countries, Sweden's reforms have come in waves. In the 1970s the payment system (based on 75% reimbursement) was replaced by one based on universal coverage with nominal user fees. In 1982 health care planning was decentralized from the national level down to the county councils, and in 1985 capitation became the most common form of paying general practitioners. Like in the United Kingdom, in Sweden the concern with cost containment in the 1980s resulted in a squeeze on health care spending. This, in turn, led to an attempt to do more with less and an emphasis on 'efficiency gains' became pronounced in the 1990s. Unlike the United Kingdom, however, in Sweden structural reforms were introduced more gradually, as each regional county council had clear authority for the provision of health care services. In Sweden, importantly, the majority of health care funds are raised at the regional and municipal level. While the national government does transfer funds directly to county councils in order to limit disparities between regions, both county councils (eighteen in total, plus two amalgamated regional bodies and one autonomous municipality) and municipalities within the county councils can levy their own taxes to pay for health care in their areas. There is some division of responsibility between county councils and municipalities: under the 1992 ÄDEL reforms, county councils devolved long-term inpatient care and care of the elderly to the municipalities, while retaining responsibility for most other regular health care services.

Between 1988 and 1992 the first major purchaser-provider system was developed. The large urban county of Stockholm was the first to separate hospitals (as providers) from the purchasers of health services (which is why the internal market in Sweden is often referred to as the 'Stockholm Model') and to offer choice of provider to patients. By 1994 over half of the county councils had introduced some form of internal market. There was evidence that efficiency gains were made: 'Improvements in both service volume and financial efficiency have been confirmed in a report from the Federation of County Councils (2002). Expenditure and also – in some categories – employee reductions across Sweden occurred simultaneously with substantial service expansions in surgical areas such as corneal lens replacement and hip replacement. Overall, operating efficiency increased substantially with no indications of decreased medical quality' (Saltman and Bergman 2005: 265). One of the main reasons for this was the shift from funding based on perceptions of need to funding based on performance. As one hospital official in Stockholm commented, 'when I started here we had a waiting list of almost one thousand patients. My understanding was that for hospitals to get more money, they had to show that they had patients waiting for a long time' (quoted in Quaye 2007: 28).

But reaction against the reforms was soon to follow. The Stockholm Model required hospitals, as public providers, to become managerially independent institutions. This, in turn, meant that they were responsible for their own budgets and had to compete for purchasers' contracts. Some counties, including Stockholm, designated certain of their hospitals as 'public companies,' with stock held by the county council. But as locally owned enterprises, hospitals were viewed as alienable property; and when Stockholm County Council 'sold' the operating capacity of one major hospital, St Göran's (St George's), to a private for-profit company that was soon taken over by foreign interests, the national Social Democratic Party acted to limit what was seen as creeping privatization within the Swedish health care system. By the mid-1990s, mirroring changes in the United Kingdom, Sweden shifted the rhetoric surrounding health care reform from 'competition' to 'cooperation,' although the underlying internal market structures were not substantially transformed.

How successful have these market reforms been in Sweden? On the one hand, several micro-studies confirmed efficiency gains after the introduction of internal market mechanisms. In Stockholm, for example, service volume improvements of 11 per cent were found with no increase in expenditure (Saltman and Bergman 2005: 266). On the other hand, there is much debate about whether these efficiencies were *caused by* the internal market structures. Some comparative studies, for example, found that similar efficiency gains were made in both counties with internal markets and those without, while others found similar efficiency gains across a number of European countries (ibid., 267). Others have pointed out that the internal markets were introduced concomitantly with a strengthening of the primary health care system, and they argue that it is the enhanced capacity of the primary care system rather than the internal market itself that has been responsible for more efficient health care utilization. Thus the same kind of confused ambivalence over the internal market that has characterized public policy in the United Kingdom also informs the administration of health care in Sweden.

Swedish health care policy reflects an ongoing tension between market-oriented policies and those grounded in solidaristic principles. Even before 2006, when a centre-right coalition won control of the government, far more emphasis was being placed on using 'real' rather than 'mimic' private providers. Again, this is similar to Britain's recent encouragement of private health care providers that compete with public ones for purchaser contracts. Like in the United Kingdom, in Sweden this embrace of the private sector was largely due to accessibility issues. In 2005 the Swedish government announced the '0-7-90-90' rule on waiting times: citizens were ensured immediate contact with the health care system, an appointment with a GP within seven days, an appointment with a specialist within 90 days, and no longer than 90 days between diagnoses of a condition and treatment for it. But by 2008, Sweden's National Board of Health and Welfare discovered that almost 45 per cent of patients exceeded this guarantee despite a $42 million surge in health care funding (Mason 2008: 130).

Like in the United Kingdom, the current vision in Sweden is that the private sector can alleviate these accessibility issues. Currently, Sweden has nine fully private for-profit hospitals. But unlike the United Kingdom, it also has a substantial number of private *primary* care clinics. Between 2000 and 2008, the number of private clinics increased from 146 to 250, although the proportion of private to public clinics varies substantially from county to county. Many of them are funded by the public system at set costs (to register for the Swedish equivalent of a 'billing number,' GPs simply negotiate the relationship with their individual county council). Interestingly, Sweden was one of the countries used by the majority of Canadian Supreme Court judges in the *Chaoulli* case when citing the viability of a public-private hybrid system. However, while one-tenth of all health care in Sweden is now provided privately, there is in Sweden very little interest for private health *insurance,* which was what the judges in *Chaoulli* were ostensibly discussing (see Chapter 4).

What Can We Learn from Britain and Sweden?

What can Canada learn from the experiences of Britain and Sweden with the internal market? All three countries have a general tax-based health care system, and all three see the provision of equitable public health care services as a long-standing political principle. All three are relatively effective in maintaining cost control, yet all three suffer problems of accessibility based on long waiting times. To what extent is an internal market a policy direction that Canada should consider?

Julian LeGrand writes that one lesson for other systems that Britain can offer is that 'putting budgets for purchasing secondary care under the control of family practitioners can work in terms of improving hospitals' responsiveness, encouraging innovation, and improving efficient resource use' (1999: 35). When LeGrand became the Labour government's new health adviser in 2004, much emphasis was placed on the principle of practice-based commissioning in which GPs were to use their front-line expertise to make efficient market decisions in purchasing health care services from providers. But GPs themselves have been less enthusiastic about this policy, holding that the entrepreneurial skills expected of them, added to the poor quality of information and training provided to them, simply do not make the role of 'front-line decision maker' an attractive one.

In Sweden the utilization of general practitioners to bring costs to heel is impaired by the fact that there is no national policy of GP gatekeeping as there is in Canada and the United Kingdom. Patients with a cough, for example, are free either to consult a GP or a respiratory specialist (although some Swedish counties do utilize GP gatekeepers). Rather, Sweden utilizes a system of graduated user fees (it costs twice as much to consult a specialist than a GP) in order to dissuade individuals from choosing high-cost specialists over GPs. But given the relatively small difference between the two fees (fifteen to twenty dollars more will allow you to see a specialist), and given the substantially increased cost to the state for the use of specialists, there is little indication that this mechanism of patient responsiveness supports the efficient use of resources.

A second lesson noted by LeGrand bears much more careful consideration. 'Incentives to encourage dramatic behaviour change by health professionals or managers,' he states, 'must be greater than those offered under the British internal market' (1999: 35); or, one might add, the Swedish internal market. The view that internal markets have not worked particularly well simply because they never were applied emphatically enough has been echoed by Klein's analysis of Britain (2006) and Hogberg's account of Sweden (2007). In both cases providers did not depend completely on securing the business of purchasers, and so could survive without competing. In both cases providers that failed to compete were not heavily penalized. In other words, the market reforms were not really markets at all, as they did not permit failure. There was good reason for this, as the political costs of failure would be borne not just by the players and patients but also by the politicians. The question, then, is whether the internal market can operate in an environment where political actors are insulated from the political responsibilities of market failure (as the current U.K. model now attempts to do), or whether the public and private features of such a hybrid simply cancel each other out. One should ask, too, whether political actors *should* be protected from the performance of components of the health care system: isn't the idea of public responsibility for health care the very point of having a public health care system?

Another related question is the extent to which it has been the adoption of measures used to balance or correct for market-based instruments, as opposed to the market principles themselves, that have produced constructive results. Both the NHS and Swedish counties have increasingly utilized performance indicators and regulatory devices to monitor performance and to limit distortions. Interestingly, a case study of Sweden's Jönköping County Council as a world-class high-performing health care system noted the importance of long-term continuity in leadership, transparency, and trust between health officials and the health care workforce, a culture of financial discipline, and the use of audit and measurement tools as well as principle of total quality management (Baker et al. 2008). Nothing was said about the importance of ensuring competition in the provision of health care services. Further, in the case of Britain, Chris Ham (2009b: 1118) has observed that 'independent assessments have shown that targets and performance management, together with increased investment, have made the biggest contribution to the improvements in the NHS.' It would seem that the features of health care system management that worked in this case could as easily be applied to a more centralized regulatory health care framework as they could be to one based on an internal market.

A fourth, and less salubrious lesson, to be learned from the experiment undertaken by Britain and Sweden is that too many attempts at finding a reform with bite can simply lead to reform fatigue. Of Sweden, Saltman and Bergman write that 'what was once a static, bureaucratic structure has seemingly spent the past ten years in a condition of permanent transformation, leading to staff burnout and a longing among both patients and personnel for organizational stability' (2005: 259). Moreover, of the United Kingdom, Klein observes that 'medical morale remains brittle' as 'the oscillations of policy over the past decade have severely tested the capacity of NHS managers to absorb and adapt to change' (2006: 412).

Of course, questions of comparison must always take into account the extent to which the entities being compared are similar enough to make policy transfer viable. One considerable difference between Britain and Sweden, on the one hand, and Canada, on the other, is the sheer geographical size of the latter compared with the compact nature of the former. To the extent that the idea of an internal market depends on the willingness of patients to travel beyond their local catchment area, too much geographical distance between purchasers and providers may limit the effectiveness of competition (even in Britain and Sweden the preference of many to choose longer waiting times over travelling for quicker service is well documented). Likewise, the introduction of user fees in such an egalitarian political culture as Sweden has been remarked on by many Canadians. However, it is precisely *because* Sweden is such an egalitarian society that user fees do not have the pernicious effect that they might in countries with a greater gap between socioeconomic classes. Those who are most economically vulnerable will always be more hesitant about using medical services when user fees exist. But when the lower socioeconomic classes exist in a more decommodified environment, where many necessary services are already heavily subsidized (e.g., day care, housing, transportation), they are more able to afford the user fees charged for health services. A more ephemeral, but potentially significant, variable in thinking about policy transfer is the influence of a strong set of homogeneous, socially embedded values underlying public support for a particular health care policy. Sweden, for example, has historically supported policy based on 'the two dominant and transcending Swedish national social values: *jamlikhet* (equality of all citizens) and *trygghet* (security)' (Saltman and Bergman 2005: 261). Similarly, polling has shown that Americans are loath to give up the room for choice in the provision health care services, even at the expense of efficiency (Alakeson 2008: 721). The question is the extent to which these cultural predilections constrain the adoption of new policies. Social values are not immutable: both the United Kingdom (in the 1940s) and Canada (in the 1980s) developed a deep attachment to public health care that had not existed previously. But it is extraordinarily difficult to determine before the fact the extent to which these social values might translate into a palpable political force.

The final observation to be made here is that there is no evidence that internal markets have allowed health care systems to achieve a broader set of objectives. Public tax-based systems such as those of Britain and Sweden have historically been strong in cost containment and equity and weaker in efficiency and responsiveness. Internal market mechanisms have, to a greater or lesser extent, made them both more efficient and responsive, but only through weakening cost control and equity. Internal markets diminish the capacity for cost containment for two reasons: first, cost efficiencies for providers depend on volume. Those providing services attempt to increase demand (both in the number of patients and in the number of treatments per patient). Second, expanding choice and competition requires spare capacity. The only way to control public costs while expanding capacity is to involve the private sector in the provision of health care services. This is precisely what is currently happening in both Britain and Sweden. However, this move simply increases total spending on health care. It also has potential consequences for equity. Where private services are offered side by side with public services, the possibility of a two-tier service model arises. Health care providers, given the option of greater remuneration in the private sphere, may be pulled out of the public sector, leading to further erosion in the quality and accessibility of services. 'We could then,' surmises Diderichsen, 'expect greater public demand for tax deductions for the premiums paid and eroding loyalty to the entire universal welfare system and the high taxes it demands' (2000: 934). The internal market, in sum, merely trades off one set of valuable characteristics for another – it does not provide a means of accommodating them all.

10   Bismarck Systems: France, Germany, and the Social Insurance Model

In recent years there has been substantial interest in looking to Europe for an alternative to the Canadian health care model (e.g., see Flood, Stabile, and Tuohy 2008). British Columbia Premier Gordon Campbell toured European states in 2006 to investigate some of these alternatives, while Canadian Medical Association (CMA) president Robert Ouellet did the same in 2009. However, if there are lessons to be learned from Europe, they are complex ones that do not promise easy solutions for Canada. It is important to remember that there is no such thing as a 'European model': all European states have distinct health care systems built on their own particular historical circumstances, culture, and political dynamics. What is frequently referred to as 'the European model' is generally some blend of public and private financing. Yet *all* systems are characterized by some combinations of public and private funding: Canada itself has a 70/30 public-private spending ratio in health care expenditure. In the two systems most frequently touted as alternatives to the Canadian model – Britain and France – there is a considerably higher ratio of public-to-private health care funding than in Canada.

What makes several European states so distinctive from Canada is that they are based on a social insurance system rather than a tax-based system. In Canada (like Britain) public health care funds are raised primarily through the general tax system. This has many advantages: it is administratively simple, it is more equitable (as long as the taxation system is progressive), it provides universal coverage, it is an effective means of cost containment, and it provides a very wide pool to 'spread the risks' so that the ill do not have to bear the burden of high insurance premiums. But social insurance systems like those in France and Germany seem to have advantages that Canadians can only envy: there are no long waiting times, for example, and there is more comprehensive coverage of services.

What is a 'social insurance' model? It is, primarily, one based on payroll taxes rather than general taxation. Employees (and employers) are 'mandated' (i.e., required) to pay into 'sickness funds' or 'mutual assistance associations' which are frequently administered jointly by representatives of both employee and employer groups. They are non-profit entities, and while they are generally considered to be 'private' or autonomous entities they are also highly regulated by the state. These sickness funds (*mutuelles* in France, *Krankenkassen* in Germany) are based historically on principles of solidarity between workers, and individuals enrolled in these plans are generally not rated according to their risk of illness or utilization of services (as in private plans) but rather their income level (as in a general taxation system). Several of the best health care systems in the world are based on the social insurance model. The question, again, is the extent to which these systems have useful lessons for Canada. Are the successes transferrable, or are they firmly embedded in a particular political culture or institutional context? Even if they could be applied to Canada, would we just be trading one set of headaches for another?

France's Health Care System

Those unfamiliar with Canada's health care system might find it frustratingly complex. But it is much simpler than that of France. Despite the complexity, however, France's system tends to work well: notwithstanding the flaws inherent in the 2000 WHO survey (which placed France at the top), France does have one of the most exemplary health care systems to be found anywhere. Yet it is not without its own problems. How does France's health care system work?

Statutory Health Insurance

What is often referred to as France's system of 'public health insurance' is actually a form of statutory (or obligatory) health insurance based on a web of discrete, independent, highly regulated, not-for-profit health insurance organizations known as *mutuelles*. France's system of mutuelles, or employee-based mutual benefit associations, goes back to the nineteenth century. Mutuelles were absorbed into the formal social security system after the Second World War, and still form the backbone of the health insurance system in France. Because these health insurance funds are financed through payroll tax, the early beneficiaries were only workers and their families. Universal coverage had been an early objective of those constructing the postwar social security system, but it was effectively undermined by occupational groups who already had advantageous independent health insurance plans. These included bank employees, miners, railway workers, clergy, civil servants, and seamen, among others (Sandier, Paris, and Polton 2004: 8). Health insurance coverage was expanded through separate health insurance associations to agricultural workers (in 1961) and to the self-employed (in 1966). Currently, the largest health insurance fund (the *régime général*) covers about 84 per cent of the population, the farmers' plan covers 7.2 per cent, and the scheme for self-employed covers approximately 5 per cent of the population. The remainder of the population is covered by much smaller mutuelles.

For legal purposes these associations are given the status of private enterprises, but they are also under the direct supervision of the Department of Social Services. This ambivalent status is the source of considerable (and increasing) political conflict. Historically, the state was responsible for policy regarding public hospitals and pharmaceuticals, while the mutuelles negotiated agreements with independent doctors and both public and private hospitals. However, one significant weakness of a social insurance model is that the fragmentation of the system makes it difficult to control costs. Moreover, there is a sense of 'ownership' by those who pay into these funds which makes it difficult politically to decrease or eliminate benefits. Contributors view their benefits as 'earned' and they therefore expect them to be delivered when required (Marmor 2008). France's health care system is one of the most expensive in the world, and the French government for years has been attempting to control health care expenditures. This has led to open conflict with the health insurance funds, who perceive that the state is transgressing on their jurisdiction. Because of this fractious institutional conflict, health care policy making in France has become exceptionally difficult (Sandier et al. 2004).

Another problem with an employment-based system is that health care benefits depend on one's employment status. During the period of high unemployment throughout the 1980s, this flaw became quite pronounced, as many were left without substantial health care coverage. In consequence, France introduced the Couverture Maladie Universelle (CMU), or the Universal Health Coverage Act, in 2000. This provides basic health insurance to the poorest subpopulation (about 1.8% of the population), and it is financed through general taxation.

An additional problem with payroll-based health insurance is that it does not provide as wide a contribution base as does one funded by general taxation. For this reason, a discrete national income tax was created in 1990 (the *contribution sociale generalisée*) to broaden the payroll tax base. By widening the source of health care contributions in this way, the statutory health insurance system has become more resistant to fluctuations in employment while remaining highly equitable (i.e., progressive) and maintaining its comprehensiveness. But in doing so, interestingly, it is moving away from a social insurance system and towards one based on general taxation (like Canada's). Funding for health care also comes from taxes on alcohol, tobacco, and cars. Additionally, a tax on the advertising money paid by pharmaceutical companies is earmarked for the public health care system.

In sum, France has universal health care coverage through a combination of mandated, mostly occupation-based health insurance for those who are employed (or retired) and state-financed health insurance for those with no access to the mutuelles. No one is without statutory health care insurance. Unlike Canada, this health insurance is quite *comprehensive:* it covers not only primary care, hospital care, and diagnostics, but it is also applied to pharmaceuticals, dental care, and optical care. But statutory health insurance does not cover the *entire* cost of *any* of these services. One of the principal ways in which French health care differs from that of Canada is that all health care costs are shared by the individual being treated. This cost-sharing takes several distinct forms.

Voluntary Complementary Health Insurance

The most significant mode of cost-sharing in France is that of voluntary complementary health insurance. The statutory health insurance system only covers a certain percentage of each health care service: for example, statutory health insurance (the rates for which are set by the French government, even though they are covered by the individual mutuelles) will cover 80 per cent of a hospital visit or 50 to 70 per cent of a GP visit. Statutory health insurance will also cover a certain proportion of prescription costs, depending on the effectiveness and relative expense of the drug (generally 35% to 65%). Eye care and dental care are covered, but usually only for a small percentage of costs.

Thus individuals are expected to shoulder a relatively significant proportion of the costs incurred. There are exemptions from the expectation of cost-sharing. These include persons with severe chronic illness (such as cancer, AIDS, or diabetes), severely disabled persons, pregnant women, veterans, newborns, and residents of nursing homes. Some procedures (such as infertility treatments) are exempt from cost-sharing, as are certain goods and services such as particular vaccines and some cancer screening. About 8.5 per cent of the population in total is exempt from co-insurance.

To address the remaining costs not covered by statutory health insurance, a system of *complementary* health insurance has evolved in France. This form of health insurance is optional, rather than mandated, but almost 90 per cent of the population has some type of complementary health insurance. There are three options for the provision of voluntary health insurance. The first is through the same mutuelles that provide statutory health insurance. These institutions provide approximately 60 per cent of voluntary health insurance. Private for-profit companies, which have the freedom to adjust for risk, account for about 20 per cent of the voluntary health insurance, while provident associations (which are jointly run by employers and employees, and often focus on retirees) comprise just under 20 per cent.

It is important to remember that this form of optional private insurance historically has not provided access to better or to faster health care (which is the function of private health insurance in Britain). Rather, it simply reimburses for services that are already covered (to various degrees) by statutory health insurance. Private health insurance 'tops up' the fees that remain once the statutory allowance is used up. Patients generally pay these remaining fees out of pocket and are reimbursed by their private providers soon after. In recent years, for-profit companies have begun to push the envelope by offering direct payment to providers or to offer coverage for services that are not covered by statutory health insurance (i.e., supplementary health insurance). These experiments are not always well received politically, as there is a deep suspicion in France that the system based historically on solidarity is being passively privatized.

There is good reason for this fear. One of the few means France has to contain costs is to restrict or decrease the amount of coverage provided by statutory health insurance (even though it is a political battle to accomplish this). Historically, complementary health insurance has picked up the slack when this happens. When this occurs, private health insurance premiums increase (or coverage decreases). The growing for-profit health insurance market encourages healthy individuals to choose commercial (for-profit) health insurance options, as their own risks and premiums are lower, which in turn, decreases the pool of healthy contributors in the not-for-profit plans (effectively making them more expensive). This has clear implications for the level of equity within the French health care system. Politically, France has been relatively successful in maintaining a reasonable level of equity for all residents. Because the French system of statutory health insurance only covers a proportion of health care fees, it was clear that implementing a system of statutory health coverage for the very poor would not be sufficient to allow them to enjoy the benefits of statutory coverage, as they would likely be unable to afford the co-payments. Thus, when the Couverture Maladie Universelle was introduced in 2000, a parallel system of complementary health insurance for the very poor was also established. This program, called the CMU-Complémentaire (or CMU-C) is a public scheme that covers the co-payments required by most health care services. It is annual, renewable, and means-tested; and it is sent directly to health care providers rather than reimbursed to patients. Moreover, since 2005, France has assisted those just above the cut-off level for the CMU-C by establishing L'Aide Pour Une Complémentaire Santé, a similar means-tested complementary health insurance program for low-income individuals not eligible for CMU-C. Health care equity between classes is more considerable since 2000 than it ever has been, but the price for achieving equity has been substantial overall cost increases.

France has, in this way, been able to provide good quality services for the whole of its population in a relatively equitable manner. But there are concerns that this will change. Complementary health insurance varies considerably across plans, and there is increasing evidence showing that 'the quality of coverage purchased (in other words, the extent of reimbursement) varies by income group' (Durand-Zaleski 2008). Nine out of ten individuals in France have complementary health insurance coverage, but wealthier individuals have better complementary coverage. The concern is that the more costs are shifted from the statutory health insurance to the voluntary complementary system, and the more healthy individuals sign with private for-profit (risk-assessed) plans, the more social solidarity in health care will be undermined.

Other Forms of Payment for Health Care Services

The point of having limited statutory health insurance coverage was originally to make individuals responsible for some costs and, in this way, to keep overall costs low. The portion of health care costs not covered by statutory health insurance was originally known as the *ticket modérateur*, as the principle was that such co-payments would *moderate* health service usage. But as the system of complementary health insurance has expanded to cover almost all of these co-payments, the point of having a co-payment in the first place – moderating demand – has effectively been negated. And, 'by negating the effect of cost sharing required by the Social Security system, private insurance induces more consumption, which drives up public and private spending on health care' (Buchmueller and Couffinhal 2004: 24). To address this dynamic, France introduced in 2008 the *participation forfaitaire*, a levy of one Euro per visit (capped at 50 Euros per year), which cannot be covered by complementary insurance plans.

There are, in addition to the coverage offered by statutory health insurance and complementary health insurance, out-of-pocket costs involved in health care expenditure. In 2000, for example, 75.5 per cent of total expenditure on health care was covered by statutory health insurance, 12.4 per cent was covered by complementary voluntary health insurance, and 11.1 per cent came from out-of-pocket spending (Sandier et al. 2004: 43). These out-of-pocket expenses are incurred in a number of different ways, but usually they stem from the wide variety of choice offered to French health care consumers. For example, the treatment costs charged by general practitioners are negotiated by physicians' associations and health care funds. This fee schedule is the *tarif de convention*, and approximately 70 per cent of these fees are generally covered by statutory health insurance, with the remaining 30 per cent covered by complementary voluntary health insurance. But physicians are not obliged to limit their fees to those set out in the tarif de convention, and they can extra-bill as long as their fees are clearly set out. Extra-billing doctors are referred to as *non-conventionés*, and patients using non-conventionés must pay the additional charges themselves.

Another form of extra-billing is the *depassement*, which is a supplemental fee that experienced physicians are allowed to charge by virtue of their extra training. It is discretionary and is more common in the wealthier regions such as Paris and the Cote d'Azur. The French government has attempted to introduce a form of (voluntary) GP gate-keeping both as a form of cost control and as a way to integrate primary and secondary health care services. Financial incentives are provided both for patients and GPs in this system. Physicians must ensure continuity of care for patients, participate in preventive programs (such as screening), comply with practice guidelines, and prescribe a certain minimal ratio of cheap and effective drugs. In return, they receive a sum of €46 for each patient they sign up. Patients must agree to use their gatekeeper GP (*médecin traitant*, or treating physician) in the first instance and follow their doctor's advice on illness prevention. Patients who do use a médecin traitant are reimbursed by statutory insurance at the full 70 per cent, while those who do not are only reimbursed at 60 per cent. This has not been a popular option, but the French have grudgingly accepted the médecin traitant in increasing numbers.

Out-of-pocket costs are also incurred in the purchase of items not covered, or poorly covered, by both forms of health insurance. This usually includes eyeglasses and orthopaedic devices, dental care, pharmaceuticals, thermal (spa) treatments, physiotherapy, and private hospital accommodation. Historically, voluntary health insurance coverage has been limited to topping up the cost of goods and services partially covered by statutory health insurance. Increasingly, however, private health insurance is beginning to cover services (such as laser eye surgery) that are not covered by statutory health insurance at all. In other words, France's system of *complementary* health insurance (which covers the same services, by the same providers, for the same populations) is beginning to develop into a system of *supplementary* health insurance (which covers alternative or additional services for those willing to pay for them). In relation to other countries, France's proportion of out-of-pocket health expenses is quite low (less than half of that in Canada), but when insurance premiums and deductibles are calculated, France's level of household spending on health care increases considerably. A simplified model of health care financing and provision in France is set out in Figure 10.1.

Evaluating France's Health Care System

Does France live up to its reputation as one of the best health care systems in the world? And should Canadians attempt to emulate it? France's great achievement has been to develop a universal, comprehensive, and responsive high-quality health care system without sacrificing

Figure 10.1. Health care service funding in France

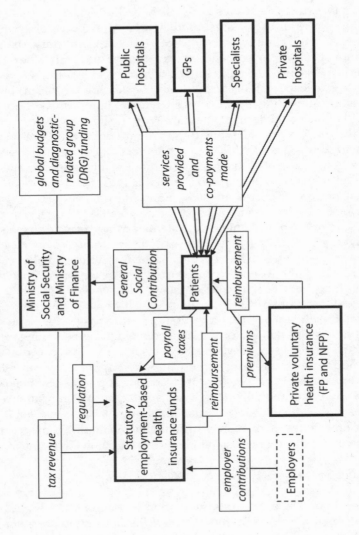

its historical commitment to solidarity and equity. But this has come at the price of severe overexpenditure, a condition that France's political officials characterize as critical and unsustainable.

The French health care system offers extensive choice to health care consumers: all residents have statutory health insurance, and most choose to purchase complementary private health insurance. While there is little choice in statutory health insurance provider, individuals have a wide choice of health service providers and complementary insurance providers. Health care users can choose the services of any GP or specialist, and any discretionary co-payments are either covered by complementary health insurance or are relatively small. Individuals have their choice of pharmaceutical products: they can, within limits, ask their doctor to prescribe more expensive, less efficacious drugs if they are willing to pay more for them. Waiting times are not very common. At the same time, France has made sure that the very poor and the very sick have excellent access to comprehensive, good quality health care resources. The extension of complementary insurance in 2000 and 2005 to the less well off, along with earlier reforms which extended statutory coverage to the retired and unemployed, has meant that all French citizens have reasonably equitable access to the same health care resources.

But France's health care system is also beset by structural difficulties which both encourage a high level of expenditure on health care and impede any effective means of controlling it. The original mechanism designed to control costs – the *ticket modérateur*, or obligatory co-payment – has been undermined by the growth of complementary health insurance coverage. Once a service has been insured, either publicly or privately, the propensity to use the services increases (although if the services are clearly needed, this is not necessarily a bad thing). This, along with the fee-for-service payment system employed by most doctors, has led a 'tacit collusion toward overuse' that exists between patients and providers, at the expense of the state (Rochaix and Wilsford 2005: 111). Since 1997 the French parliament has attempted to legislate a ceiling on health care expenditure (through the Social Security Funding Act). However, the only year this ceiling was actually met was in its first year of operation; thereafter the French health care system has operated in perpetual debt. In 2010 the shortfall is expected to be €15 billion, or about 10 per cent of its budget (Gauthier-Villars 2009).

This has led to the articulation of another 'French paradox' as intriguing as the question of why French women don't get fat. Why does such a strongly centralized political system as France's have such a hard time reigning in costs? 'In a country as centralized as France,' note Rochaix and Wilsford, 'with rather autonomous state structures and institutions, one could legitimately expect a great leverage over reform' (2005: 98). The answer is that political centralization in France has historically (and unlike Britain) been cross-cut with the practice of corporatism, which is a form of governance that gives representatives of both labour and business a formal voice in policy making. Thus the health care funding bodies (mutuelles) that were incorporated into a system of comprehensive coverage after the Second World War were seen as autonomous administrative bodies governed by representatives of both business and labour. There was an acceptance that these bodies had to recognize the state's role in setting the overall direction of health policy, but they were understood to be relatively independent bodies. Yet because these bodies are not themselves directly accountable to taxpayers, they have no pressing interest in keeping costs down. This explains the perpetual budget overrun: health funds recognize that the state's ability to force their hand to do its unpleasant business of cost-cutting is limited by both tradition and legislation.

This has been changing. Especially since the Juppé reforms of 1996, the French government has attempted to take a more active role in health care policy making. This has led to accusations that it is interfering in areas that are under the proper jurisdiction of the health funds; and relations between the health funds and the government have been increasingly fractious and hostile. This has not made health policy making any easier. The main areas in which the French state has traditionally been able to exert direct influence – control over hospitals and the enrolment of students in medical schools – is now feeling the brunt of the cost-containment measures. President Sarkozy, in the summer of 2009, targeted hospital expenditure, and (in a novel departure for France) looked across the channel at Britain's attempt to impose business practices into hospitals. They are now expected to present business plans, develop efficiency savings, and meet balanced budgets (Gauthier-Villars 2009). This has not gone over well with health care providers, but it has not yet culminated in the turbulent strikes that followed the Juppé reforms.

Interestingly, the cutbacks in the number of doctors coming onstream, the limitations on hospital spending, and the closure of small and inefficient hospitals will likely lead to the same patient dissatisfaction and accusations of 'rationing' that are familiar to people in Canada and Great

Britain. But there is little else the French state can do. Administrative attempts at achieving economic efficiencies through organizational reforms (such as the development of permanent electronic patient health files or the system of GP gatekeeping) were met with equal measures of hostility and apathy; neither has been particularly successful. One reason for this is, again, the implicit collusion between doctors and patients noted by Rochaix and Wilsford. While doctors' associations are weak and divided as a political force, doctors have nonetheless been remarkably successful in uniting with their patients to block health care reform.

The relationship between the French state and its doctors has never been especially cordial, but since the 1996 reforms it has deteriorated considerably. In France doctors are not effectively politically mobilized. They are fragmented not only according to subspecialization, but also to political orientation. Moreover, the ease of finding a doctor in France has an unfortunate downside, as an oversupply of physicians in many areas of France means that there is some acrimonious competition between doctors (especially between the older established physicians and the younger ones). French doctors have rarely been effectively united against the state, although there is some indication that this may be changing. Notwithstanding their weak ability at active political mobilization, however, they are vocal and recalcitrant enough to provide passive obstacles to effective reform. The United Kingdom has been able to implement many reforms over the past few decades largely because it has been able to bring doctors – increasingly, the general practitioners – alongside. Until France can figure out how to convince both the health funds and the doctors that reforms aimed at cost containment are both necessary and urgent, it will have to concentrate on the hospital sector and physician supply. Neither move will please the French people, who refuse to compromise on the level or quantity of their health care. Yet unless demand can be effectively dampened, supply-side restrictions will be increasingly common.

France has a very good health care system, possibly one of the best. But something has to give. Rather than simply looking at the 2000 WHO health survey, or even the extraordinary capacity of the current French health care system to provide universality, comprehensiveness, choice, and equity, it may be useful to think hard about the current trajectory of the French health care system. If critics believe that Canada's health care system is 'unsustainable,' then France is no model to emulate. In terms of unsustainable overexpenditure France is in much worse shape than Canada. Despite the fact that the French pay higher taxes while French doctors are paid considerably less than in Canada, the French health care system is still costing more than Canada's. What lies ahead for France? Either the supply of health services will be effectively curtailed (leading to fewer services being covered, less utilization of services, fewer facilities and professionals, and – *quelle horreur!* – possibly even waiting lists), or else there will be a much larger role for private health insurance (both complementary and supplementary), which will diminish the much-vaunted role of equity in French health care. Either way, it becomes evident that France has not found a way to square the circle and provide all the objectives of an ideal health care model. If anything, it merely becomes apparent that the same political dynamic that Canadians are witnessing – either waiting lists or inequitable health care – will become much more prevalent in France.

Germany's Health Care System

Germany has the oldest comprehensive system of health insurance in the world. The concept of mandated health insurance based on employment-related groups was introduced by Bismarck in 1883 as a means of undermining political support for the increasingly powerful socialist movement. Although both voluntary and mandated insurance schemes already existed in Germany at the local level, Bismarck insisted on a comprehensive national system of coverage. Yet Germany had only been a federated state for a matter of years, and the national level of government did not have the same degree of political power as it did in France or Britain. Regional governments opposed the idea of expanded national influence in social security, while business and agricultural interests (as well as the church) opposed a general tax-based system of financing such policies (Busse and Reisberg 2004: 13).

This political dynamic led to the solidification of the health insurance system that still exists in Germany today. Unlike France and Britain (which introduced a small element of decentralization relatively recently), Germany's health care system has always been based on regional units. In this regard it is similar to Canada. However, the process of health policy making in Germany is quite different. Germany has two legislative bodies: the Bundestag, which would be similar to Canada's House of Commons, and the Bundesrat, which represents the regional provinces (the Länder). While the Bundesrat is structurally similar to Canada's Senate, functionally it plays a much more active role in policy making. Any proposed legislation is normally the product of active consultation between houses (and therefore between levels of government). This negotiated system makes German policy making very stable, but it is also difficult to introduce speedy or radical reforms.

Thus, while France and Germany both have social insurance systems, the first point that differentiates them is the strongly regional focus of Germany's health care system. While all Länder participate in the broad structure of health insurance, the regions have more discretion in how they wish to operationalize their programs, and they have a stronger voice in the collective negotiation regarding the governance of the health insurance system. The second point that distinguishes France and Germany is the way in which different forms of health insurance are used to provide a comprehensive system of coverage. While both France and Germany utilize statutory health insurance, in France is it provided to everyone, but always requires a co-payment. In Germany, statutory health insurance only covers about 90 per cent of the population but, until recently, generally required little or no co-payments. Like France, there is a private health insurance component in Germany. But, unlike France, the type of private insurance is primarily *substitutive* (or alternative) with some additional *comprehensive* and *supplemental* options more recently available.

Statutory Health Insurance

As in France, the statutory health insurance system in Germany is often referred to as the 'public' health care system but, again, this is not an accurate description. In a social insurance system, the national government generally sets the general legislative framework, but within this framework decisions are made by the health funds themselves (which in Germany are called *Krankenkassen*, or sickness funds). The funds are governed autonomously by representatives of both employees and employers, and they negotiate directly with health care providers within each region regarding fee schedules and other prices. The funds are thus self-regulating, but they are subject to general government oversight.

Statutory health insurance is mandatory in Germany, but only for individuals earning less than €48,000 per year. Those who earn more have the opportunity to opt out of the statutory insurance scheme completely (although many who are eligible to do so choose to stay in it).

Those who opt out generally purchase private health care. Less than 1 per cent of the population in recent years has chosen to go without coverage; and from 2009, health insurance coverage – either public or private – has become mandatory. Public employees (such as civil servants, teachers, and university professors) and the self-employed are excluded from statutory health insurance, and generally have separate private plans.

German statutory health coverage is far more comprehensive than Canadian public health coverage. In addition to physician and hospital care and diagnostic services, statutory health insurance covers at least part of dental care, drugs and devices, rehabilitation, and sick leave compensation. A separate system of statutory insurance for long-term care has existed across Germany since 1995. While co-payments for some items and services (such as prescriptions and optometry) have been common in Germany for some time, co-payments for physician visits and hospital stays were only introduced in 2004. The co-payments themselves are, like those in France, relatively small: €10 per day for hospital visits (but only for the first month), and €10 to see a doctor, although this charge is only levied once every three months. Like France, Germany's system of statutory health insurance provides a safety net to the less well-off so that (unlike the United States) the poorer populations are guaranteed access to good quality health care. Costs not covered by statutory health insurance in Germany are limited to 2 per cent of household income (or 1% in the case of the chronically ill).

There are other important differences between statutory health insurance in France and Germany. In France there is little choice between providers of statutory health insurance: most people belong to the largest statutory health insurance organization, and the other, smaller statutory insurance bodies are based on either occupation or region. This was also the case in Germany until 1993. But, while the three largest French health funds cover 95 per cent of the population, Germany had close to a thousand discrete sickness funds. This changed following a major round of health care reforms, when Germans were given the right to choose between statutory health insurance funds (although certain small funds, such as those specifically designed for farmers, sailors, and miners retained their systems of assigned membership). Because funds now had to compete for customers, they began to merge and, by 2009, the number of statutory health insurance funds had fallen to 186.

A further distinction between the French and German systems of statutory health insurance is that the German Krankenkassen are held to stricter financial liability. They cannot accumulate debts. Therefore, if they experience a deficit, they are obliged to increase contributions. This pay-as-you-go model, where the level of expenditure must match the rate of contributions, is an important reason that German health coverage has remained stable over periods of economic contraction (and even wartime instability). But it is not unproblematic. To the extent that Germans demand a high quality of comprehensive health care, expenditure costs continue to rise, and thus contributions keep increasing as well. Statutory health insurance contributions averaged 13.5 per cent of gross income in 2001, 14.3 per cent in 2003, and hit 15.5 in January 2009. Legislation mandated the reduction of contributions to 14.9 per cent, but some experts have suggested that rates may hit 16 per cent at current expenditure rates. Moreover, where contributions were historically shared equally between employees and employers, the cost sharing has shifted from parity to a 46/54 per cent ratio shouldered by employees.

Other Forms of Payment for Health Services

Germany is distinct from Canada, Great Britain, Sweden, and France in its use of private substitutive health insurance. This means that 10 per cent of the German population relies *entirely* on private health insurance, rather than using private health insurance merely to cover mandatory co-payment (complementary insurance) or goods and services not covered at all by public or statutory health insurance (supplemental insurance). One major distinction between statutory and private health insurance in Germany is that the former is not based on risk assessment: the healthy subsidize the ill. This is precisely the point of a social insurance model: to maintain a sense of solidarity between all contributors. Under a private system, however, premiums are based on the health risk presented by each member: the healthy pay lower premiums, and the less healthy pay higher ones. Yet even the private health insurance sector faces a considerable level of regulation: private companies cannot, for example, severely penalize members as they get older. Private plan contributors are also protected from overwhelmingly high premiums should their incomes decrease substantially. And, since 2009, private substitutive health insurance firms – about fifty major companies – are expected to participate in their own 'risk adjustment scheme' to pool risks more widely so that those with expensive health care needs can afford private premiums. Private health care providing complementary and supplementary coverage has not been widespread in Germany historically, although this is beginning to change as co-payments increase and benefits are cut.

It is useful to remember that while there are two very clear-cut forms of insurance – private and statutory – there are *not* two distinct systems of health care *services:* 'Except for a small minority,' explains Greβ (2007: 33), 'healthcare providers – outpatient as well as inpatient – treat patients from both health insurance systems. Thus, privately insured patients and social insurance patients will be treated in the same hospital and by the same general practitioner or specialist.' Thus there is no substantial difference in quality between publicly and privately financed services. But there are three strong criticisms of Germany's system of dual insurance.

The first addresses the dynamic of adverse selection. Because private health insurance is risk-assessed, the lower premiums make it attractive to the healthy and wealthy. At the same time, those with poor health have no incentive to choose private health insurance. Thus net income to the statutory funds decreases as the healthy, high-income individuals exit the system, but the expenditures increase as high-cost cases remain with the statutory insurance funds. The higher these costs become, the more motivation those with low health risks have to exit, if they can, the system of statutory insurance. This, in turn, reinforces the lower-income, higher-expenditure pressures in statutory health funds. Currently, three-quarters of the German population are *required* to subscribe to statutory health insurance, while 88 per cent of the population actually *do* enroll in statutory health insurance (Busse 2008). This means that there is still room for movement out of the statutory insurance system. This raises questions about the extent to which relative equity between the two systems can be maintained if movement away from statutory insurance becomes pronounced.

The second concern rests with the movement towards greater co-payments and other forms of private insurance. While some forms of co-payment (such as those for pharmaceuticals) have existed since the 1980s, major reforms introduced in 1997 and 2004 significantly increased the use of co-payments for most goods and services for most individuals (although with ceilings, and with reduced rates for the less well-off). Unlike France, however, the use of complementary health insurance to cover co-payments is not widespread. And, while these co-payments are currently small, there is some discussion about increasing reliance on private sources of funding, such as co-payments, to keep the statutory system out of debt. By the first half of 2008, for example, the statutory health funds had massive deficits (€800 million) and shortages of between €7 billion and €9 billion were forecast for 2010 (*Der Spiegel* 2009; Stafford 2009). The issue of how to deal with these deficits is hotly debated, and depends largely on the political leanings of the parties in power. Germany is often governed by coalition governments, and after the parliamentary elections of September 2009 the influence of the centre-left Social Democratic Party (SPD) was reduced while that of the pro-business Free Democratic Party (FPD) increased. The position of the former has been that deficits should be covered by higher contributions by all health fund members, while the latter has been forceful in arguing that costs can only be reduced by greater reliance on private insurers.

The third focus of concern regarding Germany's dual-insurance system has been the development of a two-tier health care system based on waiting times. Historically waiting times have not been an issue in Germany (as in most other social insurance systems) because of the comfortable supply of doctors, and because doctors' remuneration from the public and private insurance systems were not considerably far apart. There was, in other words, no reason for doctors to choose to give preferential treatment to those with private insurance. But this is beginning to change. As costs begin to mount in the statutory system, supply-side constraints are increasingly imposed on the health care system. For example, the state has begun to limit the number of physicians entering the system, and it has attempted to constrain hospital expenditure by gradually phasing in diagnostic-related group financing. But statutory health funds have also imposed quarterly caps on physicians: the funds will not pay out more than a specified amount to doctors every three months. Therefore, if a physician meets her cap before the quarter, she must schedule patients with statutory health insurance into the *next* quarter (or else provide her services for free). A study published in 2008 showed that patients covered by statutory health insurance had to wait three times longer, on average, than patients with private health insurance. Moreover, the treatment of private patients is becoming more lucrative by as much as 35 per cent (Tuffs 2008). The debate over waiting lists in Germany is a sensitive one, and little information exists simply because hospitals are not required to keep formal public waiting lists on record (although many do so informally). As early as

Figure 10.2. Basic health care funding model, Germany

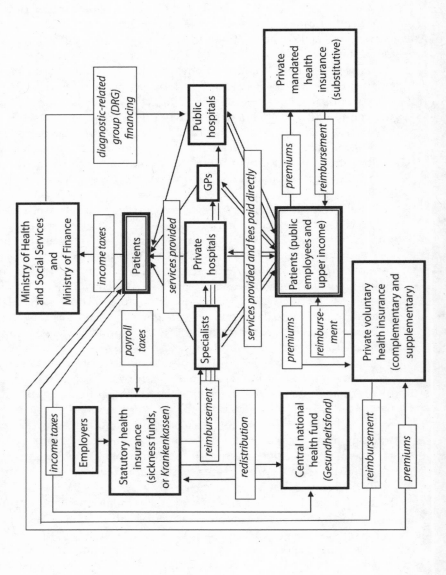

1997, many hospitals reported that 'waiting times had been prolonged and that waiting lists were not only due to limited capacities but to the hospital target budgets which render the treatment of SHI [statutory health insurance] patients financially less attractive, since regressive prices applied once the target budget had been exceeded' (Busse and Reisberg 2004: 71). In sum, the use of a prospective budget for those with statutory health insurance favoured faster access for those *without* statutory health insurance (ibid.).

Evaluating Germany's Health Care System

Germany, like France, has an excellent health care system that provides comprehensive, good quality services widely across its population (see Figure 10.2). It also enjoys considerable support from its citizens. But is it a model that Canadians should consider adopting? It is worthwhile to note that many European health care systems based on the social insurance model have been moving further away from it. France, as we saw, moved closer to the Beveridge (or British) model by integrating a general tax-based funding component into its social insurance system and by trying to implement a GP gatekeeping system. Germany has made two major changes to its own social insurance model. First, in 1993, it introduced a form of managed competition similar in principle to those enacted in both Britain and Sweden. By moving away from the system of 'assigned membership' in statutory health funds (that France still has) and allowing most individuals to choose their own health fund, the hope was that the funds, by competing for members, would actively seek efficiencies in the system through their ability to negotiate with providers. Interestingly, Germany's experience with a form of internal market is very similar to that of Britain and Sweden: it is difficult to evaluate, because it never really happened. This is especially true in Germany, where policy making in general is heavily shaped by negotiation and compromise both because of institutional design and political culture. In terms of managed competition within the health care system, write Brown and Amelung, the 'compromises that spelled creative destruction for coherence of competition as a theoretical construct' meant that managed competition had become 'manacled competition': 'To reassure the Left (and the sickness funds themselves, which worried about adverse selection), choice was balanced by risk-adjustment provisions. These would protect solidarity, but at the cost of narrowing premium differences among the funds and essentially nullifying price as a competitive consideration for all but exquisitely cost-sensitive customers. To mollify the Right, co-payments were enacted as part of the larger reform package, and competition stopped well short of such purchaser-empowering measures as selective contracting, which was anathema to providers' (1999: 84).

The second strategy, phased in from 2009 to 2011, was to integrate a centralized single-payer system (the *Gesundheitsfond*) into the current social insurance model. Thus Germany, like France, is actually moving closer towards a system like Canada's. One of the consequences of competition between statutory insurance funds was the growth of considerable disparity in premium rates for the same services between funds. This move away from social equity concerned the centre-left parties, and so attempts have been made to pool all premiums in all statutory sickness funds together to spread the risk and keep premiums equitable. This strategy began with risk equalization schemes in 1994, and culminated in 2009 with the development of the Gesundheitsfond. Now employers and employees still pay their premiums directly to their specific sickness fund, but the sickness funds must immediately forward these premiums to the Gesundheitsfond. The Gesundheitsfond amalgamates all premiums into a central fund, along with tax revenue based on income (as opposed simply to wages). The Gesundheitsfond then redistributes money back to the sickness funds using a calculation based on a uniform capitation rate (adjusted for age, gender, and existing conditions). The individual sickness funds must cover their members with the amount of money redistributed to them (this is why the funds have set caps on the number of treatments for which it reimburses individual doctors each quarter). Sickness funds do have the option of charging a small monthly supplement (of €8) on their members, and can if necessary levy an additional premium of up to 1 per cent of member income. The idea is that funds will be dissuaded from doing so because members can easily shop around between funds for better rates. Unlike Sweden, national standards are more rigorously observed, sharply limiting the disparity between regions.

The Gesundheitsfond also acts as a central fund for the direct coverage of children's health care (children were previously covered by their parents' statutory health insurance), as well as a central source for the funding of certain other social services. What this complicated reform is expected to achieve is the re-establishment of equity (and social solidarity) between members; a widening of the health care funding base (from only payroll contributions to contributions based on both payroll and other taxable income); and to contain costs by giving consumers incentives to use health care resources more efficiently. For example, if sickness funds can persuade their members to adopt a GP gatekeeping system (thereby spending less of the funds' money on more expensive specialists), then the funds are rewarded with a higher reimbursement from the Gesundheitsfond. A basic model of Germany's health care system is sketched out in Figure 10.2. It may understandably lead one to challenge health policy scholar Uwe Reinhardt's assertion that 'Germany's system is almost elegant in its simplicity' (1994: 23). But it is the system that has put the most effort into attempting to balance the objectives of comprehensiveness, quality, equity, cost containment, and (finally in 2009) universality. This is a reflection of the balance within the German political system itself between left and right, centre and regions, business and labour, and between health care users and health care providers.

But the biggest issue for Germany remains cost containment. Like other countries, Germany is using a diverse set of tools to try to contain health care spending. One example of this is the utilization of diagnostic-related group financing for hospitals. This is where reimbursement for procedures is calculated according to an established 'chart' of how much each procedure should in theory cost. If a hospital spends more per treatment than it is reimbursed for, it must shoulder the loss. This gives hospitals a clear incentive to be as economically efficient as possible in providing services. Again, like other countries, Germany is embracing the operationalization of evidence-based medicine. Germany has recently established the Institut für Qualität und Wirtschaftlichkeit im Gesundheitswesen (Institute for Quality and Efficiency in Health Care) to distinguish between effective (and cost-effective) treatments, which it accepts for coverage, and relatively useless (or unwarrantedly expensive) treatments, which it will not cover. Germany was also the first country systematically to introduce reference pricing into its statutory insurance system. This means that drugs are reimbursed according to their utility and cost-effectiveness. If patients prefer expensive, brand-name drugs over generics or older classes of drugs, then they have to make a much larger co-payment. There is a clear tension between what the population wants – free choice, immediate access, and high quality – and what recent cost containment measures will allow for. As recent reforms become more effective in shifting costs to private spending and in limiting reimbursement funds, hospital facilities, and numbers of physicians, this tension will only become more accentuated.

What Can We Learn from France and Germany?

Perhaps the clearest lesson Canadians can learn from the social insurance model is that Europeans are moving away from it, while not jettisoning it altogether. The strongest advantage of the social insurance model is political: it reinforces solidarity between individuals and contains the demand for private services by equitably distributing good quality services among the population. Because the statutory health funds have historically 'belonged' to their members, the funds are highly responsive to them. This is the main reason that the social insurance systems are so comprehensive: as members have increasingly required drugs as part of their medical treatments, the health funds have seen it as their duty to provide them (as long as the premiums were provided to allow them to do so). Social insurance models are generally quite stable for the same reason. As they are not provided by the state, but exist at arm's-length from it, any attempt by the state to implement sudden and drastic changes (like Britain did) would simply be seen as an invasive and hostile act by a body acting outside of its jurisdiction (this is especially clear in France). Comprehensiveness and equity can coexist because of the simple economic principle of risk distribution: if health risks are distributed widely enough, the sicker and less well-off are more able to afford premiums (although the worst off must be subsidized by the state).

But social insurance systems may end up as historical anachronisms. Even as health costs increase, payroll taxes account for an ever-decreasing share of countries' economic wealth. In Germany, for example, health care costs increased from 8 to 10 per cent of GDP between 1980 and 2001, while payroll contributions fell from 74 per cent to 65 per cent of GDP (Altenstetter 2003: 41). A pure system of social insurance can also be regressive, as it is based on employment, and those with long-term employment tend to be much healthier than those with long-term unemployment. The attempts to expand the financial base for health care spending and to achieve universal coverage are two reasons that European states with social insurance have been moving towards the adoption of mechanisms that employ income tax contributions and single-payer systems. But the most important reason for moving in this direction is that single-payer systems controlled as closely as possible by the state are the ones where costs are most easily (if not painlessly) contained. As health care expenditure continues to mount, the overwhelming question for all health care systems becomes how to control costs.

Many discussions of European health care systems written in English extol the superiority of European health care, whether they are based on public systems with internal markets or on social insurance (or both). But these accounts are frequently written for an American audience, and the health care system of *any* advanced European state has by most broad indicators been superior to that of the United States. Canadian readers should not be too easily seduced by these accounts, as the comparison between Canadian and European systems is much more nuanced. It is probably fair to say that they each score well according to different criteria. One measure on which all the European systems considered here draw evenly with Canada is universality (and this is one measure on which the United States has performed most poorly). European states in general tend to score higher in comprehensiveness than Canada does, and this is especially true for social insurance systems. However, the comparison is usually made between a complex system of statutory and private insurance, on the one hand, and the public system alone, on the other. If Canada, like France and Germany, was evaluated in respect to the *total* combination of coverage shared between universal public and supplementary private insurance, the comprehensiveness of coverage would look much more favourable for Canadians (as many Canadians do have some form of private insurance). Likewise, if Canada's public system were compared only with the coverage given by statutory insurance plans alone, Canada would again appear in a much more favourable light.

The consideration of equity is much more difficult to evaluate simply. Canada has a much more equitable distribution of health care *in certain sectors* as it is mandated equity: for the most part, Canadians cannot (either de facto or de jure) buy medically necessary services that their compatriots cannot afford. This unique system has had a significant impact on the development of a Canadian form of social solidarity (at least in health care). When one goes beyond primary and secondary care, however, Canada fares very poorly in terms of social equity, as many important goods and services are not even partially covered by the public system. Those who cannot afford private premiums or out-of-pocket payments must often do without, for example, prescription eyeglasses and hearing aids, completely. Canada also fares poorly in terms of accessibility and, occasionally, in terms of quality (although that is usually limited to access to technology). To the extent that primary and secondary care are not available privately, there is only a limited quantity available, and so we have discussions of explicit 'rationing.' It is noteworthy, however, that countries with universal public insurance that have a parallel private insurance sector (like Britain and Sweden) have the same irascible debate over rationing and waiting lists. It is even more worthwhile to note that when countries with social insurance (like France and Germany) attempt to address the expansionary pressures of their systems, they turn to the same tools as countries with universal public insurance systems, with the same predictable results.

France and Germany have been held up as models for Canadians to follow largely because they seem to have no accessibility issues, while Canada does. However, it is important to see this within a dynamic context, rather than as a snapshot in time taken some years ago. In recent years the political dynamic within both France and Germany has been a quiet form of creeping centralization by the state in certain areas of health policy and, somewhat paradoxically, creeping privatization in others. By making the governments (via both income tax and regulatory measures) more important players, they are more effectively able to dampen health care spending. Arguably, the reason that France and Germany have more comprehensive, accessible systems is not so much because of social insurance itself but rather because these countries impose higher taxes on their citizens, and they pay their doctors considerably less. Canada might therefore be able to improve its comprehensiveness and accessibility as effectively by raising taxes and severely cutting payments to doctors as it could by implementing a social insurance system (although few would see either strategy to be a politically viable one). Likewise, to the extent that France and Germany will be increasingly subject to cuts from the centre (caps on payments to providers, physician enrolment, number of beds available in hospitals), their people start grumbling the same litany of complaints as Canadians. From a theoretical point of view, the interesting question is not whether one system is clearly superior to any other, but rather whether these countries are increasingly converging on one basic prototype (some form of single-payer system based at least partially on income tax) distinguished by distinctive national trimmings (i.e., the particular combinations of private insurance that are largely historically determined). If this is the case, then Canadians should simply go back to the somewhat tedious but vital task of tinkering with their own system.

11 Mandated Private Insurance: The United States and the Long Road to Reform

The fascination with the comparison between American and Canadian health policy rests largely on the observation that, until relatively recently, the two systems were fairly similar. But they chose quite different paths, and the consequences have been pronounced. Canada's shift, as we have seen, began in Saskatchewan in 1957, and was solidified in national legislation in 1984. In the United States, the attempt to provide a form of national health insurance began in 1912, when Theodore Roosevelt campaigned for the Progressive Party with the promise of a system of health insurance. But, despite the efforts of Franklin D. Roosevelt, Harry Truman, John Kennedy, Jimmy Carter, and Bill Clinton, the movement to achieve a comprehensive and coordinated system of health insurance came to nothing. Except for the establishment of Medicaid and Medicare under the Johnson administration in 1965, health care in the United States has been largely decentralized, highly unregulated, and dependent on private markets. This changed dramatically in 2010 with the passage of the Patient Protection and Affordable Care Act (PPACA).

How are Americans covered? In the United States, as in Europe, health insurance is generally employment-related. Unlike Europe, however, the United States does not mandate (i.e., legally require) individuals to carry health insurance (under the PPACA, health coverage will be mandatory by 2014). While most Americans do have employment-related health insurance, employers are not required to find health insurance for their employees. Individuals also have the option of buying non – employment-related health insurance policies, but these are risk-based and can be quite expensive. All Americans over 65 are covered by Medicare. Of those under 65, 60.9 per cent have private employer-based coverage, 5.5 per cent have private non-employer coverage, 13.9 per cent are covered by Medicaid, 2.5 per cent have other public health insurance coverage (e.g., disabled individuals covered by Medicare and military veterans covered by the Veterans Health Administration, or VHA); 17.2 per cent have no health insurance at all (Tolbert 2008: 3). Rates of coverage vary considerably from state to state. Some states, such as Massachusetts, have enacted their own health reforms to minimize the number of uninsured and underinsured individuals. This is why there has been so much reference to the 'Massachusetts Model' in discussions of national health care reform. In other states, such as Texas, 32 per cent of those under 65 are without any health insurance whatsoever (compared with only 2.6 per cent in Massachusetts).

It is important to remember that there *is* considerable public health insurance in the United States, although the public programs are only available to designated groups. The two largest public health insurance programs are Medicare and Medicaid. *Medicare* is the largest program: all Americans over 65 are covered by it, as are many disabled individuals. There are actually four separate components of Medicare. The two primary parts are Hospital Insurance (Part A) and Supplementary Medical Insurance (Part B). Both are federal programs administered centrally by trust funds, but they are financed in different ways. Hospital Insurance is intended to be self-supporting, which means that it is almost entirely funded through earmarked payroll taxes. Employees currently pay 1.49 per cent of taxable earnings, which is matched by employers; self-employed individuals pay 2.9 per cent of taxable earnings (this will increase under the PPACA). Supplementary Medical Insurance is an optional program in which beneficiaries pay a monthly premium which covers only a quarter of costs. The remainder is paid through general tax revenue. From 1997, Americans have been able to receive Medicare through private fee-for-service plans (Medicare Advantage, or Part C). A prescription drug plan (Part D) was added in 2006.

Medicaid is the public health insurance program for those in the lowest income brackets. However, poverty alone does not confer eligibility. Beneficiaries of Medicaid are usually children, parents with children, pregnant women, and disabled individuals. A large number of Americans are thus uninsured because they cannot afford private health care premiums, and they are not eligible for either Medicare or Medicaid. Medicaid is also financed differently from Medicare. Both the federal and state governments share financing for Medicaid. While the federal government pays approximately 50 per cent of the costs,

Figure 11.1. How health care services are funded, United States. Changes outlined in the Patient Protection and Affordable Care Act (PPACA) will come into effect gradually until 2014.

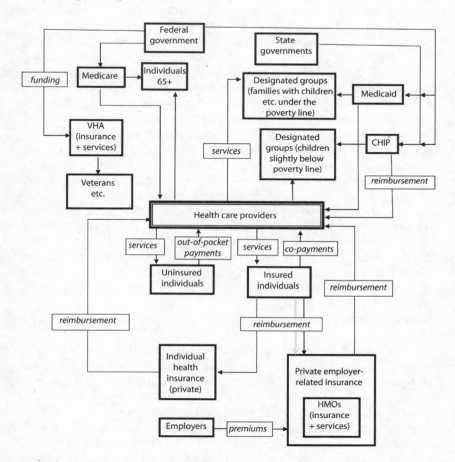

there is a formula (the federal medical assistance percentage, or FMAP) that provides states with less or more than 50 per cent depending on state income per capita (relative to national per capita income levels). This formula attempts to limit inequities in Medicaid services between states. There is nonetheless much disparity between states, as they themselves have the ability to determine (within general parameters set by the program) eligibility for Medicaid, premiums and other forms of cost-sharing to be borne by recipients, and provider reimbursement rates. As with Canadian provinces, states find that public health insurance comprises one of the highest outlays of public funds.

There are two other forms of public health insurance in the United States. Veterans Health Administration (VHA), as part of the U.S. Department of Veterans Affairs, is provided for American veterans and their families. VHA is a combination of government-funded health insurance (provided to beneficiaries without premiums), government-run hospitals, and a publicly funded network of outpatient services. The VHA is the closest that the United States has to 'socialized medicine,' and it is also notable for being one of the most highly rated health care systems in the country. VHA hospitals are consistently ranked above private for-profit hospitals, and other VHA health care outcomes frequently surpass those in the private health care system (see, e.g., Longman 2005). The Children's Health Insurance Program (CHIP) was established in 1997 in the wake of the failed Clinton health care reforms. The program provides matching federal-state funding for children who are not eligible for funding through Medicaid (i.e., in households with incomes slightly above the cut-off for Medicaid eligibility). The nature of American health care insurance and service provision as it currently exists is outlined in Figure 11.1 (several changes stipulated by the PPACA will kick in by 2014).

The Push for Reform

What explains the health care trajectory of the United States? As in any country, health policy making in the United States has been the result of a particular constellation of interests, institutions, processes, and values. Nevertheless, health policy in the United States has been the product of a passive-aggressive political dynamic, in which powerful interests have been more concerned with preventing change than with prompting it. Because there has been no centralized political control over health policy in the United States, the country has been singularly incapable of addressing many of the social and economic challenges in the provision of health care that have confronted all of the developed countries.

The Need for Reform

Compared with other OECD states, the United States has been a significant statistical outlier for a number of reasons (and not in a good way).

Two major flaws characterize the American system: first, a considerable proportion of the population does not have any health insurance coverage. Access to health services (excepting Medicare, Medicaid, and CHIP) is largely dependent on one's income level. Second, health care costs (both for services and for insurance) are considerably higher in the United States than in any other OECD country, and increasing more rapidly.

INEQUITY IN COVERAGE

In 2008, 46.3 million American were uninsured, up from 45.7 in 2007. Thirty per cent of these were young people between the ages of 19 and 29 (Schwartz and Schwartz 2010). Many of the uninsured were unemployed, and therefore unable to access either affordable insurance through their employer or more expensive health insurance available through the open market. But an expanding number of middle-class families were also finding health insurance to be increasingly unaffordable relative to household income. This is because private health insurance premiums have doubled in the past ten years, and deductibles have increased. At the same time, benefits are becoming increasingly restricted. The number of claims that are denied is also rising considerably. In consequence, approximately one in five of the uninsured in 2008 lived in households with incomes at or above U.S.$75,000, an increase of over 8 per cent from 2007 (Davis 2009).

The number of *under*insured Americans is also increasing (the definition of 'underinsured' is paying more than 10 per cent of income on out-of-pocket medical expenses, or 5 per cent for those under the poverty level). Between 2004 and 2007, the number of underinsured individuals climbed from 16 million to 25 million (Collins 2009). In the past few years, lack of insurance and underinsurance have shifted from being just an issue for low-income groups to becoming a middle-class problem: 72 million Americans under 65 had problems paying their medical bills in 2007 (up from 58 million in 2005), regardless of whether they had insurance or not; while 46 per cent of the underinsured used up all of their savings for medical bills, 33 incurred credit card debt to pay medical bills, and 29 per cent reported that they could not pay for food, heat, or rent because of medical bills (Collins 2009). Two-thirds of all personal bankruptcies in 2007 were due to illness or medical bills (Himmelstein et al. 2009). The push for health reform, then, was partly driven by middle-class Americans who were increasingly finding both health insurance and health services to be unaffordable. This effect was exacerbated by the economic recession that began in September 2008, as rising unemployment rates meant even more individuals lost afford-able coverage.

In the United States, the issues of coverage and cost containment are twisted together like a double helix, with each influencing the other in a spiral race to the bottom. Coverage declines because premiums and other co-payments are increasing so dramatically; premiums and co-payments keep rising because the cost of health care services contin-ues to climb with few tools to control it. Yet effective cost containment controls are not enacted because they are seen as 'too expensive' and too threatening to established interests. As the costs of an increasing number of services themselves increase, those who provide health care insurance must recoup these expenditures. Public health plans can meet these expenditures by shifting costs to beneficiaries (e.g., through co-payments), by limiting the kinds and amounts of services that will be reimbursed, by taking advantage of economies of scale and purchas-ing power, or by shifting costs to taxpayers more widely. Single-payer plans have the additional benefits of limiting administrative costs and, in some cases, negotiating advantageous deals from providers. In the case of Canada, costs can be kept down as well by limiting oversupply: if you do not need a service, you cannot receive it, even if you can pay for it. But a system that depends largely on private health insurance can only employ the first two of these mechanisms: increasing costs or lim-iting benefits to health insurance recipients. Both are occurring in the United States. Because so much health insurance is employment-based, insurance companies pass the costs on to the employers. Employers must then either absorb the costs, or pass the costs on to employees, or refuse to provide any health insurance at all. There is clearly a decline in the number of employers offering coverage: since 2000, employment-based coverage has fallen by 10 per cent. The number of employers cov-ering the full cost of health insurance fell over the same period from 29 to 17 per cent for individuals, and 11 to 6 per cent for families (Hacker 2006: 139). The level of health care costs passed on to individuals has also increased dramatically: out-of-pocket spending on health care for those with employer-sponsored coverage increased by 34 per cent between 2004 and 2007; but out-of-pocket costs rose most (42%) for the 1 per cent of adults with the largest medical expenses (Gabel et al. 2009).

A further problem with private health insurance is that when the pri-mary purpose of it is to make profits, dubious practices may emerge that limit coverage in order to secure profit margins. Insurance plans are increasingly offering fewer benefits and imposing more stringent conditions on reimbursement. But insurance policies are not necessarily designed to be readily accessible for those buying them. An investigative study undertaken by *Consumer Reports* found that many dubious practices were employed by private insurance companies regarding coverage. This included 'policies that didn't cover prescription drugs or outpatient chemotherapy but didn't say so anywhere in the policy document – not even in the section labeled "What is not covered"' (May 2009: 25). *Consumer Reports* also found that some policies do not count co-payments for doctors' visits or prescription drug charges towards the maximum amount paid out of pocket before expenses are totally covered, which 'can be a catastrophe for seriously ill people who rack up dozens of doctors' appointments and prescriptions a year.' (ibid). There is also the problem of 'random gotchas,' such as hospital coverage that only kicks in on the second day (the first day is usually the most expensive, as it normally involves surgery and diagnostic tests). It is also extremely difficult for the average person to determine exactly how much coverage is 'adequate.' Most people simply do not know how much cancer treatment, or a heart attack, or any other of a myriad of different conditions actually would cost them, and how much insurance coverage they should therefore have.

The most notorious example of the behaviour of health insurance companies is the practice of 'rescissions,' or 'post-claim underwriting,' in which insurance companies will minutely examine a policy for trivial errors after an individual has submitted a large claim, solely in order to refuse payment. House subcommittee hearings held in July 2009 found that 'during the previous five years, three health insurers – Assurant Health, WellPoint, and Golden Rule – had saved more than $300 million by rescinding nearly 20,000 policies based on omissions policyholders made in filling out enrollment forms' (Noah 2009a). Cynics would add that the practice of rescissions should be reviewed with an eye on the 2008 salary levels of CEOs of major health insurance firms: U.S.$9,844,212 for WellPoint's Angela Brady (the same company that increased premiums by 39% in 2009), U.S.$12,236,740 for Cigna's Edward Hanway (*after* it had been cut in half), and U.S.$24,300,112 for Aetna's Ronald Williams (Kapp 2009). Thus the issue is not simply a matter of the total number of individuals who are not covered, but rather that the increasingly higher costs of health care per se are being shouldered disproportionately by those least able to afford them.

INABILITY TO CONTAIN COSTS

All countries have experienced cost drivers in the past decade, but these tend to be more pronounced in the United States. Throughout the late 1980s and early 1990s, private employer-based health insurance reconfigured itself into a system of 'managed care' (distinct from 'managed competition') in which large health providers and insurers developed large integrated care programs to manage costs. However, this system proved to be spectacularly unable to contain health care costs. In 2007 the United States spent U.S.$2.2 trillion on health care, or approximately 16.2 per cent of the country's GDP. This works out to U.S.$7,421 per person. This is about 90 per cent higher than most OECD countries (Canada, e.g., spends about U.S.$3,500 per capita on total annual health care). Again, these figures must be held against the statistics for health outcomes, which show that the United States has no better health outcomes (and often *worse* ones) than countries that spend half of what it does on health care.

Why are health care costs so much higher in the United States than in any other OECD nation? Higher costs are to a large extent due to the interplay of two factors: there is more disposable personal income in the United States than in many other countries, and there is less capacity for the government to control health care costs directly. Historically, the U.S. federal government was not involved in providing health services (Medicare and Medicaid were only established in 1965), and therefore it did not have the incentive that other nations did to become involved in cost containment strategies much earlier. The supply of private sector services will continue to rise as long as there are individuals who can afford to buy them. The advance of medical technology is, according to many, the 'principal driver' behind the growth of health care spending (Aaron and Ginsburg 2009). Thus the scope and number of services continue to expand. Where these technologies and services are widely available in a private market to a critical mass of consumers who can afford it, costs will increase significantly.

In Canada, Sweden, Great Britain, France, and Germany, there are negotiations between governments and providers on the fees set on health care services (e.g., a routine doctor's visit, or a hip replacement, or an appendectomy). Many countries also set prices for prescription drugs. In the United States, and in the United States alone, these costs are determined by the market (except for Medicare rates). Thus a routine doctor's visit costs approximately $30 in Canada, $31 in France, and $22 in Germany. In the United States the price for such a visit ranges from \$59 to \$148 (with Medicare rates set at \$72). Total hospital and physician costs for an appendectomy are \$2,436 in Canada, \$2,700 in France, \$2,500 in Germany, and \$2, 634 in the United Kingdom. In the United States the cost for an appendectomy ranges from \$11,997 at the low end and \$26,373 at the upper, with a set Medicare rate of \$10, 400. Total costs for a hip replacement show the same pattern: \$8,483 in Canada, \$8,200 in France, \$8,500 in Germany, and \$8,347 in the United Kingdom. Costs for a hip replacement in the United States range from \$32,093 to \$67,983, with Medicare setting fees at \$17,5000 (all U.S. dollars; International Federation of Health Plans 2009). Those defending a free market in health care argue that competition between providers will naturally drive prices down (because that is what a free market does). In many cases (e.g., electronics) this is generally true. Demand for electronics, however, is limited: how many flat screen television sets does one consumer normally buy? Demand for health care services, on the other hand, is more elastic, especially when preventive care is sought or when appealing new technologies overwhelm common sense (e.g., if you exercise properly and lose weight, you probably won't need the sophisticated new forms of back surgery).

This basic flaw in the provision of health services is reinforced by a number of other factors. The way in which health services are reimbursed to providers – usually fee-for-service – rewards providers merely for supplying the service and not for improving the health outcome of the patients. It also provides incentives for providers to overtreat individuals. This is why the United States is characterized both by *oversupply* and *undersupply* in health care: those who can afford health services consume more than they need, and those who cannot afford them do not receive what they require. The United States also pays its physicians considerably more than physicians get paid in any other country, and reimburses them according to a 'relative value scale' that privileges complicated procedures (e.g., heart or back surgery) more than primary care or preventive treatments. This means that medical school graduates are inclined more and more to specialties that provide greater remuneration, and away from general practice or preventive services. Typical incomes for radiologists and orthopaedic surgeons are three times higher than for physicians working in primary care and, unsurprisingly, by 2009 family medicine had the smallest percentage of positions filled by American medical school graduates (Steinbrook 2009). The problem from a systemwide perspective is that outpatient visits that monitor cholesterol and blood pressure levels or provide nutritional guidance, smoking cessation programs, and fitness advice are often just as effective as the more expensive and invasive surgical options. But if the relative value of complicated procedures is much more lucrative, those procedures will be what 'rational' health care providers will offer; for an excellent general discussion of this phenomenon see Gawande (2009b).

Key Players

To an extent, then, lack of access to good quality, affordable health care was the driver that put health reform on the political agenda in the United States. But health care has rarely been the main focus of concern for the electorate, and it is frequently surpassed by the issues such as the economy, unemployment, and military deployment. The second reason that health reform became a major policy area in the United States was the commitment of a small but critical number of officials (elected and unelected) in the new Democratic administration. These individuals (including such key figures as Nancy Pelosi, Harry Reid, Rahm Emanuel, and the late Ted Kennedy in addition to Barack Obama) perceived a window of opportunity and were prepared to expend what political capital they had in order to achieve health reform. But perhaps the most important variable during the reform process was that many powerful political interests in the health care sector were for various reasons no longer opposed to the idea of reform: the issue then became the *type* of reform rather than the principle of reform per se.

Historically, the physicians' lobby has been instrumental in blocking the introduction of government-run plans which could place limitations on both their income and their capacity for professional self-regulation. The political power of physicians in the United State has fluctuated considerably over time. Medical doctors in colonial America had a relatively low status due to the panoply of itinerant healers, homeopaths, and hucksters that abounded because of poor professional regulation. By the late nineteenth century, American physicians imported the German model of rigorous training, licensing, and accreditation. This, combined with a massive infusion of capital to universities by wealthy industrialists, led to the creation of the discipline of modern medicine, imbued as it was with the authority of scientific standards (Starr 1982; Pescosolido and Martin 2004). The manifestation of 'medical doctor as independent practitioner' was, in fact, relatively shortlived, although the idea lives on in American society as a cultural simulacrum. By the middle of the twentieth century, political influence began to shift in favour of large corporations and away from physicians as independent providers.

The most powerful of these corporate interests is the health insurance sector. Health insurance in the United States was a consequence of the labour shortages that existed during the Second World War due to conscription. Wage and price controls (the 1942 Stabilization Act) meant that businesses were not allowed to compete for workers by offering them higher wages; thus, the obvious strategy for employers was to offer competitive benefits, including health insurance. At this time, the health insurance industry itself was relatively new: Blue Cross (which covered hospital services) and Blue Shield (which covered physician services) were only established in the 1930s. During the 1940s, the combination of high demand for health insurance and the success of Blue Cross and Blue Shield led to an explosion of commercial health insurance in the United States. These employer-based plans were attractive to both workers and businesses as unions were allowed to negotiate for favourable health plans as part of the collective bargaining process, and neither employers nor employees had to pay taxes on their contributions to the health insurance plans. The American Medical Association (AMA) was also satisfied with this arrangement, as it forestalled a government-run plan which, it feared, would place too many restrictions on the profession.

It was precisely the success of the AMA in maintaining professional autonomy that led to the declining influence of doctors. Ultimately, it was not government which undermined physicians' collective power but the expansion of the health service and health insurance industries. By the mid-1970s inflationary pressures across the board had led policy makers to focus especially sharply on the health sector, where many of these cost increases were considered to be especially high. This, in turn, led to the establishment of health maintenance organizations (HMOs), private (and usually, but not necessarily) for-profit organizations that enrolled individuals in comprehensive plans that offered a wide range of health services. The logic was that enrolling a high number of individuals would create a wide risk pool that would permit companies to offer competitive premiums to a wide proportion of the population. But throughout the 1980s, insurance premiums skyrocketed. This was partly because of the cost-shifting practised by health service providers who were faced with the new 'prospective payment system' that reimbursed Medicaid and Medicare patients according to diagnostic-related groups (DRGs) rather than actual costs. To recoup funds lost by treating patients according to the new limited reimbursement schedule, providers raised the costs charged to their private patients.

As a means of limiting high insurance costs, corporations began to embrace the model of 'managed care' based on the HMO structure. Many varieties of managed care emerged (e.g., doctors could be employed directly by hospitals or insurance companies or they could be individual contractors), but by the mid-1990s the majority of people with employer-based health insurance were signed on to managed care plans. Costs were initially kept down not only by attracting a large pool of subscribers, but also by controlling the clinical practices of health care providers. The managed care model led to a considerable level of both horizontal integration (hospitals merging with other hospitals) and vertical integration (insurance companies running hospitals directly). In this way, prescribing and treatment choices made by physicians (either employed directly or under contract) could be controlled by those paying the costs (the insurance companies). There was, as Tuohy comments, no little irony in this strategy, for 'in seeking to preserve a policy framework that shielded both their entrepreneurial discretion and their clinical autonomy from state incursion, the medical profession over time created the conditions in which entrepreneurs unconstrained by considerations of professional objectives or collegial modes of decision-making would come to play a more and more dominant role' (1999: 161). It also meant that policy holders were locked into contracts with specific HMOs, and had much less say in selecting their health service provider than the rhetoric over 'free choice' suggested.

It is thus the large corporate lobby, and not the AMA, which now holds the most considerable influence in health policy making in the United States. Indeed, most members of the AMA now accept public health insurance (Keyhani and Federman 2009), and the AMA officially endorsed a 'public option' in health care reform in 2009. Private insurers, on the other hand, are vociferously against this for a number of reasons. Unsurprisingly, the health sector as a whole experienced the highest level of lobbying in the United States in 2008 and 2009. The biggest spenders in this area are the pharmaceutical and health products manufacturers, the health insurance industry, health professionals' associations, and the hospital sector. The non-partisan Center for Responsive Politics, compiling data from the American Federal Election Commission, has found that the 'drugs and devices' industry has spent U.S.$1.6 *billion* on lobbying in the past ten years (U.S.$20.2 million in

2008 alone), while the health insurance industry has spent U.S.$586 million over the past decade (U.S.$74.2 million in 2008). Spending figures for 2008 and 2009 are presented in Table 11.1.

Special interests have two main strategies. One is to influence public opinion, with the hope that public polls and direct pressure on elected officials by constituents will push decision makers in a particular direction. In the summer leading up to congressional deliberations on health reform (June through August 2009) one million dollars (U.S.) *per day* was spent on television commercials regarding health care reform (Liberto 2009). The other strategy is to target specific elected officials who have key strategic positions (such as committee chairs) or who are considered 'soft' or 'swing' politicians whose vote could go either way. In the most recent debate over health reform, they were generally the 'Blue Dog' Democrats. These individuals tend to hold more conservative political views, and they often overlap with Republican policy positions on many issues (such as opposing government health insurance). The Center for Responsive Politics has tracked a marked rise in direct campaign contributions to Blue Dog Democrats from employees and political action committees (PACs) affiliated with health care corporations, relative to other Democrats throughout 2009, as the Blue Dogs' strategic importance on key votes became apparent (Liberto 2009). When all health sector lobbying is combined, the total over the past decade is U,S.$3.5 billion, which works out to six lobbyists and half a million dollars for *each* member of Congress (Kapp 2009). It should be noted that the mere fact that campaign donations are provided by special interests to particular candidates does not always mean that the recipients will act at the behest of their sponsors. The most notable example of this is Senator Chris Dodd of Connecticut, whose constituency is home base to several of America's large private insurance companies, such as Aetna. Dodd, who has received one of the highest levels of contributions from the private insurance industry (U.S.$774,491 over ten years), was nicknamed 'the Senator from Aetna' due to his support of the private insurance industry. Yet he became one of the most vocal and active supporters of public health insurance. Unsurprisingly, Democrats have, since 1989, received an average of 70 cents of every dollar of their campaign contributions from labour interests (employees of unions and PACs), and 30 cents of every dollar from corporate health-related industries (employees of commercial enterprises and PACs). Republicans have raised five cents for every dollar raised from labour interests, and 95 cents for every dollar raised from corporate health industries (Beckel 2009b).

Table 11.1. Lobbying and Contribution Expenditures, U.S. Health Sector (all U.S.$)

Players	Lobbying, 2008 and 2009	Contributions, 2008 and 2010 cycles
Pharmaceutical and Health Products	$839,722,151	$38,461,715
Pharmaceutical Research and Manufacturers of America (PhRMA)	$45,680,500	$282,209
Biotechnology Industry Association	$15,747,500	$226,979
Pfizer	$27,400,000	$2,245,564
Eli Lilly & Co.	$22,750,750	$1,267,283
Insurance	$1,252,021,842	$23,357,616
Blue Cross/Blue Shield	$28,938,412	$3,190,805
America's Health Insurance Plans	$12,815,000	$552,820
MetLife Inc	$9,275,000	$1,352,436
UnitedHealth Group	$10,505,000	$1,625,028
Health Professionals	$235,807,529	$113,005,969
American Medical Association	$30,335,000	$2,011,416
American Dental Association	$3,410,398	$2,658,490
American Nurses Association	$1,960,386	$915,641
American Association of Orthopaedic Surgeons	$3,109,000	$1,260,353
Hospitals/Nursing Homes	$321,378,826	$28,747,136
American Hospital Association	$32,504,860	$2,561,016
Alliance for Quality Nursing Home Care	$6,001,246	$53,500
American Health Care Association	$3,308,000	$1,472,920
Federation of American Hospitals	$6,311,000	$624,787
Advocacy		
American Association of Retired Persons	$37,374,000	$56,172
Health Care for America Now	$150,000	$500
Families USA Foundation	$57,000	$81,485
Business (PACs only)	$7,260,907,179	$445,702,504
U.S. Chamber of Commerce	$123,077,000	$288,162
Wal-Mart	$13,055,000	$2,072,078
National Federation of Independent Business	$5,790,402	$863,797
Labour (PACs only)	$119,761,828	$95,599,416
AFL-CIO[a]	$5,320,000	$1,564,318
SEIU[b]	$5,112,950	$2,961,803
AFSCME[c]	$3,240,000	$3,274,004

Source: Center for Responsive Politics, 2009.

[a]The American Federation of Labor and Congress of Industrial Organizations (AFL-CIO) is a voluntary federation of 57 national and international labour unions.
[b]Service Employees International Union
[c]American Federation of State, County, and Municipal Employees

Institutions and Processes

Polls taken during the legislative debate in 2009 over health reform showed that a clear majority of Americans favoured not only health care reform, but also that most favoured reform that involved a public health insurance option (Kaiser Foundation 2009). Americans have, since 1948, six times elected presidents committed to universal health care. Why, then, has health reform been so elusive? A major reason is that public opinion is filtered through a very complex system of policy making, one that is quite distinct from the relatively streamlined parliamentary system of government in Canada. Like Germany, the United States has a system of democratic decision making that was set up for negotiation and compromise. Decisions are made by discussions between many different groups, and it is easier for organized interests to influence decision makers at several different levels. In the United States, the legislative bodies – the House of Representatives and the Senate – are relatively independent of each other and of the President. However strongly a President may wish to pursue health reform, he must have the support of both the House and the Senate to pass the required legislation. Party discipline is much weaker in the United States than in a parliamentary system: elected representatives are more likely to support the views of their constituents (or organized interests within their constituencies) than party policy, even if both the House and the Senate are dominated by the same party that represents the President.

Policy making begins with debate within relevant committees in both the House and the Senate. These committees are run by powerful senior politicians, and organized interests focus much of their campaign contributions and other forms of lobbying on these individuals. There are five committees that have relevance to health reform (three in the House, and two in the Senate). In the House, the Energy and Commerce Committee plays an important role because several existing health care programs for targeted groups are paid through general taxation. The House Ways and Means Committee oversees health programs that come from payroll deductions, and the House Education and Labor Committee has an interest in health through its oversight role in pensions and benefits. In the Senate, the powerful Finance Committee is responsible for any general-tax funded social policy, including Medicaid, Medicare, and the Children's Health Insurance Program. The final committee, the Senate Health, Education, Labor, and Pensions (HELP) Committee focuses on health policy through employee benefits. The Senate committees are an especially difficult stage for progressive legislation, as the Senate is itself more heavily weighted in favour of the smaller, conservative, rural states (each state has two seats regardless of size), and the Senate committees reflect this particular bias.

At the committee stage, each of these five committees draws up its own bill. This means that each committee holds hearings and feedback sessions ('walk-thoughs'), drafts a formal bill, submits the bill for a cost estimate from the Congressional Budget Office, then debates and amends the bill ('mark-ups'). As a point of reference, members of the Senate Finance Committee *alone* submitted 564 amendments on their own 2009 health reform bill. If the committee passes the bill, it is forwarded to the full House (or Senate) for consideration. At this point, the three House committee bills are combined into one single bill for the House, and the two Senate bills are combined into one bill for consideration in the Senate. Each arm of Congress addresses its bill rather differently. In the House, the Rules Committee sets the terms for debate (e.g., how much time will be allotted for discussion). The House votes on the terms of debate set by the Rules Committee. If passed, the House bill is debated by the full House. After the time allotted for debate has passed, the House votes on the bill, requiring only a simple majority to pass.

In the Senate, however, the bill can take two paths. With a 'regular order' bill, Senators are allowed to speak on the bill for as long as they like, or to offer indefinite amendments. This gives rise to the possibility of a filibuster, which prolongs debate on the bill and thus obstructs its passage. The only means of overcoming the filibuster is through 'cloture,' which requires the support of a supermajority of sixty votes, to impose time limits on debate before moving the bill to a vote. If, however, the Senate agrees that the legislation is a 'reconciliation' bill, then a limited amount of debate time is imposed, with no possibility of filibuster. The drawback to a reconciliation categorization, however, is that the bill must have a much narrower focus (under the Byrd Rule, it must be central to taxes or spending). If both House and Senate pass their respective bills, then the joint House-Senate conference committee writes a 'conference report' which produces a final single bill. This bill then goes back to each house of Congress, to be debated in the particular style of each chamber (i.e., it may again be subject to filibuster by the Senate if it is not given 'reconciliation' status). If this final bill is passed by both the House and the Senate, then it goes to the President, who then either signs the bill into law or vetoes it.

It is, in this way, easy to see why specific health care proposals (such as those articulated by presidential candidates during an election campaign) may bear no resemblance to any piece of legislation that may ultimately emerge. It is also clear why a policy proposal may simply not make it through the legislative process at all (and, if it does, why it becomes so diluted by 'compromise amendments'). Powerful interest groups have many opportunities to influence policy makers at different levels and at various points in time. But because of the complicated and interconnected system of policy making in the United States, elected officials' votes are sometimes cast for reasons that have nothing to do with the policy being voted on. This is known as 'log-rolling,' and means that one member of Congress will say to another, 'you support me on policy A, and I'll support you on policy B.' Occasionally, too, strategic decisions on one policy front are made because of the impact they will have on other policies. This was the case for racial segregation in the United States. As Boychuk (2008a) has documented, attempts by the Democratic Party to set up public health services and health insurance in the Unites States were closely intertwined with integrationist policies. Greater government involvement in health care meant accepting the racial integration of health care, a position that many southern states vociferously opposed. The entrenched system of legal apartheid in southern states until the mid-twentieth century meant the development of a system that gave white southern voters a hegemonic lock over electoral politics. White southern Democrats therefore did not share the same enthusiasm for desegregation as their northern colleagues; and, given both the large number of southern states and the high number of key committees chaired by southern Democrats, postwar health reform attempts were stymied as much due to opposition to racial integration as to public health insurance per se. 'Support and opposition to national compulsory health insurance was drawn along racial as well as segregationalist/integrationist lines,' concludes Boychuk, 'and opposition to national compulsory health insurance was framed in ways that both explicitly and inadvertently raised issues relating to segregation' (ibid., 41).

Values

A final variable in understanding the dynamics of American health reform is the more amorphous issue of 'cultural values.' Throughout the year of health reform debate, Americans in general did seem to support not only health reform but, more pointedly, one that involved some form of public health insurance. A poll conducted by the Kaiser Foundation in October 2009 found that 57 per cent of respondents favoured 'creating a government-administered public health insurance option to compete with private health insurance plans.' More Americans, commented one policy analyst, believe in unidentified flying objects (UFOs) than strongly oppose a public option (Noah 2009b). But numbers vary across polls depending on exactly what *kind* of government option is presented, where the money for this option will come from, and what the perceived effects on individuals' own health care will be. There is also the difficulty that many Americans (like Canadians) do not understand how their own health care system operates. Not only was there some confusion over how the system currently operates, but the proposed changes were often complex, detailed, and more than a little arcane (the Senate health bill was 2,074 pages long; the Canada Health Act, in comparison, is thirteen pages long, and that includes both English and French versions).

What a nation's public values *are* is difficult to state conclusively. However, certain observations can be made. The concept of 'social solidarity' is quite weak in the United States (with some regional variations), and there is frequently more emphasis on self-reliance. Americans also tend to demand choice in the selection of health services. Yet one should remember that many of these characteristics can also be found in the French health care system. While social solidarity still underpins French social insurance, the *ticket modérateur* (or co-payment system) was designed to reinforce the principle of individual responsibility, and to remind citizens that they were expected to carry a proportion of health care costs. Similarly, the French are very insistent that their ability to choose health care providers not be restricted (which explains their dislike of the *médecin traitant*, or gatekeeping, system). Thus the French have a very comprehensive, universal system of health service which seems to coexist reasonably comfortably with the values of individual responsibility and choice of provider. Arguably a more influential aspect of American political culture (and one that is reflected in the fragmented structure of policy making) is suspicion of 'big government.' Opponents of a public option were quick to frame it as 'an attempt at government takeover' or as the insidious manifestation of the tentacles of socialism. This particular cultural perspective has become much more pronounced over time:

When Medicaid was enacted in 1965, 69 percent of the public said that they trusted the federal government to do what is right most of the time. That figure fell to 23 percent by 1993, when President Clinton focused on health reform, and it stood at just 19 percent in February 2010.

It's no surprise, then, that health reform opponents are most likely to cite 'the government [has] too big a role in the health care system' as the reason for their opposition (80 percent). (Brodie et al. 2010: 1126)

Reform at Last: The Patient Protection and Affordable Care Act

It is widely accepted that the American system of health care is inefficient, expensive, and inequitable. So why has it been so difficult to change the way the system works? Why, after almost a hundred years of attempted health care reform, did reformers finally succeed in passing landmark health care legislation in 2010? It is important to point out that many Americans are completely satisfied with their health insurance (Brodie et al. 2010). This is one reason that health care reform in the United States is so difficult: from the perspective of those who are reasonably healthy and financially well off, the system works reasonably well, and there is considerable resistance to change. Major health insurance reforms mean a significant redistribution of wealth, and where there is economic redistribution there is always a political struggle. If lower-income and middle-class families and individuals stand to gain, then who pays?

The point of having a mandated system (either public or private), in which everyone is obliged to bear the cost of health insurance, is that the healthy who use fewer resources will help subsidize the sick who use more. Thus the young and healthy, who are more likely to choose not to buy health insurance, will, as a group, pay more under a system of mandated insurance than they currently do. Further, if health insurance payments are linked to income, then the well-off will pay more to subsidize the poor. If a public insurance option for everyone is introduced, then it may attract customers away from the more expensive private plans, and *they* will lose. And, because the American system is largely employment-based, increasing coverage would mean a distribution from the employed to the unemployed. For historical reasons, payroll contributions by both employers and employees have, for the most part, been untaxed. This is highly regressive (the better your health care plan, the higher your premiums; and the higher your premiums, the more you save on unpaid taxes). Unsurprisingly, many employers and unions disliked the idea of a payroll tax, even a progressive payroll tax (i.e., taxation of benefits over a certain income level). Thus the politics of health reform can be understood at its most basic to be the classic questions of political science: who wins? Who loses? And what is each specific actor going to do to influence the results?

Why the 2010 Reforms Succeeded

The clear starting point for health reform was Barack Obama's 2008 electoral triumph, which meant Democratic majorities in both houses of Congress. The Obama administration, however, was quickly beset by overwhelming economic crises that heightened public anxiety over excessive public spending. Moreover, as Bill Clinton had learned, simple partisan majorities are not sufficient (unlike in parliamentary systems) to guarantee policy success. Because of the fragmented and decentralized legislative process, and given the absence of the party discipline that characterizes parliamentary systems, most national health legislation in the United States has been piecemeal. The notable exception to this was the passage of Medicaid and Medicare in 1965, which is generally understood to involve the sentimental legacy of John F. Kennedy's assassination, the superior tactical ability of Lyndon Johnson in getting legislation through Congress, a large partisan majority in Congress, rising prosperity, and the enactment of the Civil Rights Act in 1964. The Clinton reforms of 1993 met an altogether different end, and contemporary political strategists attempting health reform have clearly shown that they recognize the lessons of the ill-fated Clinton plan.

As Oberlander (2010: 1113) observes, the strategy of the Obama administration was seemingly to do precisely the opposite of the Clinton strategy:

Whereas Clinton moved slowly on health care, Obama tried to push legislation through Congress quickly. Whereas the Clinton administration developed a remarkably detailed health plan, once in office Obama did not release a fully elaborated plan, instead leaving it to Congress to flesh out the details. The Clinton health plan mandated that all employers pay for their workers' health insurance and changed how most Americans with employer-sponsored insurance would get coverage. The Obama administration sought to exempt small businesses from any mandate and reassure Americans happy with their insurance that they could keep their plans. And the Obama administration successfully pressed Senate leaders to put reconciliation instructions for health reform into the budget resolution – a filibuster shortcut that the Clinton administration had not obtained. Reconciliation gave Democrats the option of passing health care legislation in the Senate with a simple majority and without any Republican support – a key advantage, given the fragility of their filibuster-proof majority and the polarized partisan environment.

The Clinton administration had a grand theory of reform and a vision of transforming the delivery system through managed competition. It also ended up embracing – partly because of pressures from the CBO – strong, centralized, and systemwide cost controls, including premium caps and a national health care budget. In contrast, the Obama administration touted incremental, friendly sounding reforms such as electronic health records, prevention, and medical homes ... Moreover, Congress and the Obama administration reversed course from 1993–94 by proposing tax increases on wealthier Americans to pay for expanding coverage. Although the 'New Democrat' Clinton had sought to avoid any new taxes, Democrats in 2010 embraced explicitly redistributive financing.

Another key difference between 1993 and 2010 was that the urgency to achieve cost containment was so much more pronounced. Skyrocketing health care expenditure affected not only recipients of health care but, more critically, large commercial stakeholders. Large employers realized that unchecked health care expenditure increased the cost of providing employee benefits. The American Medical Association publicly endorsed health reform (as long as curtailed physician payments were not on the table). In the summer of 2009, the White House negotiated a deal with large pharmaceutical companies to bring them onside with the reforms. Finally, the large insurance companies, which had in previous years undermined reform efforts, understood that they stood to gain more from working with reformers than from opposing them. A system of mandated private insurance would mean a considerable expansion of their potential client base, especially when it was subsidized generously by government funds. Thus most of the potential opponents of health reform were, in the end, successfully co-opted by Democratic health reformers.

The Democrats' strategy of co-optation, compromise, and pragmatism extended to deal making with members of the houses of Congress as well. While the Democrats had a healthy majority in the House, a number of Democrats were fiscally or socially conservative Blue Dogs who refused to support many of the more liberal provisions of the House bill. This meant that the Speaker of the House had to broker compromises on the bill that included limiting the scope and effectiveness of the public option and refusing federal funding for abortions. The political tensions in the Senate were even more pronounced, as the Democratic caucus contained only sixty members (two of whom were independents), exactly the number needed to pass legislation free from the threat of filibuster. For this reason the Senate bill had to be diluted even more in order to secure all the needed votes, and potential dissenters knew that their leverage was high. Thus Joe Lieberman successfully opposed the expansion of Medicare benefits to those above age 55 (instead of 65), and Ben Nelson of Nebraska both defeated the attempt to strip the insurance industry of its anti-trust exemption and won additional Medicaid funds from the federal government for his state, a ploy that the media immediately dubbed the 'cornhusker kickback.' The biggest casualty of the Senate negotiations was the public option: at the end it became evident that the bill could not clear the Senate unless the public option, the liberal Democrats' hope for substantial health care reform, was jettisoned.

Thus health reform was achieved, but at considerable cost. The most effective means of controlling expenditure – a single-payer public insurance option (like Canada's) was never seen as a viable possibility, but the idea of a public insurance option operating alongside private insurance plans was viewed as a reasonable alternative. The most emphatic objection to the public option was essentially that it would work too well: it could offer less expensive premiums for more comprehensive services to a wider number of people. Private insurance companies simply would not be able to compete, and the industry might even collapse, leaving a sizeable portion of the economy *in the hands of government*. Thus the well-being of corporate America had to be preserved against the 'unfair advantages' that a public insurance system could command. This resulted in moderate political support for a 'level playing field' approach, in which the public option would not be allowed to compete, or to compete so effectively, with private plans. Either the public plan would be limited to certain individuals (e.g., those who did not have employer-based plans and were not eligible for Medicaid or Medicare), or it would not be able to use its size to leverage better prices (e.g., it could not use the lower rates already set by Medicare), or both.

To a large extent, these qualifications on public insurance undermined the very point for having it: keeping total costs down by forcing providers to offer better rates, and requiring private insurers to offer better service with lower premiums. Supporters of a public plan argued that the private insurance industry had simply become too concentrated and inefficient, and that a public insurance option would oblige private plans to become 'more efficient and more effective' in controlling health care expenditure (Holahan and Blumberg 2009). A public plan 'could 'create a benchmark for private insurers, challenging them to improve the value of their product and bargain more aggressively with dominant providers; and, through innovative methods of payment and care delivery that build on approaches used by successful public programs, it would reduce costs over time' (Hacker 2009: 1618). It is equally likely like that a public plan would be disadvantaged vis-à-vis private plans insofar as it would no doubt have a much higher proportion of high-risk individuals, which would put upward pressures on the premiums it could set (the 'crowding-out' phenomenon). In the end, however, the quid pro quo for the support of the corporate insurance sector for health reform was the death of the public option; and in the end the reformers were committed more to passing an attenuated variation of health reform legislation than to preserving the public option – which, as some point out, can still be reintroduced at the state level in the future (Halpin and Harbage 2010).

Gaining the support of the AMA and the pharmaceutical industry for health care reform was equally costly. The price of getting both groups on board was the implicit agreement not to use regulatory power to limit the prices paid for products and services. While the PPACA does reduce the growth of payments to health care providers in some areas, physicians are exempt; nor will government agencies (such as Medicare) be able to use their market power to negotiate better prices with the pharmaceutical industry. This means that very effective means of cost control have been eliminated from the final piece of legislation. There is slightly more regulation of the insurance industry. These measures include preventing some of the more unscrupulous but (currently) legal practices, such as refusing coverage for pre-existing conditions (the people who need health insurance the most are the sickest, but they are also the most obvious expenditure risks) and making the practices of rescinding claims (i.e., rescissions) illegal. While there is a relatively high level of support for such policies, they accomplish little overall structural change. American health policy analysts who follow

European health policy have argued that a comprehensive regimen of closely regulated private health insurers ('all-payer regulation') can provide a comprehensive system of universal coverage (e.g., Reinhardt 2007; Oberlander and White 2009). Yet most European states depend on private *not-for-profit* insurers, which are heavily regulated, with a considerably smaller proportion of for-profit companies (which usually are subject to much less regulation). These not-for-profit mutual associations are themselves grounded on a political culture of solidarity. It is questionable whether American for-profit corporations would be willing operate within such a heavily regulated environment. Moreover, *if* the logic of regulation is that it requires insurance firms to behave in a certain mandated fashion (such as putting the health of individuals before profits) then the question arises of why it would not simply be better to have a not-for-profit system altogether.

Nevertheless, politics, the art of the possible, always trumps policy. While considerable criticism of the PPACA was exhaustive in its explanation of how much better the legislation could have been both in controlling health care expenditure and in providing fair and affordable coverage, the legislation does implement considerable and wide-ranging changes to the American health care system.

A New American Health Care System?

The best evaluation of the new PPACA was articulated by President Obama, who admitted that the new law was a major, but not radical, reform. Briefly stated, the most considerable change in American health care has been the implementation of an individual health insurance mandate, supported by 'health exchanges' (where those seeking plans can go for 'one-stop shopping') along with government subsidies that allow low-income Americans to afford to buy comprehensive health insurance premiums. The PPACA also contains less-publicized measures (especially in preventive health and health system performance improvement) which may potentially have more long-ranging, system-wide effects on the health care sector. Some of the reforms have been implemented by 2010; others will be gradually phased in by 2019.

THE INDIVIDUAL MANDATE

'Mandated individual insurance' means that all adults must buy insurance for themselves and their families, or face a fine. It encourages individuals to shop for the best plan, and it allows them to keep their insurance regardless of their employment status (as long as they can pay the premiums). Interestingly, the individual mandate was one of the most politically unpopular aspects of health reform, with far fewer Americans preferring an individual mandate to a public option. Notwithstanding such opposition, the powerful health insurance lobby was firmly in favour of an individual mandate, as it meant a large guaranteed customer base, and a subsidized one at that. There were two main objections to individual mandated insurance. The first was simply that 'it's not the American way': individuals should have the right to *choose* whether they want to be insured at all. The second was that it would be forcing individuals to bear costs that they simply could not afford. Private individual premiums tend to be quite high, and lower 'affordable' premiums generally mean considerably higher out-of-pocket costs. Even if a family has a cheap, rudimentary plan, they might still choose to go without basic or even essential health care because of onerous deductibles or co-payments. An additional problem was that, before the passage of the PPACA, private insurers were allowed to oblige individuals with pre-existing conditions to pay very high premiums, or to deny them coverage altogether. One precondition to the implementation of an individual mandate, then, was the stipulation that private insurance companies would have to provide insurance to all applicants ('guaranteed issue'), and that the amount of variation in rates offered to various risk categories would be quite limited.

The second precondition for individual mandates was a set of subsidies (as tax deductions, tax credits, or direct financial payments) that would allow low-income purchasers to buy insurance without undue hardship. (The usual figure used is that no family should have to pay more than 12.5 per cent of household income on health insurance.) But what level of subsidies should be offered? More importantly, who would pay for them? Subsidies could be financed by taxing the employer-based insurance plans, which amount to approximately U.S.$245 billion of foregone revenue per year, or they could come from general revenues (or a specific health care tax); either way, they ultimately would amount to a considerable redistribution of domestic wealth.

The PPACA mandated individual insurance by 2014. Those refusing to buy coverage would be fined the higher of either a U.S.$695 penalty (U.S.$2,085 per family) or 2.5 per cent of household income. Exceptions would be made for financial hardship, religious objections, Native Americans, anyone uninsured for less than three months, anyone for whom the cheapest plan would still exceed 8 per cent of income, and individuals with income below the tax filing threshold (U.S.$9,350). Private insurers face new regulations that forbid them from denying coverage to individuals for any reason, and which disallow them from increasing premiums due to health status or gender (prior to reforms, being female was justification for being charged higher premiums). Age, geographical region, and tobacco use are acceptable reasons for higher premiums, but only under clearly circumscribed limits. The practice of rescission is now illegal, except in cases of fraud. Moreover, premiums cannot be arbitrarily increased; they are now subject to review. Subsidies and credits will be provided to low-income Americans on a sliding scale for those between 100 per cent and 400 per cent of the federal poverty level (about U.S.$22,000 for a family of four). In addition, young people – those least likely to purchase health insurance – will be permitted to remain covered by their parents' insurance until the age of 26.

EXCHANGES

To make the process of buying insurance easier for individuals, a mandated scheme is generally articulated in conjunction with the idea of 'health insurance exchanges' (also known as 'gateways' or 'connectors'). In theory, insurance exchanges could be organized in a number of different ways to perform a number of different functions. The basic rationale for insurance exchanges in principle, however, is that

> consumers are rarely well equipped to deal with markets offering large numbers of complex, expensive, hard-to-evaluate products – products that, as in the case of health insurance policies, may nonetheless be critical to their well-being. Consumers facing complex, high-stakes choices are prone to predictable errors. They are likely to lack the skill and time to make choices based on a careful assessment of the relative costs and quality of competing health plans, tending instead to choose on the basis of anecdotal information, such as their friends' experiences. An effective intermediary could substantially improve their choices – and thereby promote competition and thus enhance quality and efficiency. (Frank and Zeckhauser 2009: 1135)

Under the PPACA, American Health Benefit Exchanges will be created at the state level (and if states choose not to do so, the federal Office of Personnel Management will coordinate private insurers to establish some choice between plans). Two separate kinds of exchanges will exist in each state: one for individuals and one for small businesses. Small businesses with ten or fewer employees (and average wages of less than U.S.$25,000 per annum) will also receive tax credits (at the same time, health insurance tax credits for large employers will be phased out). Insurance firms that offer plans on the exchanges must conform to strict requirements and minimum standards. They must offer four levels of coverage, each of which comprises a different set of premiums, out-of-pocket costs, benefits, and catastrophic coverage. There is no employer mandate (employers can, but are not obliged, to offer health insurance to their employees). However, large employers who do not insure their employees will be assessed an annual fee of U.S.$2,000 per full-time employee.

CHANGES TO PUBLIC PROGRAMS

Another key measure taken to widen coverage for uninsured individuals was the expansion of eligibility for Medicaid programs. Before the PPACA, most childless men and non-pregnant adult women below the poverty line were not eligible for Medicaid coverage. Now all those under the age of 65 with incomes up to 133 per cent of the federal poverty level will have eligibility for Medicaid. The PPACA also establishes a more uniform minimum eligibility for Medicaid (which, as a shared-cost program between state and federal governments, had previously varied considerably between states). Changes have also been made to the Medicare program, most significantly to address the 'doughnut hole' or coverage gap in seniors' prescription reimbursement. The doughnut hole is the coverage gap in prescription drug coverage through Medicare, whereby individuals are 75 per cent covered up to an annual ceiling of U.S.$2,405 and 95 per cent covered after annual expenses reach U.S.$5,016 but have no coverage between these two amounts.

OTHER MEASURES

The PPACA establishes a series of new taxes and fees, ranging from annual fees for the pharmaceutical manufacturing sector and the health insurance industry to higher taxes on medical devices and, intriguingly, indoor tanning services. The tax on wages increases to 2.35 per cent from 1.45 per cent, while a new 3.8 per cent tax on unearned income (such as dividends and interest) takes effect in 2013. The same year, new Medicare taxes will be imposed on individuals earning more than U.S.$200,000 per year (or U.S.$250,000 for couples). And, in 2018, an excise tax of 40 per cent will be levied on 'Cadillac plans', or health insurance plans valued at more than U.S.$10,200 (or U.S.$27,500 for families), the so-called Cadillac plans.

Long-term care is another policy area addressed by the PPACA. A payroll deduction scheme allows individuals to enroll in an insurance program that will permit them to purchase future community living services when necessary. While this is a voluntary program, all working adults will be automatically enrolled in it, and they must request to be delisted if they choose not to participate. This design will likely keep enrolment at a higher level than a discretionary sign-up program.

While the most widely discussed aspects of the health reform legislation have been coverage and financing, perhaps the most interesting (and promising) measures are those attempting to address systemwide changes in the way in which health care not only is provided but also the way in which 'health care' itself is considered. The first of these approaches is an institutionalized commitment to the principles of preventing illness and promoting health. To this end, several new bodies will be established (the National Prevention, Health Promotion, and Public Health Council; the Preventive and Public Health Fund; and task forces on Preventive Services and Community Preventive Services) intended to move health care away from an expensive medical model to a more preventive one. Employers are financially encouraged to provide wellness incentive programs for employees and, effective immediately, plans will be expected to provide full coverage for certain preventive services (such as immunizations) without cost-sharing. Within a year of enactment, chain restaurants and vending machines will have to disclose nutritional information on all items sold.

The second approach focuses on the effective organization of health services. Most countries have become aware that one of the most pressing difficulties in the provision of health care has been the coordination of services for patients, who often must access two or more separate 'silos' of services to obtain the care they need. Because the United States is much more decentralized and deregulated than other jurisdictions, however, it has been extraordinarily difficult to focus on the effective coordination of these elements. What the PPACA attempts to do, first, is to counteract the bias against primary care built into the American medical model. For example, the new act provides more funding for existing community health centres, school-based health centres, and nurse-managed health clinics. Second, the PPACA develops training programs that focus on primary and coordinated-care models (such as team management of chronic disease and the coordination of physical and mental health programs). Third, the act supports pilot programs for new models of health service provision that emphasize both primary care and integrated care. These include 'medical homes' which take responsibility for ensuring that patients receive all recommended care (rather than allowing patients to shuffle between discrete health services on their own) and 'accountable care organizations,' which take responsibility for both the cost and quality of health care provided to defined populations. Other pilot programs will test the use of 'bundled payments' for acute (hospital) and post-acute (rehabilitative) care. Financial assistance will also be provided under the PPACA to develop and update the use of electronic health systems (such as medical records).

What this approach attempts is to move the provision and funding of health care away from quantity and towards quality (providers are rewarded not simply for providing services, but for good outcomes). Built into the PPACA are provisions that encourage the collection of information allowing health care to be provided in the most effective and efficient way possible. Hospitals will be given incentives to monitor and improve quality in providing health care services (such as reduced Medicare and Medicaid payments for higher than average hospital readmissions and hospital-acquired infections). Comparative effectiveness research (CER) will be promoted through the establishment of a new Patient-Centered Outcomes Research Institute.

EVALUATING AMERICA'S BLUEPRINT FOR A NEW HEALTH CARE SYSTEM

What is most striking about the passage of the new legislation was how it almost never came to be. The achievement of health reform required the sustained efforts and determination of key individuals to push the bill through by any means and in any shape possible. It also meant the willingness of liberal Democrats to support the legislation as many provisions of the bill were increasingly diluted or eliminated. But while the bill was successfully enacted after a nail-biting passage through Senate, the final legislation was much different from that envisioned by its proponents. Many Americans have expressed disappointment at the final product. Certainly it will take decades to determine if the result was worth the effort, especially as many of the key provisions of the PPACA will be phased in over several years until 2019. The two types of criticism levied on the new act were, on the one hand, that 'it was too watered down' or, on the other hand, that 'it took the wrong direction entirely.' Nevertheless, very few people held that a continuation of the status quo would have been acceptable.

What constructive changes have been won? The most hopeful accomplishment is the increased level of health insurance coverage for Americans. Before the PPACA, the national average for Americans with coverage was 83 per cent (ranging considerably from state to state). By the time the act is fully operational, coverage is expected to level out at 95 per cent. Another key achievement – with luck – will be some restraint in the level of cost expansion. This was perhaps the area of greatest contention in the debate over the health reform bill. Critics argued that the expansion of coverage would result in a significant *increase* in overall costs. Indeed, the CBO estimated the new law to cost U.S.$938 billion over ten years. But the new costs, according the act's proponents, will be financed through other measures outlined in the act. These include changes to Medicaid and Medicare, new taxes and fees, the use of exchanges (choices between comparable plans – including non-profit plans – become more transparent), and laws governing the behaviour of private insurance companies (including limits on the percentage of premiums going to administrative costs and monitoring of premium increases). The emphasis on, and development of, health promotion may diminish the use of expensive acute care; while the growth of comparative effectiveness research may help to eliminate practices that simply aren't very useful. Innovative delivery and payment programs will, ideally, move the remuneration for services towards value and away from volume. The expected success of the PPACA in 'bending the cost curve' is admittedly quite theoretical (and, some would argue, highly speculative) but, given how much costs were expected to balloon in the absence of reforms altogether, the accomplishment cannot be dismissed. The Commonwealth Fund, for example, estimated that the PPACA will reduce health care spending by U.S.$590 billion over 2010–19, slowing the annual national growth rate in health care from 6.3 per cent to 5.7 per cent (Cutler et al. 2010). More broadly (and perhaps more significantly), the PPACA is the first piece of major legislation in at least thirty years to affect a major redistributive effect from the well-off to the less well-off. The 'new right' precepts of deregulation that saw the top quintile (and especially the top per cent) of Americans gain an ever-increasing relative share of the national wealth have informed policy making in the United States since the 1980s; and even the Clinton health care reforms of the early 1990s did not attempt to address redistributive issues through health care reform to such a degree.

So it's a good start. But the PPACA is still, to a large extent, a fairly conservative piece of legislation. There are no radical or systemic attempts made to control the overuse or inappropriate use of health care services. Certainly, by providing more funding for comparative effectiveness research, and by launching pilot programs in alternative delivery and payment systems that reward outcomes, the act is pointing in the right direction. But these limited and tentative incentive systems may well have no considerable outcomes within a system that permits those who can afford to buy goods and services to demand whatever they want, and those who sell goods and services to demand whatever *they* want in exchange for them. In other countries, a system of all-payer regulation, for example, imposes limits on both purchasers and providers, and a comprehensive system of GP gatekeeping (in countries such as Britain and Canada) places limits on health care consumers. Changes in the American system are voluntary, local, and piecemeal, and they will have little effect on the way in which much health care is either provided or paid for. For example, under a new pilot program groups of doctors can share the savings to Medicare if they provide better outcomes at a lower cost; but it is not Medicare (which already has a system of capped payments) that is the real cost driver in American health care. Consumers are, for many reasons, sceptical about evidence-based care, often assuming that comprehensive and expensive care is always better (Carman et al. 2010). At the same time, most physicians have no reason to deny excessive treatment (and are, instead, rewarded for it). There are, for example, already a very good set of guidelines to determine whether individuals in accidents should receive a CT scan. But most patients will insist on it, and physicians have little or no incentive to resist the demand: among radiologists, notes one physician, the joke is that the indication for getting a CT scan of your head after a car accident 'is if you have a head' (Kolata 2010: D1). Moreover, Americans' suspicion of Big Government and their desire for untrammelled choice in the marketplace mean that any attempts to impose restrictions on inefficient health care spending will immediately be attacked. The observation that spending tens of thousands of dollars on keeping a critically ill individual in late stages of life alive for a matter of days or weeks might be a poor use of health dollars, for example, was immediately labelled 'death panels for granny' in the popular press during the health reform debate. 'The minute you attack overutilization,' states Uwe Reinhardt, 'you will be called a Nazi before the day is out' (cited in Kolata 2010). An inefficient and fragmented system of reimbursement (fee-for-service payments reimbursed by a multitude of private insurance companies) is still the dominant means of financing health care. Moreover, politically, those with the most to gain at keeping costs high (such as the pharmaceutical sector) have in no way lost any of their political influence. One might even argue that, by becoming key players within the newly reformed system, they are even better placed to prevent systemic changes that would permit effective cost containment in the future.

The acrimonious and exhausting struggle for health reform is over for now. But challenges remain, and discussions over the PPACA will always be considered with reference to how things *might* have been otherwise. Certainly, the act is pointing in the right direction, but there is less certainty that there will be much actual movement in this direction. Politically, the question is whether the new approaches introduced by the act will be the thin edge of the wedge allowing incremental changes to arise over time, or whether the conservative design of the PPACA which reinforces the influence of powerful stakeholders means a condition of path dependency that makes radical evolution even more difficult to achieve. Ultimately, it is important to acknowledge that real changes will be made under the act, both at a more abstract level and in the everyday lives of countless Americans. Regarding the former, the PPACA recognizes – at least symbolically – the need to change the way that Americans think about the nature of health care as well as health care delivery. This is a victory in itself. Regarding the latter, near-universal health care coverage will mean, at the very least, that we can now see 'a glimpse of American health care without the routine cruelty' (Gawande 2009a: 33). That is an even greater victory.

12 Conclusion

This book has attempted to explain, in some detail, how the Canadian health care system works, why it works this way, and how it compares with health care systems in other countries. What overarching conclusions can be made about health care systems, in general, and health care in Canada, in particular? Six points: first, there is no one ideal health care system; second, reform in any one direction usually has consequences for other aspects of health care; third, the Canadian system isn't that bad, but could be improved; fourth, the changes needed in Canadian health care are widely known and relatively uncontroversial; fifth, the question of *how* to achieve these changes at a system-wide level is more enigmatic and subject to a great deal of dispute; and sixth, the knowledge we *do* have about what ought to be done is filtered through a viscous mire of interests that can potentially derail, distort, or suppress possible solutions, strategies, or even articulations about what the real problems are.

There Isn't a Holy Grail of Health Care

We should not think of health care systems on a linear scale, running from best to worst. Certain countries do some things well; other countries excel in other areas. The qualitative and quantitative difficulties in attempting to line them up in a rigorously hierarchical manner simply isn't helpful. This isn't to invoke unrestrained relativism: it is useful to look more carefully at countries that tend to do many things well (as well as to understand why other states do so many things so badly). But the structural and procedural contexts of each country vary considerably; this both explains why jurisdictions do things in a particular way, and suggests that there may be a certain efficiency in constructing health policy in one country that may not exist in another. The financial and technical capacity of jurisdictions varies as well. More importantly, and more elusively, each country seems to have an amorphous but potent set of values (most often some articulation of 'choice' or 'equity') that simply seems to matter a great deal to the citizens of that particular country. No comprehensive formula will be able to rank health care systems satisfactorily when nations expect their systems not only to protect the health of the people but also to do so in a manner that reflects the norms that each jurisdiction highly values.

Health care is not just about acute care. It should not be surprising, however, that the medical model has proved to be so resilient: it addresses clearly defined causal effects requiring concrete goods and services, from which specific individuals or groups may benefit. The contemporary mind is the product of several hundred years' worth of Enlightenment thinking, which stressed objective observation and logical construction of rational ideas as the basis of legitimate knowledge. Thus, clear causal relationships remain the foundation of thinking about the provision of health care; and these are reinforced within bureaucratic cultures that emphasize accountability, efficiency, and outcomes. But this approach cannot easily be reconciled with increasing evidence that both broad social and physical factors (e.g., education, employment, environment, geography) and very subjective psychological states of mind (including self-esteem and a sense of control over one's life) also play an undeniable role in the overall state of one's physical health. The health of entire populations is determined not only by the existence of pathogens but also by social inequality. Thus the debate over 'what the ideal balance of health services is' has become increasingly dated; considerations of the trade-off between *kinds* of health care are being surpassed by debates over the trade-off between kinds of social policies and health care *itself*.

There is, then, a strange multiplicity of ideal types in health care systems; for what is best for each jurisdiction depends largely on factors that have, on the face of it, nothing to do with making ill people better. Social redistribution has little to do with cutting-edge Internet technology; but both are seen as ways to facilitate better health care. This is why an Aristotelian model is the best hermeneutic device for understanding health care systems. 'The good,' wrote Aristotle, 'is not some common element answering to one Idea,' but rather a set of goods 'that are attainable and achievable' (I.6.1096b). The way to achieve the best potential good of each individual (or system) is first to understand the particular nature of that individual (or system), and to understand the particular balance of qualities that will develop 'excellence of character' (or, in modern parlance, 'high-performing health care systems').

All Actions Have Reactions

If the best way of understanding how we ought to think about health care systems per se is Aristotelian, the most useful hermeneutic in thinking about health care *reform* is Newtonian. Certainly Newton's first law of motion – the law of inertia – is familiar enough to those wishing to reform large, unwieldy health care systems. But the second and third laws – that an object will move in the direction of the strongest forces acting on it, and that pushing hard in a particular direction will cause some considerable reaction – are perhaps more relevant for health policy analysts. Newton's second law – the summation of forces – will be discussed in a section below, with reference to political interests. The third law – the direction of forces – is especially relevant with respect to current discussions about the kinds of directions in which health care systems ought to move. For what nations are increasingly discovering is that any attempt to improve a health care system by focusing on one particular variable will likely have other consequences (either unintended or predictable) on other dimensions of the system.

The most recent example of this has been the shift in private insurance coverage in the United States. Even with the Patient Protection and Affordable Care Act reforms that come onstream in 2014, many shifts in the way insurance is offered will still be driven by the market. Similar to the managed care experiments of the 1990s, consumer demand for lower premiums has once again led the major health insurance providers – Cigna, WellPoint, Aetna, and UnitedHealth Group – to offer 'narrow network' plans that restrict the number of doctors and hospitals that those individuals that they insure can visit. By ensuring that these individuals only use services that provide good quality care for reasonable prices, the lower costs to insurers are passed on as lower premiums to enrollees. The point is that there is a trade-off: less choice for lower costs. The interesting thing about the American case is that the trade-off between choice and cost is not made by state policy makers but by individuals and businesses interacting through the market. Nonetheless, the trade-off remains.

The same dynamic exists across countries. Indeed, what has characterized much European health care reform in the past decade or so has been the shift in 'Beveridge,' or tax-based, systems (such as the U.K. and Sweden) towards increasing choice and decreasing waiting times, and the trend in 'Bismarck,' or insurance-based, systems (such as France and Germany) towards controlling costs through restrictions on choice (see, e.g., Or et al. 2010). But citizens commonly seem more aware of the qualities that are lost through reforms than of the limited gains made; rarely is either attempt at reform an unmitigated success. This is because the general characteristics of a desirable health care system cannot always be easily reconciled. Some principles – like universality and equity, or universality and cost control – are more consonant; others – like equity and responsiveness, or equity and cost control – are less congruous. No matter what shape a health care system takes, someone will be able to argue that it could be doing a better job in some respect (and that there is another country that *is* doing a better job in this area).

One of the most importunate issues currently facing all health care systems is cost containment. Health care costs are increasing dramatically everywhere. But some countries are doing a better job at controlling health expenditure than others, and one very important factor seems to be some degree of centralized state control over setting prices. This does not necessarily require public ownership (although it is, unsurprisingly, easier for public systems to control pricing). The past two decades have focused very specifically on increasing the efficiency of health care provision, and they have tended to look to the market for inspiration, as the discipline of market competition can be good, in many cases, at providing more for less. But the experiment with new public management has not been a particular success (nor has it been a complete failure). Efficient unit costs can most easily be procured by economies of scale: Adam Smith's famous observation was that one could make pins much cheaper if several people focused on only one aspect of pin-making, thereby increasing volume. But one can only use so many pins. Health care is different. Focusing on efficient production through competition tends to encourage higher volumes; and higher volumes increase total costs. Moreover, markets at the best of times are only truly efficient at finding the equilibrium between price and demand. If the market is the only determinant of demand, then price and demand may indeed find an optimal resting point. But allowing the market to be the only determinant of distribution for health services means that there would certainly be no room for either equity or universality. Once values like fairness and compassion interfere, then the efficiency of this market mechanism becomes irrevocably distorted.

Comprehensiveness and responsiveness can, however, be served well by having a number of competing providers in a health care system. These can put upward pressures on total costs (there's no point, e.g., offering services unless people buy them). But these providers can be not-for-profit as well as for-profit, and even for-profit entities can be subject to regulation. This explains why the Netherlands, which depends heavily on private health insurance, is able to attain universal coverage with much better cost containment than the United States, which is also highly dependent on private health insurance. A system with more private choices can work, but not without its own disadvantages. In addition to the tendency to respond primarily to wealth (obviously the *point* of the market), having a significant level of health services in the private sphere means that there are complex and often unpredictable political dynamics that can affect the shape of health care in unanticipated and possibly unwanted ways (one example of this has been the role that the European Court of Justice has taken in restricting public health care services if they are seen to present 'unfair advantages' to private ones.) What this means is that each country will have to decide which particular constellation of characteristics it wishes its health care system to exhibit, and what price it is willing to pay by foregoing others. As Weale (1989: 410) has explained, the pursuit of competing health care ideals 'threatens to become what logicians call an inconsistent triad; a collection of propositions, any two of which are compatible with each other but which, when viewed together in a threesome, form a contradiction. Perhaps we can have only a comprehensive service of high quality, but not one available to all. Or a comprehensive service freely available to all, but not of high quality. Or a high-quality service freely available to all, but not comprehensive. Each of these three possibilities defines a characteristic position in the modern debate about healthcare costs and organisation.'

We're Not Bad, but We Could Be Better

Canadians tend most often to compare their own system with that of the United States simply because of proximity. But Canada's health care system performs reasonably well on a number of measures compared with OECD member states in general. One aspect of this is cost containment, which is generally measured using the rate of spending considered over a number of years. Looking at recent OECD statistics, Canada is on the high end in general, but lower than several G8 countries. But what statistics themselves do not show is the *institutional capacity* of states to control health spending: in other words, does the way in which political institutions are structured facilitate the ability of countries (such as Great Britain) to control costs directly, or are states more reliant on a more tenuous combination of regulation and negotiation in order to limit cost increases (as in the case of France)? The fact that health care spending in Canada was kept down relative to other countries between 1996 and 2000 shows that (for better or worse) overall spending can be receptive to direct political decision making. The institutional capacity to turn the taps off is a crude policy tool that by itself does little to secure the efficient utilization of health care resources, but it is a powerful policy tool nonetheless. The simple fact that it can be exercised at all provides some window for long-term planning, but, more importantly, direct political control over spending makes the state an immediate 'player' in the system. This encourages the state to use its influence in order to attempt more sophisticated means of restricting cost increases (including coordinating systems, facilitating administrative and technological improvements, establishing national collaborative programs, employing economies of scale in purchasing, funding data collection, research studies, pilot programs, and so on). In other words, the more directly involved the state is in health care expenditure, the more motivation it has to keep costs down (and the more ability it has – electoral pressures notwithstanding – to do so).

Canada also does fairly well in terms of basic health outcomes, including healthy life expectancy and mortality amenable to health care. This can be attributed to a number of factors, including the system of public insurance set up between 1957 and 1972. As noted in Chapter 5, the statistical gap in health indicators between the United State and Canada began to grow noticeably after the introduction of universal public health insurance across Canada (in 1961, life expectancy in Canada was less than a year greater than that in the United States; by 2007 it was almost three years greater). Canadian health indicators have also been correlated with variables such as higher educational outcomes. More ephemerally, political support for a system of universal public health insurance remains strong. A 2009 Nanos poll, for example, showed that 86.2 per cent of Canadians preferred 'public solutions to make our public healthcare stronger' (Nanos 2009). It is this sense of social solidarity, more than any more concrete set of institutional structures, that has sustained the public health insurance system in Canada (and, critics would add, which has prevented any substantial reorientation of health care in the country).

But the problems and challenges are undeniable. On the most basic level, expenditure on health care is continually increasing, easily outpacing spending on every other service area. This rate of spending is simply not met by improvements in outcomes. A recent Commonwealth Fund survey ranked Canada second to last on a number of indicators, including quality care (services which are effective, safe, coordinated, and patient-centred), access (timely and cost-appropriate), efficiency, and equity (Davis et al. 2010). Critics might respond that this study was simply based on the subjective opinion of a random sample of patients and physicians; but the results nonetheless reflect other, more objective indicators (such as waiting times, IT usage in health systems, and rates of medical errors). A comparative survey on palliative care ranked Canada as only ninth (out of 40) as 'the best place to die' (Economist Intelligence Unit 2010).

That system-wide flaws exist is only underscored by the observation that a decade of extra money poured into the health care system has not been able to secure the kinds of changes other countries have been making: it is certainly arguable that so much unconditional funding has allowed health care systems to *avoid* having to make difficult choices about restructuring. This reflects an interesting paradox about the Canadian system: while its system of tax-based funding gives it a centralized structure (that permits some level of control over spending decisions, as noted above), Canada's health care system is highly decentralized in a number of other ways, which means that crucial elements of the health care system are simply not accountable for the outcomes they produce. The most obvious instance of this is the relationship between provinces and the federal government; for example, despite the rhetoric of meeting national standards for waiting times in exchange for additional money, meeting performance targets was never a condition for receiving federal funds. The provinces simply are not accountable to Ottawa for health care outcomes and, on principle, it is doubtful that a critical mass of them would cede their autonomy in this area for any amount of conditional cash. But decentralized decision making and the lack of systemwide accountability can be found in other relationships as well. Physicians, as self-regulating professionals, have a considerable degree of autonomy within the Canadian health care system. Thus it is unsurprising that a considerable amount of resources find their way to Canadian physicians, who have one of the best rates of relative remuneration in the world: according to the OECD, for example, Canadian GPs' remuneration rates are 3.2 times higher than the average national wages; this is quite similar to the ratio of 3.4 in the United States and 3.3 in Germany; but contrasts strikingly with the ratio of 2.6 in France and Switzerland, and 1.8 in Iceland (see Fujisawa and Lafortune 2008). At the same time, the majority of physicians in Canada are still paid according to fee-for-service, have in most cases few outcome-related performance expectations, and retain control of all qualitative training and performance evaluations. In terms of strict accountability, then, individual doctors are answerable only to the profession itself. A third form of decentralization is the dependence on the market for publicly uninsured goods. Pharmaceuticals, long-term care, dentistry, and rehabilitative services such as physiotherapy are primarily purchased through the private market, either out-of-pocket or through private insurance. In the latter case there is some cost accountability (higher costs mean higher premiums, which can mean fewer subscribers) but private insurers do ultimately have the option of simply passing costs on to consumers. The move by the government of Ontario to limit private pharmacies' practice of billing full amounts of prescription costs to insurers and pocketing the rebates given to them by pharmaceutical companies illustrates the unwillingness of private actors to become directly involved in cost accountability.

We Know What to Do

There is good news. Clinicians, policy analysts, and policy makers are increasing converging in their views of how health care should be provided. There is considerably less dispute regarding the overarching direction in which we should be going than there has been in the past, and most health reforms in most countries have increasingly coalesced around some variation of these models. The vision for the future of modern health care systems is based primarily, although not exclusively, on the following six objectives:

1. *More emphasis on primary care.* The common buzzwords here are 'medical homes,' 'collaboration,' 'coordination,' 'chronic health care management,' and 'patient-centred care.'

2. *Adopting principles of preventive care.* Important here are the concepts 'health promotion,' 'population health,' 'social or non-medical determinants of health,' and 'socially embedded health.'
3. *Better utilization of electronic health information technology.* This includes 'electronic medical records,' 'technology-enabled solutions,' 'clinical knowledge platforms,' and 'computerized provider order entry.'
4. *Payment systems that reward high-quality care.* Here we will be seeing 'performance management,' 'pay-for-performance (P4P),' 'outcomes over outputs,' 'needs-based funding,' 'money following patients,' 'choice,' and 'responsiveness.'
5. *More application of evidence-based care.* This will involve 'meaningful use' and 'comparative effectiveness research.'
6. *Long-term care.* This includes 'home care,' 'continuing care,' 'living in place,' and 'assisted living.'

These objectives are interlinked rather than free-standing – it can be easier to achieve one objective when others are in place – but, depending on the country, there tend to be diverse strategies for achieving each objective.

One of the key objectives is to strengthen primary care. Systems that use GP gatekeepers tend to work well; and countries that did not have gate-keeping systems in place a decade ago are, like France and Germany, are implementing them now (and countries that have used them effectively for years, like Britain, are reinforcing this system even more). Gate-keeping systems keep costs down by limiting access to more expensive specialized services to those who need them and by denying unnecessary treatments to those who do not need them. Because efficient health care provision depends on meeting an objective need rather than simply the desires of consumers, and because extensive training is required to determine how best to align needs with services (e.g., which patients should be given MRI scans?), the use of market mechanisms to determine supply and demand is suboptimal (this is one reason that health care is usually seen as an example of market failure). Primary care is also efficient in providing preventive services (such as immunizations) so that more expensive interventions (such as hospitalization) are avoided. Primary care can be especially useful in coordinating care across a range of services for patients. This is particularly important for achieving the effective and inexpensive management of chronic health conditions. Not only can primary care providers ensure that those requiring chronic care can navigate the health care system seamlessly, but it also facilitates the self-management of chronic conditions by, for example, making sure that patients have written post-discharge plans or a contact person for any questions or problems that arise after discharge from hospital. But, in contrast to the past, the new primary care model is not necessarily based on GPs. Rather, it is grounded in the collaborative efforts of a wide spectrum of health care professionals (nurses, psychologists, physiotherapists, nutritionists, pharmacists, and so on) who contribute their skills and expertise as required. Where large-scale, collaborative practices exist, patients have timely access to the services they need; and health care systems remain less dependent on having a sufficient number of GPs available to treat patients. This is why health policy analysts increasingly ask whether individuals have access to a 'medical home' rather than to a GP: primary services can, according to this approach, be provided by a number of health care professionals, depending on the nature of the medical condition. Proponents of this approach argue that it may not be uncommon in the future to see private practices run by teams of nurses who may employ one or two GPs to serve their practice.

The second objective is better utilization of preventive care. In the three and a half decades following the publication of the Lalonde Report there has been an increasing amount of evidence showing that health outcomes are clearly linked to social and environmental factors; there has been very little tangible backlash against the *concept* of 'non-medical determinants' of health. Nevertheless, the translation of this knowledge to public policy has been grindingly slow. The political barriers to change are discussed in Chapter 5. It is unlikely that radical changes will be made to overarching social or economic systems on the grounds that they have health-related benefits; but it is nonetheless heartening to know that policy makers have not dismissed preventive health care altogether. The idea that massive cost savings can be attained through prevention is powerful enough to remain in the political consciousness of decision makers. Further, while it is doubtful that exhaustive changes will be made at a systemwide level, basic preventive care (such as immunizations, diagnostic tests such as Pap smears and mammograms, and a focus on lifestyle issues such as diet, exercise, and tobacco use) remain key health care components. Indeed, one of the principles underlying the use of 'medical homes' is that preventive services become both *more* accessible and economical (e.g., nutritionists rather than GPs providing dietary guidance, or psychologists rather than GPs providing smoking cessation clinics.) How effectively these preventive services are used, however, depends on numerous other variables. It is instructive, for example, that the American Patient Protection and Affordable Care Act explicitly prohibits privately insured preventive services from applying any co-payment schemes (to ensure that individuals will have no barriers to utilization), while Quebec at the same time proposed a health service fee of $25 per visit (paid via income tax returns rather than at 'point of contact' with a health care provider) for all but the very poorest individuals that would apply to all preventive services secured though the public health care system.

One way of facilitating better preventive health care is through the use of electronic health records. A computerized system, for example, can easily determine whose annual tests or immunizations are due; while easy access to each patient's file by numerous health care providers more efficiently assists the monitoring and treatment of chronically ill patients. Electronic health information technology is used extensively in Britain, Australia, and the Netherlands; it lags considerably in Germany, the United States, and Canada. For example, only 20 per cent of Canadian doctors polled received computerized alerts regarding potential problems with drug doses or interactions, compared with 95 per cent in the Netherlands (Davis et al. 2010: 6).

In 2001 Ottawa established Health Infoway Canada to assist provinces in establishing electronic health record systems. The goals of this agency were

> delivering superior quality care across the system through timely access to accurate information and improved decision-making support; enhancing ongoing disease management for chronic and longer-term care by facilitating systematic follow-up; a higher level of patient involvement and education, and more guideline-compliant treatment; providing critical elements of the information required to manage wait times and improve patient access by triaging patients and scheduling according to urgency across the entire domain of qualified providers; ensuring the system's long-term sustainability through enhanced performance management of cost, quality and access, as well as management of critical resources; enabling patient self-care and remote care; and controlling system risks to the population from pandemics or other health issues. (Canada Health Infoway, n.d.)

The cost savings to be gained through the use of electronic health records are potentially very high: Canada Health Infoway has stated that the $12 million diagnostic imaging system established in eleven British Columbia hospitals has resulted in at least $4.5 million in cost reductions each year. One estimate for cost savings through the use of electronic health records for Ontario alone is $2.4 billion per year (6% of Ontario's $42.5 billion health care budget), with greater savings over time as patient outcomes improve (Webster 2010). But the cost outlay required to achieve such potential savings is also considerable, and progress implementing electronic health record systems across Canada has been hampered by federal-provincial disagreements over funding levels, issues with new privacy legislation, and a scandal over the billion dollars of funds mismanaged by eHealth Ontario. It is perhaps worth noting that countries with federal systems, in general, tend to have much lower utilization levels of electronic health technology compared with those with unitary systems (although Australia is an interesting exception).

The fourth objective of health reform is the reorientation of health care remuneration to reflect quality over volume. This is to a certain extent a reaction to NPM principles which, based on business models, quantified and monitored the production of outputs. Outputs, however, are not always as clear-cut in service industries as they are in shoe factories, and especially so in the health care industry. The current fee-for-service system, for example, simply rewards the number of patients seen rather than the number of patients cured. Thus, as Evans, Barer, and Schneider (2010: 17) point out, merely discussing health provision with respect to greater *productivity* would potentially be counterproductive as the 'proliferation of beneficial, harmful, or simply unnecessary services would all be recorded as "productivity growth."' The issue, of course, is precisely *how* to implement a system in which only the results (or 'outcomes'), rather than outputs, are rewarded. Numerous tools already exist, including capitation (which also potentially lowers the number of patients that GPs are willing to see); population-based (or needs-based) funding models; diagnostic-related group funding, which expects all health care providers to supply their services at a set cost; performance targets; and rating. All of these techniques have detractors; and some of them threaten established political interests. They have also had some positive effects. Britain, one country that has had considerable experience in this area, has noted significant results through the use of outcome-based remuneration (Ham 2009b). Nevertheless, the development of outcomes-based health policy is highly technical and dependent on an IT infrastructure that can record, monitor, and compare health outcomes across jurisdictions. It depends on agreement over what comprises an acceptable 'outcome' and it can, without careful monitoring, lend itself to distortions (if only crude outcomes are measured, all providers would want to treat colds, and no one would treat chronic conditions).

The literature analysing the success of 'pay for performance' (P4P) design is growing, but the verdict remains inconclusive. A major problem in evaluating pay for performance systems is that they vary considerably in design: Which clinical conditions are addressed? Which agents (patient, doctor, or hospital) are targeted? What is the optimal bonus size? How important is the timing of the financial rewards? (See Petersen et al. 2006.) Another problem is attempting to determine before the fact what kinds of adverse consequences can arise from a particular system design: will rewarding individual providers undermine the movement towards health care provider teams? Or will targeting particular conditions result in the neglect of conditions that are not subject to incentives or bonuses? (See Campbell et al. 2007.) The concept of pay for performance is intuitively persuasive, but a great deal depends on system design, and a large part of effective system design depends on local realities. Despite the current enthusiasm for pay for performance, caution Rosenthal and Dudley, 'it has become clear that it should not be a foregone conclusion that these programs will benefit patients or even significantly assist providers who want to improve care' (2007: 740).

The success of an outcomes-based approach depends, in turn, on a considerable body of knowledge that can tell us which kinds of treatment work *effectively*, and which do not. Comparative effectiveness research (CER) is the attempt to collect and distribute evidence-based research that examines the clinical and cost effectiveness of current treatments and procedures. The most striking example of this is perhaps the Antihypertensive and Lipid-Lowering Treatment to Prevent Heart Attack Trial (ALLHAT), which determined that cheap, old-fashioned diuretics were just as effective (and much more cost effective) than recent, expensive blood pressure medication (see http://allhat.sph.uth. tmc.edu/). Several nations have established comparative assessment agencies within the past decade, including Britain (the National Institute of Clinical Excellence in 1999); Germany (the Institut für Qualität und Wirtschaftlichkeit im Gesundheitswesen in 2000); and France (the Haute Authorité de Santé in 2004). Australia's Pharmaceutical Benefits Scheme, or PBS, was established in 1948. While Canada does not have a national body examining the relative effectiveness of all therapeutic or diagnostic options, it does have a national drug assessment agency (CADTH) and a small number of provincial quality assessment units (including Impact BC and the Saskatchewan Health Quality Council). Even the Obama administration has declared an intent to establish a CER agency, earmarking U.S.$1.1 billion in the 2009 American Recovery and Reinvestment Act. Why has there been so much emphasis on CER? Many health care experts hold that the scientific basis for much current medical treatment is weak, and that almost half of all care in the United States is unsupported by adequate evidence. 'As a result,' note Gerber and Patashnik, 'decisions about the tests and treatments to use are routinely made on the basis of anecdotes, local customs, and the personal experience of individual physicians' (2010: 3).

Finally, a key objective for Canada specifically is long-term care. Almost all states are being forced to confront an aging demographic; but some of them have been doing so much more admirably than others. The long-term care crisis in Canada is especially acute. The primary reasons are the same as those underlying the failure substantially to reform mental health care in Canada: the structure of federalism and the character of the Canada Health Act (CHA). Long-term care is a provincial responsibility, and each province has its own way of managing long-term care, with little coordination between provinces. Most long-term facilities in most provinces are privately run (but publicly regulated), and provincial funding assistance for individuals in long-term care varies considerably. The one constant across the country is the effect of the Canada Health Act. Because the CHA was only designed to fund hospital use, it was economically rational to treat long-term patients in a hospital setting despite the cost involved. As health care costs skyrocketed, the inefficient use of hospitals for long-term care became increasingly pronounced. But because long-term care facilities were dominated by private interests, the inability of (mostly elderly) individuals to pay high residence fees, even with subsidization, meant that physicians were reluctant to discharge dependent individuals from hospitals where no familial care system was in place. The result is that hospital beds are utilized by those who do not require acute care, leading to shortages that have a domino-like effect throughout wards and emergency departments. At the same time, the effort and stress of caring for dependent adults at home has had an equally adverse (although much more silent) effect on providers at the domestic level.

So we do know how to solve the health care crisis, at least at a very broad level. The problem, it would seem, is in getting to there from here.

We Just Don't Know Exactly How to Do It

The problem is not that Canadian researchers are slackers. Excellent clinical work is being produced; and numerous pilot programs (such as Alberta's Bone and Joint Institute or Ontario's Cardiac Care Network) have been remarkably successful in achieving excellent outcomes. One problem, however, is that we 'lack a way to generalize the successful approaches developed by pilot projects and the will to act on them widely' (Bégin et al. 2002: 1185). Another problem is that what may seem like a simple solution from a distance (more collaboration) may become more intractably difficult once the details get in the way. While the idea of 'getting along to get more done' might seem self-evident, there are frequently good underlying reasons (such as the way in which the demand for hierarchical accountability impedes such directives) that collaborative action can be so difficult to implement. A second problem with 'getting to there from here' is the implementation of knowledge transfer in the interface between clinicians and those who design the policies. We *know* that we can use health care professionals more efficiently, and that many of them are doing tasks for which they are expensively overqualified. But the reasons that they are used in this way may differ across unit, region, profession, and so on. There is often no one-size-fits-all way of implementing policy approaches that, on the face of it, may seem very straightforward. The gap between 'global evidence' and 'local realities' can be so diverse that each attempt to implement a single policy may require a great deal of patience and experimentation to get it right in each case. Or there may be systemic issues (like free-rider problems) which make it difficult to establish commonsensical solutions. For example, the utility of comparative effectiveness research has been known for some time; yet few wish to invest heavily in it because of its very nature as a public good (as soon as a result is produced, everyone is a beneficiary). In other words, the more successful institutes like Britain's NICE become, the less likely other countries may be to establish their own versions ('we'll just use the British guidelines; they're quite rigorous').

There are also numerous qualitative issues that remain even after the data gathering is done. We know, for example, that having access to CT machines is a good thing (it gives us superior diagnostic information). But we also know that having access to too many CT machines is a bad thing (it leads to overutilization with marginal to zero gains in real outcomes). But we don't know exactly where this point is (and it probably depends on how the resources are distributed as well: even if Canada had as many MRI machines as the United States, the results would be suboptimal if, e.g., they were all in Moose Jaw). Thus 'the number of CT scans' (or MRI scans) has become a highly politicized issue that, in the end, tells us little about the quality of health care per se. Critics have used Canada's relatively low rate of MRI and CT scans to illustrate the poor quality of health care service in this country (e.g., Simpson 2010). However, Canada's use of MRI imagery was 41 exams per thousand population, which is close to the OECD average of 48.5 per thousand. This contrasts to the U.S. rate of 91 per thousand, the Australian rate of 21 per thousand, and the Dutch rate of 35 per thousand (CIHI 2010). Yet, as Davis et al. (2010) found for the Commonwealth Fund, on a basket of indicators, the Netherlands and Australia had the *best* health care systems of those considered (first and third respectively) while the United States had the *worst*. How, then, are we to interpret the importance of the number of MRI scans to a high-performing health care system?

Another example is the increasing focus on 'choice' as a key objective in health care systems. If given the option between 'having a choice' and 'not having a choice' in the provision of health care, it is simply common sense for individuals to choose the former. But what do we mean by choice? Choice between providers in the public system? Choice between public and private providers? Choice of insurers? How much choice? At what cost choice? And is *too* much choice a good thing? As Schlesinger (2010: 367) points out, 'choice is never simple from the patient's perspective': 'The stakes are too high, making the choices fraught with anxiety. The consequences are impossible fully to anticipate, rendering judgments at best semi-informed guesses. And the circumstances are never really amenable: either the patients are healthy – and therefore can not be bothered to dwell much on medical matters – or they are sick, which often limits their capacity to process a lot of complicated information.' Knowing the direction one ought to take is a considerable step. But having a sense of where one should go is still just a step. The full commitment to policy reform requires a great deal of nuanced detail that is especially difficult to nurture within a fragmented federal system. This knowledge is admittedly not essential for change – it certainly did not stop Margaret Thatcher from embarking on the NHS's most dramatic reform – but it does make the journey of reform less bumpy and more tolerable. There is a final variable: politics. Knowing what set of objectives to embrace, and how to operationalize these goals within the framework of policy making, are necessary but not sufficient variables in achieving health system reform. Knowing how to identify political barriers, and how to accommodate (or neutralize) political interests, is perhaps the most difficult aspect of any policy process; and health care systems particularly are not lacking in the number of established interests that can potentially subvert, undermine, or even assist, in the development of new policy directions.

We Must Understand the Political Landscape

Newton's second law of motion notes that the direction in which an object moves is the result of the forces acting on it. The strongest forces will dictate the ultimate direction and velocity of the object's movement. This is also true for the political context surrounding health policy reform: institutions and systems will take the form preferred by the strongest interests, and more powerful interests will have a greater impact. To understand health care as a dynamic process rather than as merely a static system (why does the system change? why *doesn't* it?) one must consider the political context of policy making.

Here is where the political scientist's toolbox comes in handy. There are two kinds of tools. The first set addresses the standard questions about power that have been used for a long time to understand the dynamics of political engagement from military battles to municipal elections:

- Who are the key actors?
- What are their interests?
- What kinds of power do they have at their disposal?
- How willing are they to use their power?
- How able (and willing) are other interests to counter or block their attempts?
- How can strategic alliances either facilitate or hinder particular objectives?
- How do institutional or legal obstacles either facilitate or impede particular interests?

The second set of questions was introduced during the political and intellectual upheaval of the 1960s and 1970s. Taking issue with the observable interplay of orthodox institutional actors, both theorists and activists presented alternative accounts of power that began to examine why things *didn't* happen as well as why they did. These accounts attempted to explain the non-observable dynamics of power: how were perceptions and preferences shaped so that the lack of articulated opposition was seen as singularity of interest? This approach could be found within many discrete investigations of power. Foucault, for example, wrote many discourses (on madness, on health, and on sexuality) premised on the nature of power as something much more diffused and multidimensional than orthodox accounts assumed. Feminist and post-colonial theorists attempted to understand how dominant value systems were internalized and reinforced within entire societies. Marxists moved away from materialist analyses and focused on the reproduction of dominant ideologies within bourgeois institutions. As Steven Lukes argued in his seminal text on the nature of power, a flattened understanding of power severely truncates a more encompassing understanding of power as a fluid, nuanced, and often invisible social relationship. The problem for political science ever since has been how persuasively to present an account of power within a context where little or no overt coercion seems to exist. This has been especially important in a world where the standard of legitimacy regarding public policy is whether a decision conforms to the democratic imperative: a policy is the right thing to pursue simply because enough people believe it to be. As democratic norms conquer the world, power slips on a cloak of invisibility and takes on a new, much more subtle, quality. The analytical focus is no longer simply *why did an event occur?* but also *why did people allow (or want) this event to occur?*

The second set of tools, then, tends to be more controversial, though certainly no less interesting. These questions focus on the way in which power is used to shape preferences (or to reshape opposition) in order to secure compliance:

- How do key political actors use ideas and values as a means of enlisting widespread support for their interests?
- How do they use images, symbols, words, and categories to further particular interests?
- How do they use the construction of knowledge (and the standards of legitimacy based on the objectivity of science) for their own ends?
- How are certain identifiable groups disadvantaged by specific policies, and why may they nonetheless *not* oppose such policies?

The examination of health care policy making should incorporate both kinds of analyses. The orthodox tools of political analysis have lost none of their sharpness, and they are a good place to begin. To understand why particular policies or reforms are implemented (or blocked), the first step is to identify which interests may be involved. Who has the most to gain (and to lose)? Why, exactly, is any change in the status quo preferable or disadvantageous? How well organized are the players? How well funded? How well informed? What resources can they muster (or withhold)? How effective at making alliances (or calling in favours) are they? What are the networks of connection between interests? In the field of health care, the standard players are usually health care providers (especially physicians), health care consumers (either individually or as special-interest groups), taxpayers (in any system with some public provision of services), policy makers, and those who stand to gain commercially (such as drug and device manufacturers and insurance companies). The particular form these interests take will differ from jurisdiction to jurisdiction. Because many of the health care politics in Canada play themselves out on a provincial (or regional, or municipal) level, and because different interests will become involved depending on the policy in question, this book has not attempted to provide an exhaustive list of players (an analysis of policy shifts in cancer care should look at the role of tobacco companies, whereas an examination of the restructuring of emergency services probably will not). Orthodox policy analysis looks at the context within which interests jostle for primacy: what laws provide the base rules for legitimate activity? How does the particular design of relevant decision-making institutions privilege some interests over others? Traditional policy analysis may also focus on leadership: does a particular policy initiative have a 'policy champion' who has the political heft and the personal willingness to push that policy through a thicket of political apathy or opposition?

As health care becomes more sophisticated, the idea of 'health' itself moves away from simple physical mechanics (stitching up wounds, eliminating pathogens) to much more complex mind-body-society relationships. Further, as health becomes a more social construction, the nature of health *care* becomes more firmly embedded in the way in which social relationships are maintained. Health care moves away from treating visible illness to achieving a state of physical and mental perfectability (continual happiness, ever-present erections, and perfect complexions); a daunting shift from traditional ideas of health into the realm of individual identity. Finally, even as health care becomes more technical and complex, the democratic imperative means that individuals are expected to become more involved in their own health care (and that of their community). This social dimension of health is usefully understood through the application of the second set of analytical tools.

The use of pharmaceuticals, and specifically the nexus of profit-based pharmaceutical production and clinical evaluation or utilization, raises many issues that can be understood especially well with reference to this second set of questions. This includes the use of language ('impotence' become 'erectile dysfunction,' 'bipolar depression' becomes a 'mood disorder'); the use of images and symbols (why have women become the face of psychotropic medication?); and the expansion of analytic categories ('pre-Alzheimer's,' 'pre-dementia,' 'osteopenia'). Choices are constructed as 'either-or' options, rather than as more complex alternatives that may run along a spectrum or be situated on a multidirectional axis ('either have surgery, or take this drug'). Voices and interests are co-opted ('our company will fund your support group'), leading to self-censorship or voluntary adherence ('no one's told us anything, but if we undermine the company's message they'll probably remove our funding'). 'Scientific standards' are either distorted (burying negative results) or politicized (scientists funded by commercial interests set the standards for clinical use). How interests intersect with values is more difficult to determine conclusively, but is no less relevant a question (private insurance companies were able to use Americans' documented distrust of big government to push a public option off the table; Canadians' support for public health care has so far stalled attempts to achieve greater privatization in some provinces; individuals' attachment to social values in both countries diminishes considerably when their own personal interests are affected).

Both sets of tools are more useful in explaining why past events occurred as they did than at predicting how future events will unfold. Political behaviour is the result of far too many variables for us to be able to anticipate outcomes with assurance. But a solid analytical framework can at least present us with a considered set of possibilities. In the short term, the trajectory of health policy will depend on the resolution of specific issues such as the judicial decisions on *Chaoulli*-like Charter cases before the courts in British Columbia, Alberta, and Ontario; the end of the intergovernmental funding model established by the 2003 Health Care Accord and the 2004 *10-Year Plan to Strengthen Health Care*; and whether any provinces decide, to introduce user fees for health services (as Quebec proposed and then rejected in 2010). In the longer term, much will depend on the relative success in restructuring primary and preventive health care, and in establishing effective electronic health systems and long-term health care programs.

In many respects health care is a policy area sui generis. It consumes the largest proportion of provincial spending; it is a sector with which almost all individuals will engage at some point in their lives; it encompasses issues of both national and personal identity; and it raises complicated questions about economic efficiency and social justice. But health care in the twenty-first century is also characterized by an increasingly stark dialectic between technical complexity and democratic expectations. As medicine itself becomes more complex and specialized, the more individuals are exhorted to get involved, become informed, take control, and share the power. We demand clearer accountability, but we want the system to become more integrated. We want system-wide efficiencies, but we will not let efficiencies be made where they threaten our own particular interests. We expect choice and quality, but resent the cost. It's a confusing dialectic. What health care is, and what we want it to be, is mediated by politics. Until we, as citizens, understand the political dynamics underlying it, the health care system will always be shaped by those who *do* understand the politics of health care.

Appendix A: Glossary

Accountable care organizations (ACOs). Health care organizations providing services for patients across a continuum of care, and which are held responsible for the cost and quality of care provided to a defined population.

Adverse selection. The tendency of a health system or insurance plan to attract individuals who have worse than average health.

All-payer regulation. The establishment of a coordinated set of standard fee schedules for health care providers. While jurisdictions may permit exceptions, the regulated fee schedule is generally seen as the appropriate reimbursement rate for public (and often private) insurers. This serves to keep overall health care costs down.

Ambulatory care. Health care provided on an outpatient basis.

Analgesic. A drug used to reduce pain.

Bending the cost curve. In debates over U.S. health care reform, this phrase referred to the need to reduce the rate of increase in health care spending.

Beveridge system. A health care system funded through general tax revenues.

Biologics. Unlike chemical-based drugs, biologics are therapeutic substances derived from living organisms. They include such things as vaccines, blood products, and gene therapy.

Bismarck system. A health care system based on social insurance funds, primarily co-financed by employees (through payroll deduction) and employers.

Block grant. A lump sum of money given to provinces by the federal government for specific purposes.

Byrd Rule. In the U.S. legislative process, this is a stipulation in which bills allowed to proceed under reconciliation in the Senate must be limited to provisions that directly affect revenues.

Cadillac insurance plans. Very generous private insurance plans with total annual premiums of U.S.$8,000 per individual or U.S.$21,000 per family and with few or no co-payments, deductibles, or limitations. Some CEOs in the United States have plans that average U.S.$40,000 per annum.

Capitation. A system in which health care providers receive a fixed sum per patient per year, rather than a fee for each service provided.

Catastrophic health insurance. Insurance limited to severe illnesses that require high expenditure for uninsured medical services.

Centers for Medicare and Medicaid Services (CMS). Agency in the U.S. Department of Health and Human Services that regulates Medicare and Medicaid.

Cherry-picking. Actively selecting only healthy individuals for enrolment in health plans (also known as cream-skimming).

Children's Health Insurance Program (CHIP). A joint federal-state health insurance program in the United States for children whose families do not qualify for Medicaid but cannot afford private insurance.

Chronic care. Health care services for individuals with long-term or recurrent illnesses.

Clinical guidelines. Formal precepts and protocols designed to help health care providers make decisions in treating patients with specific conditions.

Co-insurance. The proportion of treatment costs paid directly by patients rather than by the insurance provider.

Community-based services. Services that allow individuals with specific health care needs to live at home.

Community health centres. Health care institutions run by not-for-profit community boards which provide both primary care and other community services through integrated teams of providers.

Community health councils (or boards). Groups of individuals either elected or appointed by government to advise health authorities on policy-making for their community.

Community rating. A method of setting insurance rates by charging all individuals the same premium regardless of health status or risk.

Comparative effectiveness research (CER). The systematic development of evidence that compares the relative advantages and disadvantages of various treatment methods for similar conditions.

Complementary health insurance. Additional voluntary insurance (usually private) that 'tops up' the statutory insurance coverage that only covers a set proportion of total health care costs.

Compulsory licensing. Limitations on the rights of patent-holders to exclude others from using patented information. In the field of health care, the patents on pharmaceuticals and medical devices are generally limited to a specified number of years before they expire.

Computerized tomography (CT) scan. Computer-generated images of structures within the body based on data taken from multiple X-ray pictures.

Congressional Budget Office. An independent, non-partisan U.S. federal agency that provides economic information, such as budget estimates, to Congress.

Continuing care. A range of services provided over an indefinite period of time to those with specific health needs so that they can maintain a relatively independent lifestyle.

Continuing medical education (CME). Programs and courses offered to medical professionals that help them maintain and increase their skills and knowledge in their particular fields of expertise.

Continuum of care. A comprehensive range of services designed to meet all the health care needs of individuals (and especially those who are frail or chronically ill).

Contract research organizations. Private firms that provide services to the pharmaceutical and biotechnology industries. These services may include clinical trial management, the preparations of submissions to drug regulatory agencies, and product evaluation.

Co-payment. A fixed fee paid to a health care provider by a patient in addition to the coverage provided by an insurance plan.

Cornhusker kickback. Political concessions won by Nebraska Senator Ben Nelson in exchange for his support of the American health care reform bill. Seen as an instance of cynical Washington deal-making, the concessions were removed in the later reconciliation bill.

Cost-sharing. Any form of contribution (such as deductibles or co-payments) made by individuals towards the cost of their health care goods or services. The remainder is generally covered by public or private insurance plans.

Cost shifting. The process of moving the costs of providing health care from one sector or demographic to another (e.g., public to private sector; or wealthy to less well-off incomes group).

Crowding out. The movement of people with employer-sponsored health insurance into public health insurance programs in the United States. This is regarded as an undesirable phenomenon as it increases the cost to governments of expanding health insurance coverage without any overall reduction of the numbers of uninsured individuals.

Deductibles. Fixed amount paid for goods or services by individuals directly before their health insurance plan begins to cover other goods or services.

Diagnosis-related group (DRG). The classification of similar medical conditions into formal administrative categories. Individuals within these groups will be allotted the same amount of funds for treatment regardless of what the actual treatment costs are.

District health authority (DHAs). Mid-level health authorities governing health care systems within a defined regional area; also known as regional health authorities (RHAs).

Double-blind. A protocol for clinical experimentation in which neither the subject nor the experimenter can differentiate between active materials and control substances.

Doughnut hole. The coverage gap in U.S. prescription drug coverage through Medicare. Individuals are 75 per cent covered up to an annual ceiling of U.S.$2,405 and 95 per cent covered after annual expenses reach U.S.$5,016; but there is no coverage between these two amounts.

Employer mandate. A requirement that employers must provide health insurance coverage for their employees.

Epidemiology. The study of factors governing the health and illness of large populations.

Evidence-based medicine. Basing medical treatment on research proving the effectiveness of specific interventions, rather than simply on traditional practices.

Fee-for-service. A payment system in which health care professionals bill for each individual service provided.

Fee schedule. The list of fixed prices for goods and services provided by medical professionals and reimbursed by public or private insurers.

First-dollar coverage. Health insurance plans that do not have deductibles.

Formulary. The list of therapeutic products (generally drugs) covered by public or private insurers.

Foundation Trusts. Hospitals in the U.K. which have a special status making them independent of the NHS. These hospitals still are considered not-for-profit, and are generally accountable (through governing boards) to the local community.

Fund holding. A system of health care delivery in which GP practices in the U.K. were given financial allotments directly in order to purchase services (e.g., from hospitals) for their patients.

Gatekeeping. A system of health care provision in which access to expensive diagnostic and treatment services are controlled by primary care professionals (generally GPs or nurse practitioners).

Generics. Pharmaceutical products, identical to brand-name drugs, that are manufactured after the original drug patent expires.

Gesundheitsfond. The umbrella health insurance fund in Germany that collects health insurance contributions from employers and employees, then redistributes the cash back to sickness funds according to specific criteria. This procedure helps to maintain a broad risk pool across the numerous sickness funds.

Ghost writing. In medical writing, the practice of submitting to journals scientific papers that have been anonymously written by one person but have other individuals named as authors. The high-profile individuals given authorship may change certain aspects of the paper before submission, or they may simply read the paper and append their name to it for publication.

Group health insurance. Private health insurance offered to any group of people, including employees of a company or members of a union. The main alternative to group health insurance is individual insurance, where people buy health insurance policies directly from a company.

Guaranteed issue. A regulation that obliges health insurance plans to accept all those wishing to enroll, regardless of their health status or risk.

Health human resources. The study and practice of providing the appropriate levels and balance of health care professionals for the effective provision of health services across a population.

Health insurance co-operative. Not-for-profit health insurance organizations that are owned by the individuals holding policies with them.

Health insurance exchange. A marketplace created by governments or independent agencies to provide a selection of comparable (and clearly explained) plans to individuals and small businesses. These plans may be private for-profit, private not-for-profit, or public.

Health maintenance organization (HMO). A form of managed care organization in which health insurance companies use a network of health care providers to give their members access to comprehensive health care services. By using a gatekeeping system, and by using only selected health care professionals who provide good quality services for competitive prices, overall costs are kept down.

High-risk insurance pools. Public or private health insurance plans established by state governments in the United States to provide coverage for high-risk individuals who are refused private coverage because of existing medical conditions.

Individual mandate. A system that requires individuals by law to carry health insurance (either public or private, individual or group insurance).

Internal markets. A public health care system in which 'purchasers' (generally GPs and district health authorities) are given funds by the government to buy services from public or private health care providers (also known as quasi-, mimic, managed, or regulated markets).

Key opinion leaders (KOLs). Specialist physicians or leading academic scientists whose authority is seen to influence other physicians' treatment decisions (especially in prescribing drugs).

Licensed practical nurses (LPN). Nurses whose qualifications enable them to provide basic nursing services. They generally have less training than registered nurses.

Long-term care. A wide spectrum of services provided over an indefinite period to individuals with chronic illnesses or permanent disabilities. These services are generally provided in an institutional setting.

Magnetic resonance imaging (MRI) scan. A diagnostic tool utilizing radio or magnetic waves rather than X-rays to collect detailed images of structures within the human body.

Managed care. A system of providing health care services designed to promote the efficient use of health care resources. This is generally done by requiring patients to see primary care providers before they are referred to specialists, ensuring that preventative health services are fully utilized, and closely monitoring chronic conditions.

Managed care organization. A system of health care provision in which health insurance companies establish contracts with a network of health care professionals to provide services to their clients.

Managed competition. A system of health care provision in which a set of independent, competing health care services are overseen or monitored by a central authority. Purchasers have a more limited selection of choices, and the conditions under which the providers offer their services are more restricted than in the open marketplace.

Means-testing. The practice of determining whether an individual's or family's income falls below a certain level before access to specific programs is granted.

Medicaid. A system of public health insurance run jointly by U.S. state and federal governments. Until the Patient Protection and Affordable Care Act was passed, only specific categories of low-income Americans (children, pregnant women, disabled individuals) were eligible for coverage. Beginning in 2014, all Americans who fall below 133 per cent of the federal poverty line will be eligible for Medicaid.

Medical home. An institutional base, usually a primary health care clinic, which serves to coordinate the types of health services required by patients (and especially those with chronic conditions).

Medical underwriting. The determination of individuals' health risks, used by health insurance companies to set premiums.

Medically necessary. Services deemed to be appropriate and necessary for the treatment of a particular condition, determined in accordance with the standards of clinical evidence and good medical practice.

Medicare. In Canada, a term commonly used to refer to the public health insurance system (likely a shorthand term for the Medical Care Act of 1966). In the United States, a federal health insurance program for individuals 65 years of age and over.

Moral hazard. A situation in which individuals shielded from the full cost of a transaction (e.g., because they have an insurance policy that pays for part or all of the costs; or because their parents are paying for it) will behave differently than if they were responsible for total costs.

Needs-based planning. A system of resource allocation based on an assessment of the health care requirements of circumscribed populations rather than on traditional patterns of funding.

New public management. An approach to public sector administration based on market-oriented rather than command-and-control principles. The goals of NPM are generally some combination of cost control and individual empowerment, and the strategies used to attain these goals include competition, privatization, and other forms of alternative service delivery.

Notice of compliance (NOC). The authorization given by Health Canada allowing a pharmaceutical product to be placed on the market. A conditional notice of compliance (NOC/c) means that a product may only be placed on the market under certain conditions (normally, that the drug will continue to be monitored by the company for any possible long-term effects).

Nurse practitioner. A registered nurse who has received additional training and can provide many of the same services that a GP can (such as prescribing drugs, sending patients for diagnostic tests, or referring patients to specialists).

Out-of-pocket payment. Money given by patients directly to health care providers for specific services rendered.

Pay for performance. Any system in which health care providers are rewarded for providing good quality services at reasonable prices.

Pay or play. The stipulation that employers either provide health insurance to their employees directly, or else pay a set amount allowing them to find their own insurance coverage.

Physician assistant. A health care professional who can perform specific and limited medical tasks under the direct supervision of a physician.

Placebo. A treatment with no active ingredients (e.g., a sugar pill).

Population health. An approach which looks at the health outcomes of a circumscribed population. It generally focuses on health promotion, illness prevention, and non-medical determinants of health in addition to the clinical treatment of diseases.

Post-marketing surveillance. The practice of continuing to monitor drugs even after they have been approved for public use.

Practice-based commissioning. The current evolution from GP fund holding, primary care groups, and primary care trusts in Britain, in which GPs form groups and are given public funds with which to purchase services from public and private health care providers. While similar in nature to previous manifestations of GP fund holding, practice-based commissioning is more extensive both in the number of GPs involved, and in the range and level of services they are expected to purchase.

Preferred provider organization (PPO). A form of managed care organization in which health insurance companies contract with a network of health care providers to provide economical health care services to members. PPOs are generally not as tightly structured as health maintenance organizations (which, e.g., require enrollees to sign up with a primary care physician).

Premium. Regular cash payment made to insurers in exchange for insurance coverage.

Primary care. Basic, preventative, and other non-specialty health services generally provided by family doctors or nurses.

Primary care groups. In 1999, primary care groups (PCGs) replaced GP fund holders as the main commissioning agents for health care services within Britain's NHS. Mainly composed of GPs and community nurses, PCGs were larger than GP fund holders and were given a wider responsibility for community health.

Primary care trusts (PCTs). Primary care trusts (U.K.) were the next evolution of primary care groups. Similar in principle to the PCGs, they amalgamated the responsibilities of both PCGs and district health authorities, and became responsible for the commissioning not only of health care services, but also of social services.

Progressive licensing. A system of pharmaceutical regulation that facilitates the ongoing collection of data, evaluation of effects, and communication of concerns regarding a therapeutic substance before and after its approval for public use.

Prospective payment system (PPS). A system based on diagnosis-related groups, in which payment for services is determined by how many patients are in each diagnostic category (with its corresponding rate of remuneration), rather than by how much money was actually used to treat each individual patient.

Public option. In discussions of U.S. health care reform, the addition of a public insurance plan within a system of mandated insurance.

Purchasing pool. The amalgamation of uninsured individuals, or small groups of individuals, into one large group in order to give them the same purchasing power enjoyed by large entities when negotiating advantageous rates with health insurance companies.

Rating. Determining the potential risk of an individual applying for private health insurance, and setting the premiums according to the perceived likelihood that this individual will utilize health services or goods.

Rescission. The arbitrary cancellation of an individual's health insurance policy by an insurance company. If an individual's treatment costs are high, a company may decide to review the individual's policy to see if there has been any misrepresentation of past health service utilization, whether relevant to the existing condition or not, as this presents legal grounds for a company to refuse payment for all subsequent claims.

Reconciliation. A legislative process within the U.S. Senate that restricts the use of the filibuster.

Reference pricing. A practice in which insurers examine the relative effectiveness of all drugs used to treat a particular condition, and then reimburse only the drug judged to produce the best effect for the lowest cost.

Registered nurse. A nurse with full qualifications (in Canada, this is a Bachelor of Science degree in Nursing).

Revolving door. The phenomenon of influential individuals within one sector (such as business, academia, or government) moving directly to positions of influence within another field (and sometimes back again).

Risk pooling. Lowering insurance costs by spreading the risk. This is achieved by increasing the number of people or entities enrolled in an insurance plan.

Selective reporting. The practice of researchers or research-oriented firms to publicize positive results and to bury negative results of studies.

Sickness funds. Private, regulated, not-for-profit health insurance agencies that are funded by contributions provided by both employers and employees (also known as *mutuelles* in France, or *Krankenkassen* in Germany).

Silos. Discrete health care sectors that are neither integrated nor coordinated with others.

Single-payer system. A system in which health insurance is provided by a single entity (usually, but not necessarily, the state).

Social determinants of health (SDOH). Defined by the World Health Organization as 'the conditions in which people are born, grow, live, work and age, including the health system. These circumstances are shaped by the distribution of money, power and resources at global, national and local levels, which are themselves influenced by policy choices.'

Socialized medicine. A system in which the state is directly responsible for providing health insurance, funding hospitals, and paying health care professionals. The best examples of this are Cuba's system of national health care, and the Veterans Health Administration in the United States.

Statutory health insurance. A form of health insurance in which a defined population of individuals are required by law to contribute through payroll deductions and employer contributions to a regulated health insurance fund.

Subsequent entry biologics. Generic forms of biologic pharmaceuticals (also known as bio-similars or follow-on protein products).

Substitutive health insurance. A form of voluntary health insurance that defined populations may choose to purchase in place of statutory health insurance.

Summary Basis of Decision. A document issued by Health Canada which explains the scientific cost-benefit analysis underlying a decision to approve a drug. This decision is based on considerations of safety, efficacy, quality, and current regulatory requirements.

Supplementary health insurance. A form of voluntary health insurance that provides additional benefits for those with basic statutory health insurance, giving individuals enhanced service options such as access to faster services, wider treatment options, or non-medical amenities.

Underinsured. Having insufficient health insurance to cover health care needs. Although individuals may be insured, they may face high premiums or co-payments, or the level of services provided may be very limited. In the United States, insured individuals who pay more than 10 per cent of their income on health care goods or services (or 5 per cent for those under the poverty level) in addition to what is covered by their insurance plans are considered underinsured.

Universal coverage. A population that is completely covered by health insurance (either public or private).

Veterans Health Administration. The division of the U.S. Department of Veterans Affairs (VA) that operates and administers all health-related programs for veterans, including outpatient clinics, hospitals, medical centres, and long-term facilities.

Wildavsky's Law. Health care costs will increase to the level of available funds; therefore, that level must be limited to keep costs down.

Appendix B: Web Resources

Because of its interdisciplinary nature, the study of health care involves an extensive knowledge base that tends to shift quickly and erratically. Tracking these changes can be a tricky business. Online sources are invaluable for being able to follow these modulations. They also offer a great diversity of informed commentary on the possible implications of these changes. The following online resources, which are by no means either exhaustive or definitive, should be quite helpful in keeping up with current events within the field of health care. The resources range from sites presenting the official line to those that question it. Perhaps the best places to start are very general health policy websites such as the Kaiser Family Foundation and the Commonwealth Fund. While primarily addressing U.S. health care policy, they do present a wealth of comparative information as well. For Canada-specific discussions of health care policy, a good starting point would be searching for health-related topics within the general policy sites listed below. The blog spots range from the distinguished to the quirky. Most blogs focus on U.S. health care but, again, many also offer broader observations about health care policy and health politics in general. Longwood's is a good source for current information about Canadian health policy. Some websites and blogs are industry watchdogs: Open Secrets provides data on the relationship between politicians and the large financial corporations (such as health insurance and pharmaceutical firms); the American Medical Student Association reports on the relationship between academic health science centres and pharmaceutical industries; Fierce Pharma keeps an eye on the drug industry in general; and Jim Edwards offers downloadable documents from key court proceedings. The Health Wonk Review is an umbrella site that presents a bird's-eye view of what's being discussed in the health care blogosphere. Unsurprisingly, some health care bloggers have moved to Twitter, which can be worth a search (especially for breaking stories). A word of warning: websites and blogspots can be notoriously unstable; do not be surprised if you find that one of the sources listed here has been removed. Finally, a number of key health policy journals are also listed. As the contents for almost all of them are only accessible through research libraries' online portals, the webpages for the journals themselves are not listed. If you do have access to these journals, do not be intimidated by the professional journals for medicine or law: many of them (such as the *Canadian Medical Association Journal*, the *British Medical Journal*, or the *New England Journal of Medicine*) publish excellent, accessible articles on health policy on a regular basis.

Websites

1. Websites on Health: Canada

Canadian Health Services Research Foundation (CHSRF) – http://www. chsrf.
    ca/home_e.php#2
Canadian Institute for Health Information (CIHI) – http://secure.cihi.ca/
    cihiweb/splash.html
Canadian Institutes of Health Research (CIHR) – http://www.cihr-irsc.gc.ca/
    e/193.html
CHSRF mythbusters – http://www.chsrf.ca/mythbusters/index_e.php
Health Canada – http://www.hc-sc.gc.ca/english
Health Council of Canada – http://www.healthcouncilcanada.ca/splash.htm
Longwoods.com – http://www.longwoods.com/
Mental Health Commission of Canada – http://www.mentalhealth commission.ca
Public Health Agency of Canada – http://www.phac-aspc.gc.ca/index-eng.php

2. Websites on Health: International

American Medical Students' Association Scorecard – http://www.
    amsascorecard.org/
The Commonwealth Fund – http://www.commonwealthfund.org/
Direct to Consumer Advertising – http://www.csa.com/discovery
    guides/direct/review.php
Drug Promotion Database – http://www.drugpromo.info/

EU Health Links – http://homepages.gold.ac.uk/erandall/euro-links.html

Eurohealth – http://www.lse.ac.uk/collections/LSEHealth/documents/
eurohealth.htm

European Observatory on Health Systems and Policies – http://www.euro.
who.int/en/home/projects/observatory

FDA Basics – http://www.fda.gov/AboutFDA/Basics/default.htm

FDA Track – http://www.fda.gov/AboutFDA/WhatWeDo/track/default.htm

The Guardian/health policy – http://www.guardian.co.uk/politics/health

Health Action International – http://www.haiweb.org/

Health Policy Monitor – http://www.hpm.org/en/index.html

Health Systems in Transition (European Observatory) – http://www.euro.who.
int/en/home/projects/observatory/publications/health-system-profiles-hits

Healthy Skepticism – http://www.healthyskepticism.org/global/

Integrity in Science Database – http://www.cspinet.org/integrity/

Kaiser Family Foundation – http://www.kff.org/

Kaiser Permanente Institute for Health Policy – http://www.kpihp.org/kpihp/
default.aspx

The King's Fund – http://www.kingsfund.org.uk/

National Physicians' Alliance – http://npalliance.org/

No Free Lunch – http://www.nofreelunch.org/aboutus.htm

The Nuffield Trust – http://www.nuffieldtrust.org.uk/

OECD/health – http://www.oecd.org/topic/0,3373,en_2649_37407_1_1_1_1_374
07,00.html

OECD Health Data 2010: Indicators and Statistics – http://www.oecd.org/docu
ment/30/0,3343,en_2649_34631_12968734_1_1_1_37407,00.html

Open Secrets /health care – http://www.opensecrets.org/capital_eye/health_
intro.php

Pew Prescription Policy – http://www.prescriptionproject.org/

Pharmed Out – http://www.pharmedout.org/

Prescrire (in English) – http://english.prescrire.org/

Public Citizen – http://www.publiccitizen.org/Page.aspx?pid=183

Red Scrubs – http://postscript.communitycatalyst.org/

U.S. health care information site – http://www.healthcare.gov/

World Health Organization – http://www.who.int/en/

3. General Policy Sites in Canada That Include Health Care Issues

Atlantic Institute for Market Studies/healthcare – http://www.aims.ca/
healthcare.asp?cmPageID=157

Canadian Centre for Policy Alternatives – http://www.policy alternatives.ca/

Canadian Policy Research Network – http://www.cprn.org/
Fraser Institute – http://www.fraserinstitute.org/
Institute of Intergovernmental Relations (IIGR) – http://www.queensu.
    ca/iigr/
Policy.ca – http://policy.ca/

Blog/News Sites

1. Health Care

British Medical Journal – http://blogs.bmj.com/bmj/
Café Pharma – http://www.cafepharma.com/boards/forumdisplay.php?f=4
Carlat Psychiatry – http://carlatpsychiatry.blogspot.com/
The Changing NHS – http://stevepashley.squarespace.com/
Clinical Psychology and Psychiatry: A Closer Look – http://clinpsyc.blogspot.
    com/
The Commonwealth Fund – http://www.commonwealthfund.org/
    Publications/Blog.aspx
Drug Wonks – http://drugwonks.com/blog_post/
Euro Observer – http://www.euro.who.int/en/home/projects/observatory/
    publications/euro-observer
Eye on FDA – http://www.eyeonfda.com/
Fierce Pharma – http://www.fiercepharma.com/news
Furious Seasons – http://www.furiousseasons.com/
Gary Schwitzer's Health News Review – http://www.healthnewsreview. org/
    blog/
Gooznews on health – http://www.gooznews.com/
The Grossman FDA Report – http://www.fdamatters.com/
Health Affairs – http://healthaffairs.org/blog/
Health Care (at the New Republic) – http://www.tnr.com/articles/health-
    care
Health Care (at the Wall Street Journal) – http://blogs.wsj.com/health/
The Health Care Blog – http://www.thehealthcareblog.com/
    the_health_care_blog/
Health Care Policy and Market Review – http://healthpolicyandmarket.
    blogspot.com/
Health Care Polls – http://healthcarepolls.blogspot.com/
Health News Review – http://www.healthnewsreview.org/
Health Policy Hub – http://blog.communitycatalyst.org/

Health Populi – http://healthpopuli.com/
Health Reform Galaxy – http://rwjfblogs.typepad.com/healthreform/
Health Wonk Review – http://www.healthwonkreview.com/mt/
Hooked: Ethics, Medicine, and Pharma – http://brodyhooked.blogspot.com/
In the Pipeline – http://pipeline.corante.com/
In Vivo – http://invivoblog.blogspot.com/
Internet Drug News – http://www.coreynahman.com/
Jim Edwards NRx – http://jimedwardsnrx.wordpress.com/
Kaiser Health News – http://www.kaiserhealthnews.org/
Kevin MD – http://www.kevinmd.com/blog/
Longwoods – http://longwoodsblog.blogspot.com/
Maggie Mahar's Health Beat – http://www.healthbeatblog.org/
MD Whistleblower – http://www.mdwhistleblower.blogspot.com/
National Journal – http://healthcare.nationaljournal.com/
New America health – http://health.newamerica.net/blogmain
New England Journal of Medicine – http://blogs.nejm.org/now/
New England Journal of Medicine health reform – http://healthcarere form.
  nejm.org/?emp=marcom
NPR Shots – http://www.npr.org/blogs/health/
Ontario Health Association – http://www.ohatoday.com/Pages/Default.aspx
Peter Rost – http://peterrost.blogspot.com/
Pharma Gossip – http://pharmagossip.blogspot.com/
Pharma Marketing – http://pharmamkting.blogspot.com/index.html
PharmaLive – http://pharmalive.com/
Pharmalot – http://www.pharmalot.com/
Physicians for a National Health Programme – http://pnhp.org/blog/
Politico – http://www.politico.com/healthcare/
Postscript – http://postscript.communitycatalyst.org/
Prescription Action Litigation – http://blog.prescriptionaccess.org/
Prescriptions (at the New York Times) – http://prescriptions.blogs.nytimes.
  com/
The Pump Handle – http://thepumphandle.wordpress.com/
Sarah Boseley's Global Health – http://www.guardian.co.uk/society/
  sarah-boseley-global-health
Scientific Misconduct – http://scientific-misconduct.blogspot.com/
Social Audit UK – http://socialaudit.org.uk/
Tom Klosson's OHA – http://www.oha.com/News/TomClossonBlog/default.
  aspx

2. General Policy Blogs (That Include Health Care Issues)

Ezra Klein (at the Washington Post) – http://voices.washingtonpost.com/ezra-klein/
The Huffington Post – http://www.huffingtonpost.com/
Matthew Iglesias – http://yglesias.thinkprogress.org/
The Monkey Cage – http://www.themonkeycage.org/
Robert Reich – http://robertreich.blogspot.com/

Online Journals

1. Canada

Canadian Journal of Psychiatry
Canadian Journal of Public Health
Canadian Medical Association Journal
Canadian Public Administration
Canadian Public Policy
ElectronicHealthcare
HealthcarePapers
Healthcare Policy
Healthcare Quarterly
Law and Governance
McGill Journal of Law and Health
Policy Options

2. International

Administration and Policy in Mental Health
American Journal of Medicine
American Journal of Public Health
Annals of Internal Medicine
Archives of Internal Medicine
British Medical Journal
Health Affairs
Health Economics
Health Economics, Policy, and Law
Health Research Policy and Systems
International Journal of Health Services
Journal of the American Medical Association

Journal of Health Politics, Policy, and Law
Journal of the History of Medicine
Journal of Medical Ethics
Journal of Public Administration Research and Theory
Lancet
Milbank Quarterly
National Review of Medicine
New England Journal of Medicine
PloS Medicine
Prevention and Treatment
Social Science and Medicine
Women & Health

References

Aaron, Henry, and Paul Ginsburg. 2009. 'Is health spending excessive? If so, what can we do about it?' *Health Affairs* 28/5: 1260–76.

Abelson, Julia. 2001. 'Understanding the role of context in local health care decision making.' *Social Science and Medicine* 53/6: 777–93.

Abelson, Julia, and John Eyles. 2002. 'Public participation and citizen governance in the Canadian health system.' Discussion paper no. 7 for the Commission on the Future of Health Care in Canada (Romanow Commission), Ottawa.

Abraham, John. 2002a. 'Making regulation responsive to commercial interests: Streamlining drug industry watchdogs.' *British Medical Journal* 325 (16 Nov.): 1164–9.

– 2002b 'The pharmaceutical industry as a political player.' *Lancet* 360/9344: 1499–1502.

Aiken, Linda, et al. 2001. 'Nurses' reports on hospital care in five countries.' *Health Affairs* (May/June): 43–53.

Alakeson, Vidhya. 2008. 'America's health choices.' *British Medical Journal* 337 (27 Sept.): 720–2.

Alikhan, L.M., and Jeffrey Lozon. 2007. 'Canada's public health system: Is the pace of progress sufficient?' *Healthcare Papers* 7/3: 52–9.

Altenstetter, Christa. 2003. 'Insights from health care in Germany.' *International Perspective Forum* 93/1: 38–44.

Anderson, Gerard, and Peter Sotir Hussey. 2001. 'Comparing health system performance in OECD countries.' *Health Affairs* 20/3: 219–32.

Anderson, Gerard, and Patricia Markovich. 2010. *Multinational Comparisons of Health Systems Data, 2008*. New York: Commonwealth Fund.

Angell, Marcia. 2005. *The Truth about Drug Companies: How They Deceive Us and What to Do about It*. New York: Random House.

Armstrong, Pat, and Hugh Armstrong. 2002. 'Planning for care: Approaches to health human resource policy and planning.' Discussion paper no. 128 for the Commission on the Future of Health Care in Canada (Romanow Commission), Ottawa.

Arrow, Kenneth. 1963. 'Uncertainty and the welfare economics of medical care.' *American Economic Review* 53/5: 941–73.

Attaran, Amir. 2008. 'A legislative failure of epidemic proportions.' *Canadian Medical Association Journal* 179/1: 9.

Aucoin, Peter. 2005 'New public management and new public governance: Finding the balance.' Paper presented to the Institute of Public Administration of Canada, Annual Conference, Regina, 28–31 Aug.

– 2006. 'The staffing and evaluation of Canadian deputy ministers in comparative Westminster perspective: A proposal for reform.' *Restoring Accountability: Research Studies.* Vol. 1. *Parliament, Ministers and Deputy Ministers.* Ottawa: Public Works and Government Services Canada, 141–54.

Auditor General Canada. 2008. *Report of the Auditor General of Canada,* ch. 5. Available at http://www.oag-bvg.gc.ca/internet/English/aud_ch_oag_200805_05_e_30701.html. Accessed 23 July 2009.

Auton (Guardian ad litem *of) v. British Columbia (Attorney General).* 2004. [2004] 3 S.C.R. 657, [2004] SCC 78 (Supreme Court of Canada).

Baird, Patricia. 2003. 'Getting it right: Industry sponsorship and medical research.' *Canadian Medical Association Journal* 168/10: 1267–8.

Baker, G.R., A. MacIntosh-Murray, C. Porcellato, L. Dionne, K. Stelmacovich, and K. Born. 2008. 'Jönköping county council.' In *High Performing Healthcare Systems: Delivering Quality by Design.* Toronto: Longwoods, 121–44.

Baker, G.R, et al. 1998. 'Healthcare performance management in Canada: Who's doing what?' *Healthcare Quarterly* 2/2: 22–6.

Bakvis, Herman, and Luc Juillet. 2004. *The Horizontal Challenge: Line Departments, Central Agencies and Leadership.* Ottawa: Canada School of Public Service.

Banting, Keith, and Stan Corbett, eds. 2002. *Health Policy and Federalism: A Comparative Perspective on Multi-level Governance.* Montreal: Institute of Intergovernmental Relations and McGill-Queen's University Press.

Barer, Morris. 2005. 'Experts and evidence: New challenges in knowledge transfer.' In Colleen Flood, Kent Roach, and Lorne Sossin, eds. *Access to Care, Access to Justice.* Toronto: University of Toronto Press, 216–33.

Barer, Morris, and Greg Stoddart. 1991. *Toward Integrated Medical Resource Policies for Canada. Background Document.* June. Available at http://www.chspr.ubc.ca/files/publications/1991/hpru91-06D.pdf. Accessed 10 Oct. 2010.

Batt, Sharon. 2005. 'Marching to different drummers: Health advocacy groups in Canada and funding from the pharmaceutical industry.' *Women and Health Protection*. Jan. Available at http://www.whp-apsf.ca/en/index.html. Accessed 19 April 2009.

Beckel, Michael. 2009a. 'Will $1.2 Million a Day Convince Congress to Buy Big Pharma's Rx for Change?' 25 June. Available at http://www.opense crets.org/news/2009/06/will-12-million-a-day-convince.html. Accessed 26 June 2009.

– 2009b. 'Stakeholder in health insurance reform debate gave big to senators.' 24 Dec. Available at http://www.opensecrets.org/news/2009/12/stakeholders-in-health-insuran.html. Accessed 4 Jan. 2010.

Bégin, Monique. 2002. 'Revisiting the Canada Health Act (1984): What are the impediments to change?' Speech given to the Institute for Research on Public Policy, Ottawa, 20 Feb.

Bégin, Monique, Laura Eggerton, and Noni Macdonald. 2009. 'A country of perpetual pilot projects.' *Canadian Medical Association Journal* 180/12: 1185.

Bevan, Gwyn, and Ray Robinson. 2005. 'The interplay between economic and political logics: Path dependency and health care in England.' *Journal of Health Politics, Policy and Law* 30/1–2: 53–78.

Bickerton, James. 1999. 'Reforming health care governance: The case of Nova Scotia.' *Journal of Canadian Studies* (Summer): 159–90.

Black, Martha, and Katherine Fierlbeck. 2006. 'Whatever happened to regionalization? The curious case of Nova Scotia.' *Canadian Public Administration* 49/4: 506–26.

Block, Ray, et al. 2008. 'The impact of integrating mental and general health services on mental health's share of total health care spending in Alberta.' *Psychiatric Services* 59/8: 860–3.

Bouchard, Ron, and Monika Sawicka. 2009. 'The mud and the blood and the beer: Canada's progressive licensing framework for drug approval.' *McGill Journal of Law and Health* 3: 49–84.

Bourgeault, I.L., and Gillian Mulvale. 2006. 'Collaborative health care teams in Canada and the USA: Confronting the structural embeddedness of medical dominance.' *Health Sociology Review* 15/5: 481–94.

Boychuk, Gerard. 2008a. *National Health Insurance in the United States and Canada: Race, Territory and the Roots of Difference*. Washington, DC: Georgetown University Press.

– 2008b. *The Regulation of Private Health Funding and Insurance in Alberta under the Canada Health Act: A Comparative Cross-Provincial Perspective*. SPS Research Papers: The Health Series, School of Policy Studies, University of Calgary, vol. 1, no. 1 (Dec.).

– 2002. 'The changing political and economic environment of health care
in Canada.' Discussion paper no. 1 for the Commission on the Future of
Health Care in Canada (Romanow Commission), Ottawa.

Brennan, Troyen, et al. 2006. 'Health industry practices that create conflicts of
interest.' *Journal of the American Medical Association* 295/4: 429–33.

Brodie, Mollyann, et al. 2010. 'Liking the pieces, not the package:
Contradictions in public opinion during health reform.' *Health Affairs*
29/6: 1125–30.

Brown v. British Columbia (Minister of Health). 1999. [1999] B.C.J. No. 151 (B.C.
Court of Appeal).

Brown, Lawrence, and Volker Amelung. 1999. '"Manacled competition":
Market reforms in German health care.' *Health Affairs* 18/3: 76–91.

Brownlee, Shannon. 2007. *Overtreated: Why Too Much Medicine Is Making Us
Sicker and Poorer.* New York: Bloomsbury.

Bruni, Rebecca, Andreas Laupacis, and Douglas Martin. 2008. 'Public engagement in setting priorities in health care.' *Canadian Medical Association Journal*
179/1: 15–18.

Buchmueller, Thomas, and Agnes Couffinhal. 2004. *Private Health Insurance in
France.* Health Working Papers no. 12. Paris: OECD.

Buckwell, Charlie. 2008. 'Should the drug industry work with key opinion
leaders? Yes.' *British Medical Journal* 336 (21 June): 1404.

Busse, Reinhard. 2008. 'The German health care system.' In *Descriptions of
Health Care Systems.* New York: Commonwealth Fund. Available at http://
www.allhealth.org/briefingmaterials/CountryProfiles-FINAL-1163.pdf.
Accessed 8 July 2009.

Busse, Reinhard, and Annette Reisberg. 2004. *Healthcare Systems in Transition:
Germany.* Copenhagen: WHO Regional Office for Europe on behalf of the
European Observatory on Health Systems and Policies.

Cameron v. Nova Scotia (Attorney General). 1999. [1999] N.S.J. No. 33 (N.S.
Supreme Court).

Cameron, David, and Richard Simeon. 2002. 'Intergovernmental relations in
Canada: The emergence of collaborative federalism.' *Publius* 32/2: 49–71.

Campbell, Stephen, et al. 2007. 'Quality of primary care in England with the
introduction of pay for performance.' *New England Journal of Medicine* 357
(12 July): 181–90.

Canada, Federal/Provincial/Territorial Advisory Committee on Health
Delivery and Human Resources (ACHDHR). 2005. *A Framework for
Collaborative Pan-Canadian Health Human Resource Planning.* Ottawa:
ACHDHR. Revised 2007. Available at Available at http://www.hc-sc.gc.ca/
hcs-sss/pubs/hhrhs/2007-frame-cadre/index-eng.php. Accessed 29 May 2009.

Canada Health Infoway. n.d. 'EHR 2015: Advancing Canada's next generation of healthcare.' Available at http://www2.infoway-inforoute.ca/Documents/Vision_2015_Advancing_Canadas_next_generation_of_healthcare%5B1%5D.pdf. Accessed 27 Oct. 2010.

Canadian Alliance on Mental Illness and Mental Health. 2002. *A Call for Action, Building Consensus: A National Action Plan for Mental Illness and Mental Health.* Available at http://www.camimh.ca/callforaction.htm. Accessed 16 Oct. 2010.

Canadian Population Health Initiative. 2007. 'About the CPHI.' Available at http://secure.cihi.ca/cihiweb/dispPage.jsp?cw_page=cphi_about_e. Last updated 30 April. Accessed 29 June 2009.

Casebeer, Ann. 2004 'Regionalizing Canadian healthcare: The good – the bad – the ugly.' *Healthcare Papers* 5/1: 88–93.

Cassels, Alan, Jaclyn van Wiltenburg, and Wendy Armstrong. 2009. *What's in a Scan? How Well Are Consumers Informed about the Benefits and Harms Related to Screening Technology (CT and PET scans) in Canada?* Ottawa: Canadian Centre for Policy Alternatives.

Castonguay, Claude. 2008. *Getting Our Money's Worth: Report of the Task Force on the Funding of the Health Care System.* Released Jan. by the Government of Quebec. http://www.financementsante.gouv.qc.ca/en/rapport/pdf/RapportENG_FinancementSante.pdf. Accessed 11 Oct. 2010.

CBC. 2006. 'Liberal party fines Volpe $20,000.' Available at http://www.cbc.ca/canada/story/2006/09/29/volpe-liberals.html.

– 2004. 'Pharmacare FAQs.' Available at http://www.cbc.ca/news/background/healthcare/pharmacare_faq.html.

Centre for Responsive Politics. 2009. 'Health care reform: industry cheat sheet.' Available at http://opensecrets.org/capital_eye/health.php?type=O&cycles=2010. Accessed 28 Oct. 2010.

Chadwick, Edwin. 1842. *Report on the Sanitary Conditions of the Labouring Population.* Available at http://www.deltaomega.org/ChadwickClassic.pdf. Accessed 11 April 2009.

Chaoulli c. Québec (Procureur general). 2000. J.Q. n° 479 (Cour supérieure du Québec – Chambre civile).

Chaoulli c. Québec (Procureur general). 2002. J.Q. n° 759 (Cour d'appel du Québec).

Chaoulli v. Quebec (Attorney General). [2005] 1 S.C.R. 791, [2005] SCC 35 (Supreme Court of Canada).

Choudhry, Sujit. 2005. 'Worse than *Lochner*?' In Flood, Roach, and Sossin, eds., *Access to Care, Access to Justice,* 75–100.

Church, J., and P. Barker. 1998. 'Regionalization of health services in Canada: A critical perspective.' *International Journal of Health Services* 28/3: 467–86.

CIHI (Canadian Institute for Health Information). 2010. 'Use of MRI and CT exams varies greatly among provinces.' Posted 22 July. Available at http://secure.cihi.ca/cihiweb/dispPage.jsp?cw_page=media_20100722_e. Accessed 29 July 2010.

– 2009. *Supply, Distribution and Migration of Canadian Physicians, 2008.* Ottawa: CIHI.

– 2008a. *Health Care in Canada 2008.* Ottawa: CIHI.

– 2008b. *Making Sense of Health Rankings.* Ottawa: CIHI.

– 2007a. *Health Care in Canada 2007.* Ottawa: CIHI.

– 2007b. Availability of Mental Health Data, 2004–2005 (May). Available at http://secure.cihi.ca/cihiweb/en/downloads/hmhdb_hospital_mental_health_statistics_2004_2005_e.pdf. Accessed 12 Jan. 2009.

– 2005. *Health Care in Canada 2005.* Ottawa: CIHI.

CMA (Canadian Medical Association). 2009. *Statistical Information on Canadian Physicians.* Available at http://www.cma.ca/index.cfm/ci_id/16959/la_id/1.htm#mig. Accessed 15 June 2010.

Colgrove, James. 2002. 'The McKeown thesis: A historical controversy and its enduring legacy.' *American Journal of Public Health* 92/5: 725–9.

Collier, Joe. 2007. 'Inside big pharma's box of tricks.' *British Journal of Medicine* 334 (27 Jan.): 209.

Collins, Patricia, and Michael Hayes. 2007. 'Twenty years since Ottawa and Epp.' *Health Promotion International* 22/4: 337–45.

Collins, Sara. 2009. *The Growing Problem of Underinsurance in the United States: What It Means for Working Families and How Health Reform Will Help* (Testimony). New York: Commonwealth Fund. 15 Oct. Available at http://www.commonwealthfund.org/Content/Publications/Testimonies/2009/Oct/The-Growing-Problem-of-Underinsurance.aspx. Accessed 11 April 2010.

Competition Bureau Canada. 2008. *Benefiting from Generic Drug Competition in Canada: The Way Forward.* Ottawa: Publishing and Depository Services.

Connery, Robert H. 1968. *The Politics of Mental Health.* New York: Columbia University Press.

Consumer Reports. 2009. 'Hazardous health plans.' *Consumer Reports* (May): 24–9.

Coombes, Rebecca. 2008. 'Dr Nurse will see you now.' *British Medical Journal* 337 (20 Sept.): 660–2.

Courchene, Thomas. 2008. *Reflections of the Spending Power: Practices, Principles, Perspectives.* Montreal: Institute for Research on Public Policy.

– 1996. *ACCESS: A Convention on the Canadian Economic and Social Systems.* Toronto: Ministry of Intergovernmental Affairs.

Crawford, Mark. 2005. 'Truth of consequences? The law and politics of the GATS health care debate.' *Canadian Foreign Policy* 12/2: 97–105.

Crossley, T.F., J. Hurley, and S.H. Jeon. 2006. 'Physician labour supply in Canada: A cohort analysis.' SEDAP Research paper no. 162. Hamilton, ON: McMaster University.

Curry, Natasha, Nick Goodwin, Chris Naylor, and Ruth Robertson. 2008. *Practice-Based Commissioning: Reinvigorate, Replace, Abandon?* London: King's Fund.

Cutler, D.M., K. Davis, and K. Stremikis. 2010. *The Impact of Health Reform on Health System Spending.* New York: Commonwealth Fund.

Davidson, Alan. 1999. 'British Columbia's health reform: "New directions" and accountability.' *Canadian Journal of Public Health* 90/S1: 35–8.

Davis, Karen. 2009. *New Census Data on Uninsured Americans* (Testimony). New York: Commonwealth Fund. 10 Sept. Available at http://www.com monwealthfund.org/Content/News/News-Releases/2009/Sept/Statement-from-Karen-Davis-New-Census-Data-on-Uninsured-Americans.aspx. Accessed 14 Oct. 2010.

Davis, Karen, Cathy Schoen, and Kristof Stremikis. 2010. 'Mirror, mirror on the wall: How the performance of the US health care system compares internationally: 2010 update.' New York: Commonwealth Fund, pub. No. 1400 (June).

Davis, Simon. 2006. *Community Mental Health in Canada.* Vancouver: UBC Press.

De Búrka, G., and J. Scott, eds. 2006. *Law and New Governance in the EU and U.S.* Oxford: Hart.

Deber, Raisa. 2008. 'Access without appropriateness: Chicken little in charge?' *Healthcare Policy* 4/1: 23–9.

– 2004. 'Why did the World Health Organization rate Canada's health system as 30th? Some thoughts on league tables.' *Longwoods Review* 2/1: 2–7.

– 2002. 'Delivering health care services: Public, not-for-profit, or private?' Discussion paper no. 17 for the Commission on the Future of Health Care in Canada (Romanow Commission), Ottawa.

Deber, Raisa, Christopher McDougall, and Kumanan Wilson. 2007. 'Public health through a different lens.' *Healthcare Papers* 7/3: 66–71.

Decter, Michael. 2006. 'Health reform for those who really need it.' Address to St Joseph's Health Centre, Toronto, 12 May.

Delamothe, Tony. 2008a. 'NHS at 60: Universality, equity, and quality of care.' *British Medical Journal*, 7 June: 1278–81.

– 2008b. 'NHS at 60: A comprehensive service.' *British Medical Journal*, 14 June: 1344–5.

– 2008c. 'NHS at 60: A centrally funded health service, free at the point of delivery.' *British Medical Journal*, 21 June: 1410–12.

– 2008d. 'NHS at 60: A fairly happy birthday.' *British Medical Journal*, 28 June: 25–9.

Demers, Tony, et al. 2008. 'Comparison of provincial prescription drug plans and the impact on patients' annual drug expenditures.' *Canadian Medical Association Journal* 178/4: 405–9.

Der Spiegel. 2009. 'Looming shortfalls for Germany's health care system.' 10 Aug. Available at *Der Spiegel* online at http://www.spiegel.de/international/germany/0,1518,654040,00.html. Accessed 5 Sept. 2009.

Dickinson, Harley. 2002. 'How can the public be meaningfully involved in developing and maintaining an overall vision for the health system consistent with its values and principles?' Discussion paper no. 33 for the Commission on the Future of Health Care in Canada (Romanow Commission), Ottawa.

Diderichsen, Finn. 2000. 'Sweden.' *Journal of Health Politics, Policy and Law* 25/5: 931–5.

Douglas, Tommy. 2005. 'Medicare: The time to take a stand.' In Katherine Fierlbeck, ed., *The Development of Political Thought in Canada.* Peterborough, ON: Broadview Press, 113–24.

Downie, Jocelyn, and Matthew Herder. 2007. 'Reflections on the commercialization of research conducted in public institutions in Canada.' *McGill Health Law Publication* 1/1: 23–44.

Durand-Zaleski, Isabelle. 2008. 'The French health care system.' In *Health Care System Profiles.* New York: Commonwealth Fund. Available at http://www.commonwealthfund.org/Content/Resources/2008/Mar/Health-Care-System-Profiles.aspx. Accessed 22 Oct. 2010.

Dyck, Erica. 2007. 'Land of the living sky with diamonds: A place for radical psychiatry?' *Journal of Canadian Studies* (Fall): 42–66.

Dyer, Owen. 2007. 'Lilly investigated in U.S. over the marketing of olanzapine.' *British Medical Journal* 334 (27 Jan.): 171.

– 2004. 'GlaxoSmithKline faces U.S. lawsuit over concealment of trial results.' *British Medical Journal* 328 (12 June): 1395.

Economist Intelligence Unit. 2010. 'The quality of death: Ranking end-of-life care across the world.' *Economist.* Available at http://www.eiu.com/site_info.asp?info_name=qualityofdeath_lienfoundation&page=noads&rf=0. Accessed 12 Oct. 2010.

Eldridge v. British Columbia (Attorney General). 1997. [1997] 3 S.C.R. 624 (Supreme Court of Canada).

Epp, Jake. 1986. *Achieving Health for All: A Framework for Health Promotion*. Ottawa: Health and Welfare Canada.

Epps, Tracey, and David Schneiderman. 2005. 'Opening medicare to our neighbours or closing the door on a public system?' In Flood et al., *Access to Care, Access to Justice*, 369–89.

Evans, Robert G. 2008. 'Thomas McKeown, meet Fidel Castro: Physicians, population health and the Cuban paradox.' *Healthcare Policy* 3/4: 21–32.

– 2005a. 'Preserving privilege, promoting profit: The payoffs from private health insurance.' In Flood et al., *Access to Care, Access to Justice*, 347–68.

– 2005b. 'Fellow travelers on a contested path: Power, purpose, and the evolution of European health care systems.' *Journal of Health Politics, Policy and Law* 30/1–2: 277–93.

– 2002. 'Raising the money: Options, consequences, and objectives for financing health care in Canada.' Discussion paper no. 27 for the Commission on the Future of Health Care in Canada (Romanow Commission), Ottawa.

– 2000. 'Canada.' *Journal of Health Politics, Policy and Law* 25/5: 889–97.

– 1997. 'Going for the gold: The redistributive agenda behind market-based health care reform.' *Journal of Health Politics, Policy, and Law* 22/2: 427–63.

– 1984. *Strained Mercy: The Economics of Canadian Health Care*. Toronto: Butterworth.

Evans, Robert G., and Kimberlyn McGrail. 2008. 'Richard III, Barer-Stoddart, and the daughter of time.' *Healthcare Policy* 3/2: 18–28.

Evans, Robert G., and G.L. Stoddart. 1994. 'Producing health, consuming health care.' In R.G. Evans, M. Barer, and T. Marmor, eds., *Why Are Some People Healthy and Others Not?* New York: Aldine de Gruyter, 27–64.

Evans, Robert G., Morris Barer, and Theodore Marmor, eds. 1994. *Why Are Some People Healthy and Others Not?* New York: Aldine de Gruyter.

Evans, Robert G., Morris Barer, and David G. Schneider. 'Pharoah and the prospects for productivity in HHR.' *Healthcare Policy* 5/3 (2010): 17–26.

Ferris, L.E., P.A. Singer, and C.D. Naylor. 2004. 'Better governance in academic health sciences centres.' *Journal of Medical Ethics* 30: 25–29.

Fierlbeck, Katherine. 2011. 'The dialectics of law and politics: Federal health policy in Canada and the EU.' In Finn Laursen, ed., *The European Union and Federalism: Polities and Policies Compared*. Farnham, UK: Ashgate Press, 155–77.

– 2010. 'Public health and collaborative governance.' *Canadian Public Administration* (March): 1–19.

Findlay, Tammy, and Lynell Anderson. 2010. 'Does public reporting measure up? Federalism, accountability and child care policy in Canada.' *Canadian Public Administration* 53/3: 417–38.

Fingard, Judith, and John Rutherford. 2008. *Protect, Befriend, Respect: Nova Scotia's Mental Health Movement, 1908–2008*. Halifax: Fernwood.

Flood, Colleen, and Tom Archibald. 2001. 'The illegality of private health care in Canada.' *Canadian Medical Association Journal* 164/6: 825–30.

Flood, Colleen, and Sujit Choudhry. 2002. 'Strengthening the foundations: Modernizing the Canada Health Act.' Discussion paper no. 13 for the Commission on the Future of Health Care in Canada (Romanow Commission), Ottawa.

Flood, Colleen, and S. Lewis. 2005. 'Courting trouble: The Supreme Court's embrace of private health insurance.' *Healthcare Policy* 1/1: 26–35.

Flood, Colleen, Kent Roach, and Lorne Sossin, eds. 2005. *Access to Care, Access to Justice*. Toronto: University of Toronto Press.

Flood, Colleen, Mark Stabile, and Sasha Kontic. 2005. 'Finding health policy "arbitrary": The evidence on waiting, dying, and two-tier systems.' In Flood, Roach, and Sossin, eds., *Access to Care, Access to Justice*, 296–320.

Flood, Colleen, Mark Stabile, and Carolyn Hughes Tuohy, eds. 2008. *Exploring Social Insurance: Can a Dose of Europe Cure Canadian Health Care Finance?* Kingston: School of Policy Studies, Queen's University.

Flood, Colleen, Mark Stabile, and Carolyn Hughes Tuohy. 2006. 'What is in and out of medicare? Who decides?' in Colleen Flood, ed., *Just Medicare: What's In, What's Out, How We Decide*. Toronto: University of Toronto Press.

Flood, Colleen, Mark Stabile, and Carolyn Hughes Tuohy. 2004. 'How does private finance affect public health care systems?' *Journal of Health Politics, Policy and Law* 29/3: 359–96.

Flood, Colleen, and Terrence Sullivan. 2005. 'Supreme disagreement: The highest court affirms an empty right.' *Canadian Medical Association Journal* 173/2: 142.

Fooks, Cathy, et al. 2002. 'Health human resource planning in Canada: Physician and nursing work force issues.' Summary Report for the Commission on the Future of Health Care in Canada (Romanow Commission), Ottawa.

Forchuk, Cheryl, et al. 2007. 'Housing, income support and mental health: Points of disconnect.' *Health Research Policy and Systems* 5/14. Available at http://www.ncbi.nlm.nih.gov/pmc/articles/PMC2238740/pdf/1478-4505-5-14.pdf. Accessed 13 Oct. 2010.

Forest, P.G., et al. 1999. *Issues in the Governance of Integrated Health Systems*. Ottawa: Canadian Health Services Research Foundation.

Forget, E., Raisa Deber, and L.L. Roos. 2002. 'Medical savings accounts: Will they reduce costs?' *Canadian Medical Association Journal* 165/2: 143–7.

Frank, Richard, and Richard Zeckhauser. 2009. 'Health insurance exchanges: Making the markets work.' *New England Journal of Medicine* 361/12: 1135–7.

Frankish, C. James, Glen Moulton, Darryl Quantz, Arlene Carson, et al. 2007. 'Assessing the non-medical determinants of health: A survey of Canada's health regions.' *Canadian Journal of Public Health* 98/1: 41–8.

Fujisawa, Rie, and Gaetan Lafortune. 2008. 'The remuneration of general practitioners and specialists in 14 OECD countries: What are the factors influencing variations across countries?' OECD Working Paper no. 41. Paris: OECD.

Gabel, Jon, et al. 2009. 'Trends in underinsurance and the affordability of employer coverage, 2004–2007.' *Health Affairs* 28/4: w595–w606.

Gagnon, Marc-Andre, and Joel Lexchin. 2008. 'The cost of pushing pills: A new estimate of pharmaceutical promotion expenditures in the United States.' *PloS Medicine* 5/1: 29–32.

Galloway, Gloria. 2008. 'Provinces angry over drug rules.' *Globe and Mail*, 27 May: A8.

Gammon, Keri. 2006. 'Pandemics and pandemonium: Constitutional jurisdiction over public health.' *Dalhousie Journal of Legal Studies* 15/1: 1–38.

Garattini, Silvio, and Vittorio Bertele. 2007. 'How can we regulate medicines better?' *British Medical Journal* 335 (20 Oct.): 803–5.

Gauthier-Villars, David. 2009. 'France fights universal health care's high cost.' *Wall Street Journal*, 7 Aug. Available at http://online.wsj.com/article/SB124958049241511735.html. Accessed 22 Oct. 2010.

Gawande, Atul. 2009a. 'Getting there from here.' *New Yorker*, 26 Jan. Available at http://www.newyorker.com/reporting/2009/01/26/090126fa_fact_gawande. Accessed 12 Feb. 2010.

– 2009b. 'The cost conundrum.' *New Yorker*, 1 June: 26–33.

Gerber, Alan S., and Eric M. Patshnik. 2010. 'Problem solving in a polarized age: Comparative effectiveness research and the politicization of evidence-based medicine.' *Forum* 8/1: 1–13.

Gillis, John. 2008. 'Province to lease private clinic.' *Halifax Chronicle Herald*, 13 March: A1.

Gilpin, Robert. 1975. *U.S. Power and the Multinational Corporation.* New York: Basic Books.

Glazier, Richard, et al. 2009. 'Capitation and enhanced fee-for-service models for primary care reform: A population-based evaluation.' *Canadian Medical Association Journal* 180/11: E72–E81.

Glouberman, S. 2001. *Towards a New Perspective on Health Policy.* Ottawa: Canadian Policy Research Networks.

Grande, D., D. Frosch, A. Perkins, and B. Kahn. 2009. 'Effect of exposure to small pharmaceutical promotional items on treatment preferences.' *Archives of Internal Medicine* 169/9: 887–93.

Gratzer, David. 2007. 'The ugly truth about Canadian health care.' *City Journal* (Summer). Available at http://www.city-journal.org/html/17_3_canadian_healthcare.html. Accessed 11 Oct. 2010.

– 1999. *Code Blue: Reviving Canada's Health Care System*. Toronto: ECW Press.

Gray, Gwendolyn. 1991. *Federalism and Health Policy: The Development of Health Systems in Canada and Australia*. Toronto: University of Toronto Press.

Greschner, Donna. 2002. 'How will the Charter of Rights and Freedoms and evolving jurisprudence affect health care costs?' Discussion paper no. 20 for the Commission on the Future of Health Care in Canada (Romanow Commission), Ottawa.

Greß, Stefan. 2007. 'Private health insurance in Germany: Consequences of a dual system.' *Healthcare Policy* 32/2: 29–37.

Grob, Gerald. 1991. *From Asylum to Community: Mental Health Policy in Modern America*. Princeton: Princeton University Press.

Gross, Edith B. 1998. 'Gender differences in physician stress: Why the discrepant findings?' *Women and Health* 26/3: 1–14.

Groves, K.E.M., I. Sketris, and S.E. Tett. 2003. 'Prescription drug samples – does this marketing strategy counteract policies for quality use of medicines?' *Journal of Clinical Pharmacy and Therapeutics* 28: 259–71.

Groves K.E.M., J. MacKinnon, and I.S. Sketris. 2009. 'Prescribing Behavior.' In N.M. Rickles, A.I. Wertheimer, and M.C. Smith, eds., *Social and Behavioral Aspects of Pharmaceutical Care*, 2nd ed. Sudbury, MA.: Jones and Bartlett, 141–76.

Hacker, Jacob. 2009. 'Poor substitutes: Why cooperatives and triggers can't achieve the goals of a public option.' *New England Journal of Medicine* 361/17: 1617–19.

Hacker, Jacob. 2006. *The Great Risk Shift*. Oxford: Oxford University Press.

Hagan, John. 1987. 'Social science evidence in constitutional litigation.' In Robert J. Sharpe, ed., *Charter Litigation*. Toronto: Butterworths, 213–32.

Halpin, Helen, and Peter Harbage. 2010. 'The origins and demise of the public option.' *Health Affairs* 29/6: 1117–25.

Ham, Christopher. 2009a. 'The 2009 budget and the NHS.' *British Medical Journal* (29 April): 1024.

– 2009b. 'Lessons from the past decade for future health reforms.' *British Medical Journal* (28 Oct.): 1118–20.

Hawthorne, Geoffrey. 1991. *Plausible Worlds: Possibility and Understanding in History and the Social Sciences*. Cambridge: Cambridge University Press.

Health Canada. 2004. *10-Year Plan to Strengthen Health Care* (Sept.). Available at http://www.hc-sc.gc.ca/hcs-sss/delivery-prestation/fptcollab/2004-fmm-rpm/index-eng.php. Accessed 13 Oct. 2010.

– 2001. 'What is the population health approach?' Modified Dec. 8. Available at http://www.phac-aspc.gc.ca/ph-sp/approach-approche/appr-eng.php#health. Accessed 29 June 2009.

Health Council of Canada. 2008. *Rekindling Reform: Health Care Renewal in Canada, 2003–2008*. Toronto: Health Council.

Healy, David. 2002. *The Creation of Psychopharmacology*. Cambridge, MA: Harvard University Press.

Henry, David, and Joel Lexchin. 2002. 'The pharmaceutical industry as medicines provider.' *Lancet* 360 (16 Nov.): 1590–5.

Hertzman, Clyde, and Arjumand Siddiqi. 2008. 'Tortoises 1, hares 0: How comparative health trends between Canada and the United States support a long-term view of policy and health.' *Healthcare Policy* 4/2: 16–24.

Himmelstein, David, et al. 2009. 'Medical bankruptcy in the United States, 2007: Results of a national study.' *American Journal of Medicine* 122/8: 741–6.

Hogberg, David. 2007. 'Sweden's single-payer health system provides a warning to other nations.' *National Policy Analysis* (May). Available at http://www.nationalcenter.org/NPA555_Sweden_Health_Care.html. Accessed 4 Oct. 2010.

Holahan, John, and Linda Blumberg. 2009. *Is the public plan option a necessary part of health reform?* The Urban Institute Health Policy Center. Available at http://www.urban.org/publications/411915.html. Accessed 22 Oct. 2010.

Hollis, Aidan. 2009. 'Generic drug pricing and procurement: A policy for Alberta.' *University of Calgary School of Policy Studies Communique* 1/1: 1–53.

Hood, Christopher, and Guy Peters. 2004. 'The middle aging of new public management: Into the age of paradox?' *Journal of Public Administration Research and Theory* 14/3: 267–82.

Horton, R. 2004. 'The dawn of McScience.' *New York Review of Books* 51/4: 7–9.

Howard, Cori. 2006. 'ER for hire.' *Globe and Mail*, 25 Nov.: F3.

IMS Health. 2010a. Canadian Disease and Therapeutic Index, 2010. Available at http://www.imshealth.com/portal/site/imshealth. Accessed 27 March 2010.

IMS Health. 2010b. Pharmaceutical Trends. 2010. Available at http://www.jaguarpublications.com/industryupdates/pdf/1_avril_2010_AQ11_48_45.PDF. Accessed 28 Oct. 2010.

International Federation of Health Plans. 2009. *Comparative Price Report: Medical and Hospital Fees by Country*. Available at http://voices.washingtonpost.com/ezra-klein/IFHP%20Comparative%20Price%20Report%20with%20AHA%20data%20addition.pdf. Accessed 29 Oct. 2010.

Kaiser Foundation. 2009. *Health Care Costs: A Primer.* Washington, DC: Kaiser Family Foundation.

Kapp, Matt. 2009. 'The sick business of health-care profiteering.' 24 Sept. Available at http://www.vanityfair.com/politics/features/2009/09/health-care200909. Accessed 21 Oct. 2010.

Kazanjian, A., et al. 2000. *Issues in Physician Rresources Planning in BC.* Vancouver: University of British Columbia, Centre for Health Services and Policy Research.

Keelan, Jennifer, and Kumanan Wilson. 2008. 'Learning from *Listeria*: The autonomy of the Public Health Agency of Canada.' *Canadian Medical Association Journal* 179/9: 877–9.

Kent, Alastair. 2007. 'Should patient groups accept money from drug companies? Yes.' *British Medical Journal* 334 (5 May): 934.

Keyhani, Salomeh, and Alex Federman. 2009. 'Doctors on coverage: Physicians' views on a new public insurance option and medicare expansion.' *New England Journal of Medicine* (1 Oct.): e24(1)–e24(4).

King's Fund. 2010. *A High-Performing NHS? A Review of Progress 1997–2010.* Ed. Jo Maybin and Ruth Thorlby. London: King's Fund.

Kirby, Michael. 2006. *Out of the Shadows at Last: Transforming Mental Health, Mental Illness and Addiction Services in Canada.* Ottawa: Standing Senate Committee on Social Affairs, Science, and Technology.

– 2002. *The Health of Canadians: The Federal Role (The Kirby Report).* Ottawa: Standing Senate Committee on Social Affairs, Science and Technology.

Kirsch, Irving, and Thomas Moore. 2002. 'The emperor's new drugs: An analysis of antidepressant medication data submitted to the FDA.' *Prevention and Treatment*, 15 July. Available at http://alphachoices.com/repository/assets/pdf/EmperorsNewDrugs.pdf. Accessed 24 Oct. 2010.

Klein, Rudolf. 2007. 'The new model NHS: Performance, perceptions, and expectations.' *British Medical Bulletin*, 26 May: 1–12.

– 2006. 'The troubled transformation of Britain's National Health Service.' *New England Journal of Medicine* 355/4: 409–15.

– 1998. 'Why Britain is reorganizing its National Health Service – yet again.' *Health Affairs* 17/4: 111–25.

Kolata, Gina. 2010. 'Law may do little to curb unnecessary care.' *New York Times*, 30 March: D1.

Kondro, Wayne 2008. 'Industry handouts: Enough is enough,' *Canadian Medical Association Journal* 178/13: 1651.

– 2006a. '*Chaoulli* decision resonates one year later.' *Canadian Medical Association Journal* 176/1: 17–18.

– 2006b. 'Brand-name drug companies fail to meet R&D commitments.' *Canadian Medical Association Journal* 174/4: 344.

Krugman, Paul, and Robin Wells. 2006. 'The health care crisis and what to do about it.' *New York Review of Books* 53/5. Available at http://www.nybooks.com/articles/archives/2006/mar/23/the-health-care-crisis-and-what-to-do-about-it/?page=1. Accessed 29 Oct. 2010.

Krumholz, Harlan, Joseph Ross, Amos Presler, and David Egilman. 2007. 'What have we learned from Vioxx?' *British Medical Journal* 334 (20 Jan.): 120–3.

LaJeunesse, Ronald. 2002. *Political Asylums*. Edmonton: Muttart Foundation.

Lalonde, Marc. 1974. *A New Perspective on the Health of Canadians*. Ottawa: Government of Canada.

Lang, Michelle. 2008a. 'South African doctors find "blessings" of rural life.' *Calgary Herald*, 14 Dec. Available at http://www.calgaryherald.com/business/ARCHIVE+Michelle+Lang+award+winning+work+South+African+doctors+find+blessings+rural+life/2393382/story.html?id=2393382. Accessed 20 Oct. 2010.

– 2008b '"We need our doctors," South Africans plead.' *Calgary Herald*, 16 Dec. Available at http://www.calgaryherald.com/entertainment/ARCHIVE+Michelle+Lang+award+winning+work+need+doctors+South+Africans/2393360/story.html?id=2393360. Accessed 20 Oct. 2010.

Lavis, J. 2002. 'Ideas at the margin or marginalized ideas? Nonmedical determinants of health in Canada.' *Health Affairs* 21: 107–12.

Lazar, Harvey, Keith Banting, Robin Boadway, David Cameron, and France St-Hilaire. 2002. *Federal-Provincial Relations and Health Care: Reconstructing the Partnership*. Summary Report on Fiscal Federalism and Health for the Commission on the Future of Health Care in Canada (Romanow Commission), Ottawa.

Lear, Julia, and Elias Mossialos. 2008a. 'EU law and health policy in Europe.' *Euro Observer* 10/3: 1–3.

– 2008b. 'Competition law and health services.' *Euro Observer* 10/3: 5–6.

Leatt, Peggy, George Pink, and Michael Guerriere. 2000. 'Towards a Canadian model of integrated health care.' *Healthcare Papers* 1/2: 13–35.

Lee, Kirby, Peter Bacchetti, and Ida Sim. 2008. 'Publication of clinical trials supporting successful new drug application: A literature analysis.' *PLoS Medicine* 5/9: 1348–56.

LeGrand, Julian. 1999. 'Competition, cooperation, or control? Tales from the British National Health Service.' *Health Affairs*, May/June: 27–39.

LeGrand, Julian, N. Mays, and J. Mulligan. 1998. *Learning from the NHS Internal Market*. London: King's Fund.

LeGrand, Julian, and Ray Robinson, eds. 1994. *Evaluating the NHS Reforms*. London: King's Fund.

Lenzer, Jeanne, and Shannon Brownlee. 2008. 'Doctor takes "march of shame" to atone for drug company payments.' *British Medical Journal* 336 (5 Jan.): 20–1.

Lett, Dan. 2008. 'Private health clinics remain unregulated in most of Canada.' *Canadian Medical Association Journal* 178/8: 986–7.

Levitt, Kari. 1970. *Silent Surrender: The Multinational Corporation in Canada.* Toronto: Macmillan.

Lewis, S. 2002. 'The bog, the fog, the future: Five strategies for renewing federalism in health care.' *Canadian Medical Association Journal* 166/11: 1421–2.

– 2001. 'Devolution to democratic health authorities in Saskatchewan: An interim report.' *Canadian Medical Association Journal* 164/3: 343–7.

– 1998. 'Still here, and still flawed, still wrong: The case against the case for taxing the sick.' *Canadian Medical Association Journal* 159/5: 497–9.

Lewis, S., and Denise Kouri. 2004. 'Regionalization: Making sense of the Canadian experience.' *Healthcare Papers* 5/1: 12–31.

Lexchin, Joel. 2007a. 'Pharmacare: Equity, efficiency, and effectiveness – we've waited long enough.' In Bruce Campbell and Greg Marchildon, eds., *Medicare: Facts, Myths, Problems, Promise.* Toronto: Lorimer, 262–7.

– 2007b. 'Notice of compliance with conditions: A policy in limbo.' *Healthcare Policy* 2/4: 114–22.

– 2006. 'Bigger and better: How Pfizer redefined erectile dysfunction.' *PLoS Medicine* 3/4: 439–42.

– 2004. *Transparency in Drug Regulation: Mirage or Oasis?* Ottawa: Canadian Centre for Policy Alternatives.

– 2001. 'Pharmaceuticals: Politics and policy.' In P. Armstrong, H. Armstrong, and D. Coburn, eds., *Unhealthy Times.* Oxford: Oxford University Press, 31–44.

– 1997. 'After compulsory licensing: Coming issues in Canadian pharmaceutical policy and politics.' *Health Policy* 40/1: 69–80.

Liberto, Jennifer. 2009. 'Health care lobbying: Political power machine.' 8 Sept. Available at http://politicalticker.blogs.cnn.com/2009/09/08/health-care-lobbying-political-power-machine/#more-67805. Accessed 29 Oct. 2010.

Lindquist, Evert. 1999. 'Efficiency, reliability, or innovation? Managing overlap and interdependence in Canada's federal system of governance.' In Robert Young, ed., *Stretching the Federation: The Art of the State in Canada.* Kingston: Institute of Intergovermental Relations, 35–68.

Litva, A., et al. 2002. '"The public is too subjective": Public involvement at different levels of health-care decision making.' *Social Science and Medicine* 54/12: 1825–37.

Lo, Bernard, and Marilyn J. Field, eds. Institute of Medicine; Committee on Conflict of Interest in Medical Research, Education, and Practice. 2009. *Conflict of Interest in Medical Research, Education, and Practice: A Focus on Medical Research.* Washington, DC: National Institutes of Medicine and National Academies Press.

Longman, Phillip. 2005. 'The best care anywhere.' *Washington Monthly*, Jan./ Feb. Available at http://www.washingtonmonthly.com/features/2005/0501. longman.html. Accessed 12 Oct. 2010.

Lukes, Steven. 1974. *Power: A Radical View*. London: Macmillan.

MacKinnon, Neil, and Ivan Ip. 2009. 'The National Pharmaceuticals Strategy: Rest in peace, revive, or renew?' *Canadian Medical Association Journal* 180/8: 801–3.

MacPherson, Catherine, and Nuala Kenny. 2009. 'The power of "principles" in a National Pharmaceuticals Strategy.' *Healthcare Policy* 4/3: 25–36.

Maioni, Antonia. 2008. 'The Castonguay Report: Quebec's quiet revolutionary strikes again.' *Policy Options* (April): 31–5.

– 1998. *Parting at the Crossroads: The Emergence of Health Insurance in the United States and Canada*. Princeton: Princeton University Press.

Manfredi, Christopher, and Antonia Maioni. 2002. 'Courts and health policy: Judicial policy making and publicly funded health care in Canada.' *Journal of Health Politics, Policy and Law* 27/2: 213–39.

Marchildon, G.P. 2006. 'Federal pharmacare: Prescription for an ailing federation.' *Inroads* 18 (Winter/Spring): 94–108.

– 2005. *Health Systems in Transition: Canada*. Copenhagen: WHO.

Marmor, Ted. 2008. 'The comparative dimension of policy analysis: Rules of the game?' In Flood, Stabile, and Tuohy, *Exploring Social Insurance*, 185–98.

Mason, Christopher. 2008 'Public-private health care delivery becoming the norm in Sweden.' *Canadian Medical Association Journal* 179/2: 129–31.

Mathieu, Sylvain, et al. 2009. 'Comparison of registered and published primary outcomes in randomized controlled trials.' *Journal of the American Medical Association* 302/9.

Mazankowski, Donald. 2001. *Report of the Premier's Advisory Council on Health*. Dec. (Released by the Government of Alberta, Jan. 2002.) Available at http://www.premiersadvisory.com/reform.html.

McGinnis, J. Michael, Pamela Williams-Russo, and James Knickman. 2002. 'The case for more active policy attention to health promotion.' *Health Affairs* 21/2: 78–93.

McIntosh, Tom. 2006. *Don't Panic: The Hitchhiker's Guide to Chaoulli, Wait Times and the Politics of Private Insurance*. Ottawa: Canadian Policy Research Networks.

– 2004. 'Intergovernmental relations, social policy and federal transfers after Romanow.' *Canadian Public Administration* 47/1: 27–51.

McIntosh, Tom, Renee Torgerson, and Nathan Klassen. 2007. *The Ethical Recruitment of Internationally Educated Professionals: Lessons from Abroad and Options for Canada*. Research report H/11. Ottawa: Canadian Policy Research Networks.

McKeown, Thomas. 1976a. *The Modern Rise of Population*. New York: Academic Press.

– 1976b. *The Role of Medicine: Dream, Mirage, or Nemesis?* London: Nuffield Trust.

McLeod, Paul. 2008. 'Private clinics work, government says.' *MetroNews*, 13 Nov.: 5.

McMillan, Colin, and Seema Nagpal. 2007. 'The public health system in Canada: Not meeting the needs of Canadians.' *Healthcare Papers* 7/3: 60–5.

Mintzes, Barbara. 2005. *Educational Initiatives for Medical and Pharmacy Students about Drug Promotion: An International Cross-Sectional Survey*. Geneva: World Health Organization and Health Action International.

– 2004. 'Drug regulatory failure in Canada: The case of Diane-35.' Women and Health Protection. Oct. Available at http://www.whp-apsf.ca/en/documents/diane35.html. Accessed 11 Oct. 2010.

Mooney, Helen. 2009. 'Elsevier says offering $25 gift cards for positive reviews was mistake.' *British Medical Journal* 339 (14 July): 131.

Morgan, Gwyn. 2008. 'Three wishes for a better Canada.' *Globe and Mail*, 22 Dec.: B2.

Morton, F. 1999. 'Dialogue or monologue?' *Policy Options* (April): 23–6.

Mossialos, Elias, Govin Permanand, Rita Baeten, and Tamara Hervey, eds. 2009. *Health Systems Governance in Europe: The Role of EU Law and Policy*. Cambridge: Cambridge University Press.

Mowat, David, and David Butler-Jones. 2007. 'Public health in Canada: A difficult history.' *Healthcare Papers* 7/3: 31–6.

Moynihan, Ray. 2009. 'Court hears how drug giant Merck tried to "neutralize" and "discredit" doctors critical of Vioxx.' *British Medical Journal* 338 (11 April): 849.

– 2008a. 'Doctors' education: The invisible influence of drug company sponsorship.' *British Medical Journal* 336 (23 Feb.): 416–17.

– 2008b. 'Key opinion leaders: Independent experts or drug representatives in disguise?' *British Medical Journal* 336 (21 June): 1402–3.

– 2008c. 'Independent drug watchdog in Canada under funding threat.' *British Medical Journal* 336 (7 June): 1265.

Mulvale, Gillian, Julia Abelson, and Paula Goering. 2007. 'Mental health service delivery in Ontario, Canada: How do policy legacies shape prospects for reform?' *Health Economics, Policy, and Law* 2: 363–89.

Murphy, Tom. 2009. 'Pfizer fined $2.3b for illegal drug marketing.' *Halifax Chronicle Herald*, 5 Sept.: C6.

Nanos, Nik. 2009. 'Canadians overwhelmingly support universal health care.' *Policy Options* (Nov.): 12–14.

Naylor, C.D., ed. 1992. *Canadian Health Care and the State: A Century of Evolution.* Montreal: McGill-Queen's University Press.

Naylor, David. 2003. *Learning from SARS: Renewal of Public Health in Canada – A Report of the National Advisory Committee on SARS and Public Health.* Ottawa: Health Canada.

Nelson, Geoffrey. 2006. 'Mental health policy in Canada.' In Anne Westhues, ed., *Canadian Social Policy,* 4th ed. Waterloo, ON: Wilfrid Laurier University Press, 245–66.

Newhouse, Joseph, et al. 2008. 'Commentary: Attribution in the RAND health insurance experiment.' *Journal of Health Politics, Policy, and Law* 33/1: 295–308.

Noah, Timothy. 2009a. 'Why you can't trust your health insurer.' *Slate,* 27 July. Available at http://www.slate.com/id/2223680/. Accessed 28 July 2009.

Noah, Timothy. 2009b. 'Public enemy.' *Slate,* 29 September. Available at http://www.slate.com/id/2230938/. Accessed 30 September 2009.

Nova Scotia. 1994. *Nova Scotia's Blueprint for Health System Reform: Report of the Minister's Action Committee on Health System Reform.* Halifax: Government of Nova Scotia.

Nuffield Trust. 2010. *Giving GPs Budgets for Commissioning: What Needs to Be Done?* London: Nuffield Trust.

Nyman, John. 2008. 'Commentary: Health plan switching and attribution bias in the RAND health insurance experiment.' *Journal of Health Politics, Policy and Law* 33/2: 309–17.

– 2007. 'American health policy: Cracks in the foundation.' *Journal of Health Politics, Policy and Law* 32/5: 759–83.

Oberlander, Jonathan. 2010. 'Long time coming: Why health reform finally passed.' *Health Affairs* 29/6: 1112–17.

Oberlander, Jonathan, and Joseph White. 2009. 'Systemwide cost control – the missing link: The health care reform.' *New England Journal of Medicine* 361/12: 1131–3.

OECD. 2010. *Health Data 2008: How Does Canada Compare?* Available at http://www.oecd.org/dataoecd/46/33/38979719.pdf. Accessed 22 Oct. 2010.

– 2007. *Health Data 2007.* Paris: OECD.

Or, Zeynep, et al. 2010. 'Are health care problems systemic? Politics of access and choice under Beveridge and Bismarck systems.' *Health Economics, Policy and Law* 5: 269–93.

Ouellet, Richard. 2002. 'The effects of international agreements on Canadian health measures.' Discussion paper no. 12 for the Commission on the Future of Health Care in Canada (Romanow Commission), Ottawa.

Paris, Joel. 2008. *Prescriptions for the Mind*. Oxford: Oxford University Press.

Pescosolido, Bernice, and Jack K. Martin. 2004. 'Cultural authority and the sovereignty of American medicine: The role of networks, class and community.' *Journal of Health Politics, Policy, and Law* 29/4: 735–56.

Petersen, Laura, et al. 2006. 'Does pay for performance improve the quality of health care?' *Annals of Internal Medicine* 145/4 (15 August): 265–72.

Petter, Andrew. 2005. 'Wealthcare: The politics of the *Charter* re-visited.' In Flood, Stabile, and Kontic, ed., *Access to Care, Access to Justice*, 116–38.

– 1989. 'Federalism and the myth of the federal spending power.' *Canadian Bar Review* 68 (Sept.): 448–79.

Pharmaceutical Online. 2009. 'Prescription drugs market to cross $897B by 2015.' 2 July. Available at http://www.pharmaceuticalonline.com/article.mvc/Global-Prescription-Drugs-Market-To-Cross-0001. Accessed 22 Oct. 2010.

Pickett, Kate, and Richard Wilkinson. 2009. *The Spirit Level: Why More Equal Societies Almost Always Do Better*. London: Allen Lane.

PMPRB. 2010. *Patented Medicine Prices Review Board Annual Report*. 2009. May. Available at http://www.pmprb-cepmb.gc.ca/cmfiles/ar09-en-online.pdf. Accessed 15 Oct. 2010.

– 2007. *Non-patented Prescription Drug Prices Reporting: Non-patented Single-Source Drugs in Canada*. Availabe at http://www.pmprb-cepmb.gc.ca/CMFiles/nppdp-4e38JBM-12192007-5851.pdf. Accessed 15 Oct. 2010.

Pollan, Michael. 2003. 'Is corn making us fat?' *New York Times Upfront*, 8 Dec. Available at http://www.thefreelibrary.com/Is+corn+making+us+fat%3F+Michael+Pollan+argues+that+U.S.+farm+policy. . .-a0112585038. Accessed 10 Oct. 2010.

Pollock, Allyson, and Graham Kirkwood. 2009. 'Independent sector treatment centres: Learning from a Scottish case study.' *British Medical Journal* 338 (30 April): 1108–11.

Priest, Lisa. 2009. 'The million-dollar club: Losing big, losing often.' *Globe and Mail*, 5 Oct.: A4.

– 2008. 'Record costs threaten Canada's picture of health.' *Globe and Mail*, 14 Nov.: A14.

Prosser, Tony. 2009. 'EU competition law and public services.' In Mossialos et al., *Health Systems Governance in Europe*, 137–46.

Public Health Agency of Canada. 2002. *Review of Best Practices in Mental Health Reform*. Available at http://www.phac-aspc.gc.ca/mh-sm/pubs/bp_review/reves1-eng.php. Accessed 16 Oct. 2010.

Quaye, Randolph. 2007. *Recent Reforms in the Swedish Health Care System*. Lanham, MD: University Press of America.

Rachlis, Michael. 2004. *Prescription for Excellence: How Innovation Is Saving Canada's Health Care System*. Toronto: HarperCollins.

Raftery, J., et al. 2009. 'Ranibizumab (Lucentis) versus bevacizumab (Avastin): Modeling cost effectiveness.' *British Journal of Ophthalmology* 91/9: 1244–6.

Randall, Glen E., and A. Paul Williams. 2009. 'Health-care reform and the dimensions of professional autonomy.' *Canadian Public Administration* 52/1: 51–69.

Reinhardt, Uwe. 2007. 'Faith-based health policy: The urge to privatise.' *British Medical Journal* 334/7605: 1193.

– 1994. 'Germany's health care system: It's not the American way.' *Health Affairs* (Fall): 22–4.

Rice, Thomas. 1997. 'Can markets give us the health system we want?' *Journal of Health Politics, Policy, and Law* 22/2: 383–426.

Richards, John. 1999. 'Comments on Antonia Maioni's paper.' In Young, *Stretching the Federation*, 122–8.

Ritchie, Ronald. 1973. 'Sources of policy advice.' In K. Kernahagn, ed., *Bureaucracy in Canadian Government*, 2nd ed. Agincourt, ON: Methuen, 85–93.

Rivet, Christine, Bridget Ryan, and Moira Stewart. 2007. 'Hands on: Is there an association between doing procedures and job satisfaction?' *Canadian Family Physician* 53 (Jan.): 92–3.

Roach, Kent. 2005. 'The courts and medicare: Too much or too little judicial activism?' In Flood, Roach, and Sossin, eds., *Access to Care, Access to Justice*, 184–204.

Rochaix, Lise, and David Wilsford. 2005. 'State autonomy, policy paralysis: Paradoxes of institutions and culture in the French health care system.' *Journal of Health Politics, Policy and Law* 30/1–2: 97–119.

Rochon, Jean. 1988. *Rapport de la Commission d'enquête sur les services de santé et les services sociaux*. Quebec City: Government of Quebec.

Roemer, Milton I. 1982. 'Market failure and health care policy.' *Journal of Public Health Policy* 3/4: 419–31.

Romanow, Roy. 2002. *Building on Values: The Future of Health Care in Canada*. Ottawa: Commission on the Future of Health Care in Canada.

Rosenthal, Meredith, and R. Adams Dudley. 2007. 'Pay-for-Performance: Will the latest payment trend improve care?' *Journal of the American Medical Association* 297/7: 740–44.

Ross, Joseph, et al. 2009. 'Pooled analysis of Rofecoxib placebo-controlled clinical trial data: Lessons for postmarket pharmaceutical safety surveillance.' *Archives of Internal Medicine* 169/21: 1976–84.

Ross, Joseph, Kevin Hill, David Egilman, and Harlan Krumholz. 2008. 'Guest authorship and ghostwriting in publications related to rofecoxib: A case study of industry documents from rofecoxib litigation.' *Journal of the American Medical Association* 299/15: 1800–12.

Rourke, James. 1993. 'Politics of rural health care: Recruitment and retention of physicians.' *Canadian Medical Association Journal* 148/8: 1281–8.

Russell, Peter. 2005. 'Chaoulli: The political versus the legal life of a judicial decision.' In Flood, Roach, and Sossin, eds., *Access to Care, Access to Justice*, 5–18.

Saltman, Richard. 2008. 'Decentalization, re-centralization and future European health policy.' *European Journal of Public Health* 18/2: 104–6.

Saltman, Richard, Vaida Bankauskaite, and K. Vrangback, eds. 2007. *Decentralization in Health Care: Analysis and Outcome*. London: Open University Press.

Saltman, Richard, and Sven-Eric Bergman. 2005. 'Renovating the commons: Swedish health care reforms in perspective.' *Journal of Health Politics, Policy, and Law* 30/1–2: 254–75.

Sandier, S., V. Paris, and D. Polton. 2004. *Healthcare Systems in Transition: France*. Copenhagen: WHO.

Schafer, Arthur. 2004. 'Biomedical conflicts of interest: A defence of the sequestration thesis.' *Journal of Medical Ethics* 30/1: 8–24.

Schlesinger, Mark. 2010. 'Choice cuts: Parsing policymakers' pursuit of patient empowerment from an individual perspective.' *Health Economics, Policy, and Law* 5: 365–87.

Schmidt, Herald. 2007. 'Patients' charters and health responsibilities.' *British Medical Journal* 335 (8 Dec.): 1187–89.

Schoen, Cathy, Robin Osborn, Michelle M. Doty, Meghan Bishop, Jordon Peugh, and Nandita Murukutia. 2007. 'Toward higher-performance health systems: Adults' health experiences in seven countries, 2007.' *Health Affairs* 31 Oct. [web exclusive]: 717–34.

Schulz, Rockwell, and Stephen Harrison. 1986. 'Physician autonomy in the Federal Republic of Germany, Great Britain, and the United States.' *International Journal of Health Planning and Management* 1/5 (Oct.): 335–55.

Schwartz, Karyn, and Tanya Schwartz. 2010. *Medicaid and the uninsured: How will health reform impact young adults?* Washington, DC: Kaiser Family Foundation.

Scott, F.R. 1977. *Essays on the Constitution*. Toronto: University of Toronto Press.

Sanger, Matthew. 2001. *Reckless Abandon: Canada, the GATS, and the Future of Health Care*. Ottawa: Canadian Centre for Policy Alternatives.

Shiels, J., and P. Hogan. 1999. 'Cost of tax-exempt health benefits in 1998.' *Health Affairs* 18/2: 176–81.

Shortell, Stephen, et al. 1993. 'Creating organized delivery systems: The barriers and facilitators.' *Hospital and Health Service Administration* 38/4: 447–66.

Shorter, Edward. 2009. *Before Prozac*. Oxford: Oxford University Press.

– 1997. *A History of Psychiatry*. New York: Wiley.

Silversides, Ann. 2008. 'Public-private partnerships, part 2: Calculations of risk.' *Canadian Medical Association Journal* 179/10: 991–4.

Simmons, Harvey. 1989. *Unbalanced: Mental Health Policy in Ontario, 1930–1988*. Toronto: Wall and Thompson.

Simonet, Daniel. 2008. 'The new public management theory and European health-care reforms.' *Canadian Public Administration* 51/4: 617–35.

Simpson, Jeffrey. 2010. 'And the worst record on timely access to primary care goes to. . .' *Globe and Mail*, 20 July: A15.

– 2008. 'Listening to the sounds of health-care silence.' *Globe and Mail*, 19 Nov.: A19.

Singer, Natasha. 2009a. 'A birth control pill that promised too much.' *New York Times*, 11 Feb. Available at http://www.nytimes.com/2009/02/11/business/11pill.html. Accessed 30 Oct. 2010.

– 2009b. 'Medical papers by ghostwriters pushed therapy.' *New York Times*, 4 Aug. Available at http://www.nytimes.com/2009/08/05/health/research/05ghost.html. Accessed 30 Oct. 2010.

Sketris, I., E.L. Ingram, and H. Lummis. 2007. *Optimal Prescribing and Medication Use in Canada: Challenges and Opportunities*. Toronto: Health Council of Canada.

Skinner, Brett J., and Mark Rovere. 2008. *Paying More, Getting Less*. Fraser Institute. Oct. Available at http://www.fraserinstitute.org/research-news/display.aspx?id=13276. Accessed 30 Oct. 2010.

Skinner, Brett, Mark Rovere, and Marisha Warrington. 2008. *The Hidden Costs of Single Payer Health Insurance*. Fraser Institute. Sept. Available at http://www.fraserinstitute.org/research-news/display.aspx?id=13515. Accessed 30 Oct 2010.

Smith, Richard. 2007. 'Should we loosen the grip on drug companies?' *British Medical Journal* 335 (1 Sept.): 454.

– 2005. 'Medical journals are an extension of the marketing arm of pharmaceutical companies.' *PLoS Medicine* 2/5: 364–6.

Solomon, Sam. 2007. '*Chaoulli* copycat cases crop up across country.' *National Review of Medicine* 4/1. Available at http://www.nationalreviewofmedicine.com/issue/2007/01_15/4_policy_politics02_1.html. Accessed 30 Oct. 2010.

Sossin, Lorne. 2005. 'Towards a two-tier constitution? The poverty of health rights.' In Flood, Roach, and Sossin, eds., *Access to Care, Access to Justice*, 161–83.

Spurling, Geoffrey et al. 2010. 'Information from pharmaceutical companies and the quality, quantity, and cost of physicians' prescribing: A systematic review.' *PLoS Medicine* 7/10: e1000352 1–22.

Sretzer, Simon. 2002. 'Rethinking McKeown: The relationship between public health and social change.' *American Journal of Public Health* 92/5: 722–5.

Stafford, Ned. 2009. 'German health policy is likely to become more pro-doctor, expert predicts.' *British Medical Journal* (6 Oct.): 828.

Standing Senate Committee on Social Affairs, Science and Technology. 2002. *Study on the State of the Health Care System in Canada, 1999–2002* (The Kirby Report). Ottawa: Government of Canada.

Starr, P. 1982. *In Sickness and in Wealth: The Rise of a Sovereign Profession and the Making of a Vast Industry*. New York: Basic Books.

Steinbrook, Robert. 2009. 'Easing the shortages in adult primary care: Is it all about money?' *New England Journal of Medicine* 360/26: 2696–9.

Steinman, M.A., L. Bero, M.M. Chren, and S. Landefeld. 2006. 'Narrative review; the promotion of gabapentin: An analysis of internal industry documents.' *Annals of Internal Medicine* 145/4: 284–93.

Stevens, Simon. 2004. 'Reform strategies for the English NHS.' *Health Affairs* 23/3: 37–45.

Stewart, Hamish. 2005. 'Implications of *Chaoulli* for fact finding in constitutional cases.' In Flood, Roach, and Sossin, eds., *Access to Care, Access to Justice*, 207–15.

Stueck, Wendy. 2006. 'B.C. clinic abandons plan for patient fees.' *Globe and Mail*, 4 Dec.: A4.

Sussman, Sam. 1998. 'The first asylums in Canada.' *Canadian Journal of Psychiatry* 43/3: 260–4.

Tanne, J. 2010. 'Few U.S. medical schools and medical centres are disclosing industry ties.' *British Medical Journal* 340 (27 Feb.): 446.

– 2009a. 'U.S. university psychiatrist loses chairmanship over drug company payments.' *British Medical Journal* 338 (6 Jan.): 896.

– 2009b. 'Merck discloses $3.7m paid to U.S. doctors for speeches over three months.' *British Medical Journal* 339 (26 Oct.): 989.

– 2007. 'Bristol-Myers Squibb to pay $515m.' *British Medical Journal* 335 (13 Oct.): 742.

Tate, C. Neal, and Torbjörn Vallinder. 1995. *The Global Expansion of Judicial Power*. New York: New York University Press.

Taylor, M.G. 1978. *Health Insurance and Canadian Public Policy: The Seven Decisions that Created the Canadian Health Insurance System*. Montreal: McGill-Queen's University Press.

Telford, Hamish. 2003. 'The federal spending power in Canada: Nation-building or nation-destroying?' *Publius* 33/1: 23–44.

Thomson, Sarah, and Elias Mossialos. 2008. 'Internal market rules and regulation of private health insurance: Threat or opportunity?' *Euro Observer* 10/3: 7–9.

Tolbert, Jennifer. 2008. *Approaches to Covering the Uninsured: A Guide.* Washington, DC: Kaiser Family Foundation.

Tomblin, Steven. 2002. 'Creating a more democratic health system: A critical review of constraints and a new approach to health restructuring.' Discussion paper no. 3 for the Commission on the Future of Health Care in Canada (Romanow Commission), Ottawa.

Tomblin Murphy, Gail, and Linda O'Brien-Pallas. 2002. 'How do health human resources policies and practices inhibit change? A plan for the future.' Discussion paper no. 30 for the Commission on the Future of Health Care in Canada (Romanow Commission), Ottawa.

Toop, Les, and Dee Mangin. 2007. 'Industry-funded patient information and the slippery slope to New Zealand.' *British Medical Journal* 335 (6 Oct.): 694–5.

Tuohy, Carolyn. 2003. 'Agency, contract, and governance: Shifting shapes of accountability in the health care arena.' *Journal of Health Politics, Policy, and Law* 28/2–3: 195–215.

– 1999. *Accidental Logics: The Dynamics of Change in the Health Care Arena in the United States, Britain, and Canada.* Oxford and New York: Oxford University Press.

Tuffs, Annette. 2008. 'Germany has two-tier health service, study shows.' *British Medical Journal* (12 April): 796.

Tupper, Allan. 2001. 'The contested terrain of Canadian public administration in Canada's third century.' *Journal of Canadian Studies* 35/4: 142–60.

Turner, Erick, et al. 2008. 'Selective publication of antidepressant trials and its influence on apparent efficiency.' *New England Journal of Medicine* 358/3: 252–60.

Tyhurst, J.S., et al. 1963. *More for the Mind: A Study of Psychiatric Services in Canada.* Toronto: Canadian Mental Health Association.

Ubelacker, Sheryl. 2008. 'Frustration brewing among family physicians across Canada.' *Globe and Mail,* 9 Jan.: L4.

United Kingdom, Department of Health. 2004. *Code of Practice for the International Recruitment of Healthcare Professionals.* Available at http://www.dh.gov.uk/en/Publicationsandstatistics/Publications/Publications PolicyAndGuidance/DH_4097730. Accessed 10 Oct. 2010.

– 1989. *Working for Patients* (Cm. 555). London: HMSO.

Vedula, S., L. Bero, R. Scherer, and K. Dickersin. 2009. 'Outcome reporting in industry-sponsored trials of gabapentin for off-label use.' *New England Journal of Medicine* 361/20: 1963–71.

Viens, A.M., and J. Savulescu. 2004. 'Introduction to the Olivieri symposium.'
Journal of Medical Ethics 30: 1–7.

Vining, Aidan, and Anthony Boardman. 2008. 'Public-private partnerships in
Canada: Theory and evidence.' *Canadian Public Administration* 51/1: 9–44.

Waldman v. British Columbia (Medical Services Commission). 1997. [1997] B.C.J.
No. 2014 (B.C. Court of Appeal).

Wang, Amy, Christopher McCoy, Mohammed Hassan Murad, and Victor
Montori. 2010. 'Association between industry affiliation and position on
cardiovascular risk with rosiglitazone: Cross-sectional systematic review.'
British Medical Journal 340 (18 March): 799.

Watson, D., S. Slade, L. Buske, and J. Tepper. 2006. 'Intergenerational differences
in workloads among primary care physicians: A ten-year, population-based
study.' *Health Affairs* 25/6: 1620–8.

Weale, Albert. 1998. 'Rationing health care.' *British Medical Journal*
316/7129: 410.

Weatherill, Sheila. 2009. *Report of the Independent Investigator into the 2008
Listeriosis Outbreak.* Ottawa: Government of Canada, July.

Webster, Charles. 2002. *The National Health Service: A Political History.* Oxford:
Oxford University Press.

Webster, Paul. 2010. 'Ontario's plan for electronic health records is at risk, official says.' *Canadian Medical Association Journal* 182/6: E253–4.

Wiktorowicz, Mary. 2005. 'Restructuring mental health policy in Ontario:
Deconstructing the evolving welfare state.' *Canadian Public Administration*
48/3: 386–412.

Wilson, Kumanan, Barbara von Tigerstrom, and Christopher McDougall.
2008. 'Protecting global health security through the International Health
Regulations: Requirements and challenges.' *Canadian Medical Association
Journal* 179/1: 44–8.

Woolhandler, Steffie, and David Himmelstein. 2007. 'Competition in a publicly funded healthcare system.' *British Journal of Medicine* 336 (9 June):
1126–9.

World Health Organization. 2008. *Closing the Gap in a Generation: Health Equity
through Action of the Social Determinants of Health.* Geneva: WHO.

– 2000. *The World Health Report 2000. Health Systems: Improving Performance.*
Geneva: WHO.

– 1986. *The Ottawa Charter for Health Promotion.* (Nov.) Available at http://
www.who.int/healthpromotion/conferences/previous/ottawa/en/. Accessed
10 Oct. 2010.

Wright, Charles. 2005. 'Different interpretations of "evidence" and implications for the Canadian health care system.' In Flood, Roach, and Sossin, eds., *Access to Care, Access to Justice*, 220–33.

Wright, D., J. Moran, and S. Gouglas. 2003. 'The confinement of the insane in Victorian Canada.' In R. Porter and D. Wright, eds., *The Confinement of the Insane: International Perspectives, 1800–1985*. New York: Cambridge University Press, 100–28.

Yank, D. Rennie, and L.A. Bero. 2007. 'Financial ties and concordance between results and conclusions in meta-analyses: Retrospective cohort study.' *British Medical Journal* 445 (8 Dec.): 1202–5.

Young, Robert, ed. 1999. *Stretching the Federation*. Kingston, ON: Institute for Intergovernmental Relations.

Zwarenstein, Merrick, and Shaun Treweek. 2009. 'What kind of randomized trials do we want?' *Canadian Medical Association Journal* 180/10: 998–1000.

Index

national pharmaceutical strategy
53, 60
National Prescription Drug
Utilization Information System
186
national treatment 101
Naylor Report 108
needs-based planning 57, 68, 142–3,
146, 155, 307, 310
Netherlands 96, 219, 222–3, 303, 309,
314
New Brunswick 23, 69, 78, 156, 157,
199, 211
*New Directions for a Healthy British
Columbia* 69
new managerialism 68
'New Modes of Governance' 60
new public governance 78, 82
new public management (NPM)
47, 62, 64–8, 71, 73–6, 80, 84, 86,
225–8, 310
new right 63–4, 163, 296
Newfoundland 19, 22–3, 130, 154,
156–7, 159, 198, 211
Newton's laws 301, 315
NOC/c. *See* conditional notice of
compliance
non-medical determinants of health.
See social determinants of health
North American Free Trade
Agreement (NAFTA) 101–2
notice of compliance (NOC) 189
Nova Scotia 23, 24–7, 69, 76–7, 79,
133, 139, 155–7, 192, 211
nurse practitioner 138–40, 168
nurses 16, 25, 136, 137–8, 140–4,
147–50, 207, 229, 280, 294, 308;
licensed practical 138; psychiatric
201, 203, 213; registered 135,
139–40, 204

nutrition 28, 105, 115, 120, 122,
124–6, 128, 175, 205, 276, 294
nutritionists 308

Obama, Barack xii, 276, 286–7, 290,
312
obesity 127, 129, 175
objectivity of science 166, 168, 178,
193, 316
occupational therapists 135, 138, 203,
213
ombudsman 80
Ontario 17–20, 23–4, 26–7, 45, 48, 69,
71, 73, 85, 99–100, 106, 108, 117,
135, 138–40, 142, 149, 154, 156–8,
166, 174, 198–9, 204, 209, 211, 216,
306, 310, 313, 318
Ontario Cardiac Care Network 99,
313
Ontario Hospital Association 216
Ontario Health Insurance Plan 204
Ontario Medical Association 216
open federalism 114
open-label studies 180
Organization for Economic Cooperation and Development
(OECD) 14, 30–1, 123, 132, 270–1,
274, 303–4, 306, 314
orphan diseases xi
osteopenia 318
Ottawa 18–20, 22, 24, 26, 45, 47, 50–3,
55, 57–9, 61, 67, 75, 89–90, 111, 114,
120, 154, 157–8, 163–4, 174, 183,
187–9, 305, 309
Ottawa Charter for Health Promotion 120
outcomes-based health policy 310
out-of-pocket payment 9, 12–13,
19, 41
Out of the Shadows at Last 49, 209